Principles of

Community Health

Jack Smolensky, M.P.H., Ed.D.

Associate Professor of Health Education,
Department of Health and Hygiene,
San José State College, San José, California

Franklin B. Haar, Ph.D.

Professor of Health Education,
School of Health, Physical Education, and Recreation,
University of Oregon, Eugene, Oregon

W. B. SAUNDERS COMPANY

Philadelphia and London

Preface

ALL OF US who are interested in community and public health are concerned with such key words and phrases as *prevention, health education, current trends or shift in emphasis, major public health problems today,* and *evaluation.* These key thoughts are emphasized in this book.

The contents may be divided into four necessary and important sections: (1) sociological and anthropological aspects of health with emphasis upon cultural patterns and values; (2) solving community health problems with emphasis upon community planning and organization; (3) community health education methods and materials with emphasis upon communication, motivation, and leadership; and (4) basic public health problems today with emphasis upon prevention and health education, including alcoholism, water and air pollution, geriatrics, mental health, suicide, chronic diseases, radiological health, and space health.

iii

Valuable critical assistance and helpful suggestions were received from Henry M. Bockrath, M.D., M.P.H., Health Officer, Hilo, Hawaii; Merle Cosand, M.D., M.P.H., Health Officer, San Bernardino County Health Department, California; and Wayne Jepson, Assistant Professor of Health Education, San José State College. The authors also benefited from the services, interest, and experience of Dr. Marston Girard, Dr. Estes Levine, Richard Whitlock, Jean Lees, and Lyle Hansen, all of San José State College; Winea Simpson, M.D., Maternal and Child Health Director, San Bernardino County Health Department, California; and Emil Furrer, M.D., University of Oregon.

Last but not least, many thanks are extended to Patt Smolensky who gave assistance and encouragement throughout the preparation and writing of this book.

JACK SMOLENSKY
FRANKLIN B. HAAR

Contents

Appendices

Appendix II

Appendix III

Appendix IV

Appendix V

Appendix VI

Appendix VII

Chapter I

Basic Health Problems Today

THERE ARE MANY community health problems of major importance today. However, as public health and medical advances are made in certain areas, some major problems become minor and are soon replaced by others. Medical and public health officials may differ in their opinions when listing the leading community health problems during any period of time. Certain health problems may be of more concern in some areas than in others. For example, many health problems are magnified in the booming states of California, Arizona, and Florida. Furthermore, one's definition of a health problem depends upon his interests, his academic and professional background and training, his immediate and past health problems, his social and cultural heritage, his value system, and his definition and philosophy of health and community health.

One method of determining the health of a nation or community is to analyze the death rate. In Table 1 the leading causes of death in the United States in 1956 are listed and the rate per

1

Table 1.   Deaths and Death Rates for the 10 Leading Causes of Death in 1956.
(Death Rates for these Same Causes in 1900*)

CAUSE OF DEATH	NUMBER OF DEATHS 1956	RATE PER 100,000 POPULATION	
		1956	1900
All causes	1,564,476	935.4	1,719.1
1. Diseases of heart	602,995	360.5	137.4
2. Cancer and other malignant neoplasms	247,357	147.9	64.0
3. Cerebral hemorrhage and other vascular lesions affecting central nervous system	177,845	106.3	106.9
4. All accidents	94,780	56.7	72.3
5. Certain diseases of early infancy	64,546	38.6	62.6
6. Influenza and pneumonia	47,103	28.2	202.2
7. General arteriosclerosis	32,018	19.1	—
8. Diabetes mellitus	26,184	15.7	†
9. Congenital malformations	21,065	12.6	12.0
10. Cirrhosis of liver	17,924	10.7	12.5

* *Summary of Health and Vital Statistics*, U. S. Department of Health, Education, and Welfare, Public Health Service, National Office of Vital Statistics, Washington, D. C., 1958.
† Not comparable because of change in classification.

100,000 population compared with the rate in 1900. Although these statistics may change from year to year (sometimes due to classification differences), leading causes of death will remain quite consistent during the next decade. *Suicide* ranked eleventh with approximately 16,000 deaths, followed by *tuberculosis* with about 14,000 deaths. Stomach and duodenal ulcers account for about 10,000 deaths each year. Many of these deaths could have been prevented; many lives could have been prolonged. Most of these leading causes of death are discussed in this book; prevention is stressed in each case.

Another approach in determining the health of a community or nation involves the incidence of diseases and any physical, mental, social, emotional or economic impairment of individuals within a community caused by these diseases. Such problems include suicide, alcoholism, dental decay, diabetes, communicable diseases, mental illness and degenerative diseases. One or more major community health problems in each age group are discussed in this chapter; most of them are preventable. (See Table 2 for the five leading causes of death in each age group in 1956.)

Conditions that influence the incidence of disease in community health are: tremendous population increase (see Figure 1),

Table 2.   Deaths and Death Rates for Five Leading Causes of Death in Specified Age Groups, 1956.

AGE AND CAUSE OF DEATH	NUMBER	RATE PER 100,000 POPULATION
All causes (1–4 Years)	16,603	110.4
1. All accidents	4,675	31.1
2. Influenza and pneumonia	2,312	15.4
3. Congenital malformations	1,978	13.2
4. Cancer and other malignant neoplasms	1,669	11.1
5. Gastroenteritis	571	3.8
All causes (5–14 Years)	14,899	46.9
1. All accidents	6,316	19.9
2. Cancer and other malignant neoplasms	2,247	7.1
3. Congenital malformations	886	2.8
4. Influenza and pneumonia	736	2.3
5. Rheumatic fever	261	0.8
All causes (15–24 Years)	24,587	114.0
1. All accidents	13,545	62.8
2. Cancer and other malignant neoplasms	1,839	8.5
3. Homicide	1,290	6.0
4. Diseases of heart	1,050	4.9
5. Suicide	859	4.0
All causes (25–44 Years)	104,892	224.2
1. Diseases of heart	21,175	45.3
2. All accidents	20,986	44.9
3. Cancer and other malignant neoplasms	18,798	40.2
4. Cerebral hemorrhage and other vascular lesions affecting central nervous system	4,860	10.4
5. Suicide	4,821	10.3
All causes (45–64 Years)	401,182	1,178.7
1. Diseases of heart	162,520	477.5
2. Cancer and other malignant neoplasms	92,450	271.6
3. Cerebral hemorrhage and other vascular lesions affecting central nervous system	34,306	100.8
4. All accidents	19,207	56.4
5. Cirrhosis of liver	9,133	26.8
All causes (65 Years and Over)	893,156	6,199.9
1. Diseases of heart	417,190	2,895.9
2. Cerebral hemorrhage and other vascular lesions affecting central nervous system	137,596	955.1
3. Cancer and other malignant neoplasms	129,978	902.2
4. General arteriosclerosis	30,128	209.1
5. All accidents	26,417	183.4

* *Summary of Health and Vital Statistics*, U. S. Department of Health, Education, and Welfare, Public Health Service, National Office of Vital Statistics, Washington D. C., 1958.

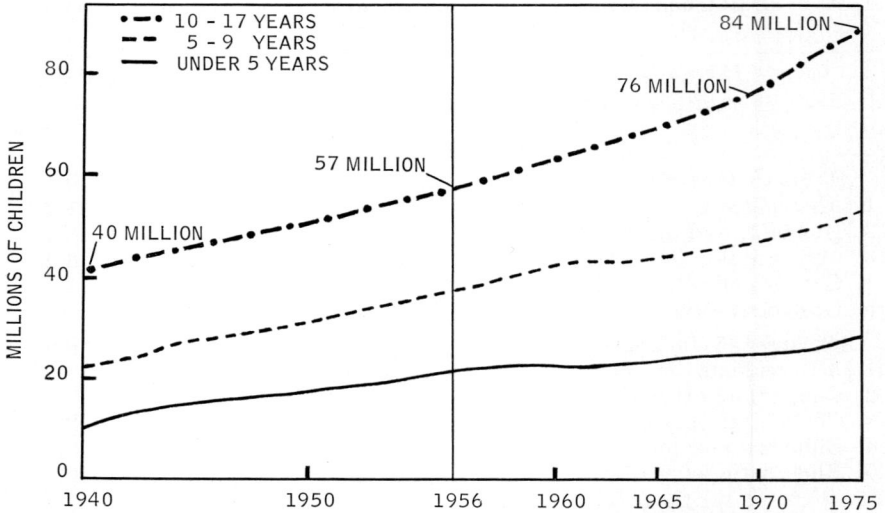

Figure 1. Estimated trend in child population to 1975.

The number of children in the United States has been increasing not only because of higher birth rates but also because of continued progress in reducing infant and child mortality. Population experts predict, if present fertility and mortality trends continue, further rise in numbers in each group under 18 in the next decade or two to: 70 million by 1965, 76 million by 1970 and 84 million by 1975. Children under 18 in 1956 make up a third of the nation's total population. By 1975, according to this outlook they will comprise 37 per cent of the United States population.

air and water pollution, environmental sanitation. Each of these conditions is discussed in this book; prevention is stressed in each case.

COMMUNITY HEALTH PROBLEMS OF INFANCY AND CHILDHOOD

Prematurity

A major cause of death in the United States today is associated with birth. In 1955, deaths occurring at birth numbered an estimated 165,376; 1,901 of these were maternal deaths; 86,124 were deaths of infants before or during birth; and 77,351 were deaths of live-born infants in the neonatal period.[1] Similar statistics have been recorded each year since 1955. Statistically, these figures replace those for accidents as the fourth leading cause of death in the United States. The seriousness of this problem is magnified when we consider that in addition to the death toll, many mothers survive only to suffer from chronic ailments, and many babies survive only to be plagued with congenital malformations or central nervous system disorders.

Prematurity is the leading cause of death in infants under one year of age. Premature delivery increases the possibility of death in the newborn twenty times.[2] A premature baby is defined as a baby weighing five and one half pounds (2,500 grams) or less at birth. Although there has been a marked reduction in infant and maternal mortality during the past 60 years, most infant mortality reduction has been in a decrease of deaths after the first month of life; the death rate during the first month of life has decreased very slowly. The most hazardous periods to the baby are immediately after birth and during the first three days of life.

PREVENTION. Since more than half of the early infant deaths occur in babies born prematurely, we must learn more about the nature and causes of premature births. Adequate prenatal care is considered the best known way to prevent premature births, but many prenatal clinics are overcrowded and understaffed, have too few physicians in attendance, and often lack adequate obstetrical supervision. There is need for clarification and recording of causes of death, for development of new drugs to arrest premature labor, and for further research on congenital malformations and other aspects of infant deaths; for better care and more adequate facilities for the premature infant and for special attention to certain socioeconomic groups and rural areas. Finally, this problem, like all community health problems, requires better teamwork among physicians, nurses, scientists, educators, voluntary and official health agencies and others.

Congenital Malformations

Congenital malformations are the third leading cause of death among persons from birth to 15 years of age. Approximately 300,000 infants are born with congenital malformations each year. A congenital malformation is a structural defect that is present at birth, and may occur in any of the body systems or organs. The cost of treating and rehabilitating these youngsters is very large when we consider that about 30 per cent of those under treatment in state agencies for crippled children have congenital malformations or birth injuries.

Research indicates that there are many causes of congenital malformation, and it is seldom possible to attribute the defect to a single cause. It is now believed that some congenital anomalies may be acquired during fetal development as well as inherited. German measles, toxoplasmosis, or syphilis may be responsible for

CAUSES OF INFANT DEATHS

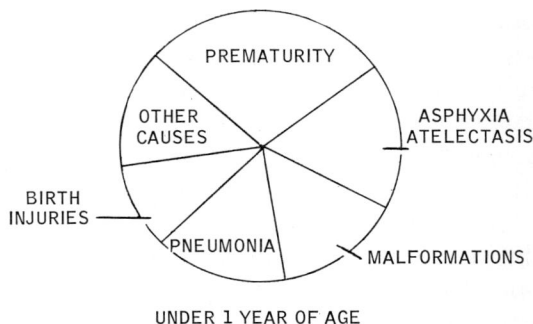

UNDER 1 YEAR OF AGE

PREVENTION--PREMATURITY

1. Prenatal care

2. Adequate facilities

3. Cooperation

4. Coordination

5. Research

6. Education

PREVENTION--
CONGENITAL MALFORMATIONS

1. Protection against maternal infections

2. Prenatal care

3. Education

4. Cooperation

5. Coordination

6. Research

Figure 2.   Causes and prevention of death among infants under one year of age.

congenital anomalies. Other causes of congenital malformations include maternal and fetal radiation, poor maternal diet, chromosome variations, blood incompatibility (Rh factor), birth injuries due to difficult and traumatic deliveries (dystocia), and lack of oxygen to the fetus (anoxia).[3]

The greatest incidence of congenital malformations involves the central nervous system causing musculoskeletal, cardiovascular, and genitourinary defects.[4] It is estimated that approximately 315,000 children have cerebral palsy, 310,000 have epilepsy and 1,500,000 children are mentally retarded.[5]

PREVENTION. Further research is necessary to shed more light on this problem. Prematurity and congenital malformations may be interrelated and thus may be studied together. At any rate, teamwork is necessary to solve these major public health problems.

The Children's Bureau of the United States Public Health Service and the state and local health departments are to be commended for their part in saving crippled or handicapped children from becoming dependent adults. Since the Crippled Children's Service Program was started in 1927, thousands of children whose parents were unable to pay for the necessary medical attention or who could pay for only part of it, have had their handicaps corrected and have grown into normal, functioning adults. The largest percentage of children cared for under the program include orthopedic cases, ear conditions that affect hearing, disease and deformities of the eyes, cerebral palsy cases, and rheumatic fever cases.

The National Foundation is now directing its attention to congenital malformations and defects of the nervous system.

Childhood Accidents

Accidents are the leading cause of death among persons one to 25 years of age. There are approximately 15,000 accidental deaths per year among children from one to 15 years of age; most of these accidents could have been prevented. Accidents occurring most frequently in the one to 15 year-old age group include, in order, motor vehicle, drowning, fire burns, falls, firearms, and poisons. Motor vehicle accidents are responsible for approximately one-third of all accident fatalities in this age group. Males consistently outnumber females in statistical compilations of accidental deaths and injuries in all categories except fire burns.

New dangers have arisen with scientific and technological advances. For example, the power lawn mower, plastic swimming pool, and plastic laundry bag have added sorrow as well as happiness to the lives of many people. Increased interest in rockets and space travel has led to many accidents among amateur rocketeers who insist on mixing their own propellants. Television has inspired young "fast-draw" experts, who, upon finding Dad's loaded gun within easy reach, accidentally shoot their friends, relatives, or themselves. The large number of new and potentially lethal products used in our farms and homes raises further problems. The increasing number of available medicines reveals a corresponding increase in the number of accidental poisoning cases.

PREVENTION. Education is the key to accident prevention. We must teach children the facts, help them develop positive safety attitudes, and guide them in channeling these basic factors into everyday practices. Supporting elements must include parental supervision and guidance, legislation, coordination of community safety activities, cooperation of community agencies, and continued research.

Table 3. Childhood Accidents*
What You Should Know—What You Should Do

AGE	TYPICAL ACCIDENT	NORMAL BEHAVIOR CHARACTERISTICS	PRECAUTIONS
1st year	Falls	Rolls over at about 4 months; creeps, stands and may walk between 6 and 12 months	Do not leave alone on tables, beds or bathinette; keep crib sides up
	Burns	Is helpless to leave source of burn such as burning house	Keep electric cords and appliances away; do not leave in house alone; test water in bath
	Inhalation or ingestion of foreign objects Poisonings	Puts everything into mouth	Keep small objects and poisons out of reach
	Drowning	Is helpless in water	Do not leave alone in bath
2d year	Falls	Is able to walk; can manage stairs	Keep screens on windows and gate at stairs
	Burns	Reaches for any utensils on stove or table	Keep handles of pots and pans on stove out of reach, hot foods away from edge of table; keep electric cords out of reach; cover unused electric outlets; do not leave alone in house
	Drowning	Is helpless in water	Keep in enclosed space when outdoors or not in company of adult
2-4 years old	Poisonings	Has great curiosity; puts everything into mouth. Is able to open doors; can run and climb, can throw ball, ride tricycle	Keep medicine, household compounds out of reach
	Falls		Keep doors locked where danger of falls—cellar, screens on windows; teach risks of throwing sharp objects
	Drowning	(See above)	(See above)
	Poisonings	Investigates closets and drawers	
	Burns and cuts		Keep knives, electrical equipment out of reach
	Firearms	Plays with mechanical gadgets	Keep firearms locked up
5-9 years old	Motor vehicle		Teach safety in street and driveway
	Motor vehicle	Is daring and adventurous	
	Bicycle accidents	Control more advanced over large than over small muscles	Teach traffic and bicycle safety
	Drowning		Encourage but do not push swimming skills
	Burns	(See above)	
	Firearms		Keep firearms locked up
	Falls	Loyalty to group makes him willing to follow other leaders	
10-14 years old	Motor vehicles	Need for strenuous activity	Teach rules of pedestrian and traffic safety; prepare for driving by setting good example
	Drowning Burns Falls	Plays in hazardous places. Need for approval of those his age leads to daring or hazardous feats	Provide safe and acceptable facilities for recreation and social activities

Parade, August 2, 1959, Reprint from The New England Journal of Medicine. Boston, Massachusetts.

Leukemia

Cancer is the second leading cause of death in school age children. *Leukemia,* or "white blood," a form of cancer in which the red blood cells are crowded out by an overproduction of white blood cells, accounts for about one-half of the deaths from all forms of cancer in children between the ages of one and 14. For example, approximately 4,000 children from one to 14 years of age die from cancer each year; 50 per cent, or 2,000 of these children die from leukemia.

A number of generally accepted or strongly suspected causes of leukemia are known. Suspected causes include x-rays, radium, viruses, and certain chemical compounds; experts believe, however, that the prime or determining causes have not yet been identified. Although there is no known cure for leukemia, recent advances in medicine have permitted over one-half of all leukemia patients to live a year or more after the illness begins, and certain vaccines look promising.

PREVENTION. The American Cancer Society is currently spending over $3,000,000 per year for research related to leukemia. Millions of dollars more must be invested to defeat this enemy which kills 2,000 children and over 12,000 adults each year. It is interesting

LEUKEMIA DEATH RATE BY AGE GROUPS   ▮ 1940   ☐ 1956

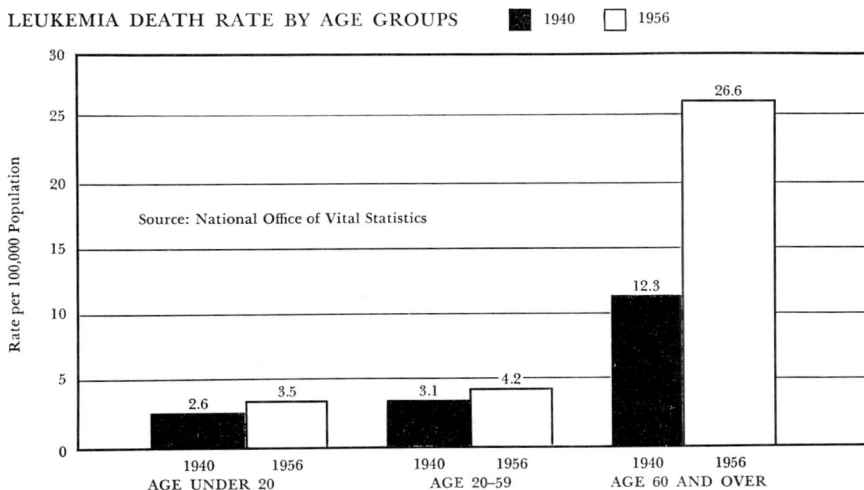

Figure 3. A question puzzling medical science and cancer researchers is why the alarming increase of leukemia deaths among the over-60 age group since World War II, while mortality rates in children and mid-life age groups—though showing some increase—remain relatively unchanged? (*From 1960 Cancer Facts and Figures.* American Cancer Society.)

to note that there has been an alarming increase of leukemia deaths among the over-sixty age group since World War II. Although more research is necessary to determine the exact nature and underlying causes of leukemia, it seems wise at this time to guard against over-exposures to x-rays, radium, or certain chemicals such as *benzol*.

Dental Health

Dental decay is the most prevalent disease of childhood. While dental disease is constantly at epidemic proportions in our total population, it is most serious in children. In our nation's children it is estimated that less than one-half of the teeth that need dental repair have received proper care. Dental decay in children is occurring at a rapid rate and if all dentists worked day and night and only on children, they could not repair the damage as fast as it is appearing. Prevention is a must!

Innumerable factors have been related at one time or another to the development or lack of development of dental caries. Major suspected causes include: pregnancy, chronic debilitating diseases such as diabetes and tuberculosis, disturbance of various endocrine glands, radiation, psychic trauma, nutritional deficiencies, inadequate dental cleansing, enzymes, saliva, bacteria, and inherited or acquired immunity or susceptibility.

Pyorrhea, a disease of the gums known medically as periodontal disease, is responsible for the loss of more teeth than all other causes combined, including tooth decay; 21 million Americans have had to resign themselves to being toothless or to wearing dental plates. The disease attacks without pain, and thus the symptoms are easy to ignore. Although gingivitis, an inflammation or bleeding of the gums, is the first sign of pyorrhea, the infection is ignored until the fibers and bone surrounding the tooth are destroyed.

PREVENTION. It is difficult to identify any single cause of tooth decay, but science has provided a method of preventing about two-thirds this decay in children. In 25 years of research it has been proved that about one part per million of fluoride in community water supplies will reduce dental decay in children up to approximately 65 per cent and will give life-long improved dental health. (See Figure 4.)

Although the fluoridation program is supported by the American Medical Association, the American Dental Association, and the

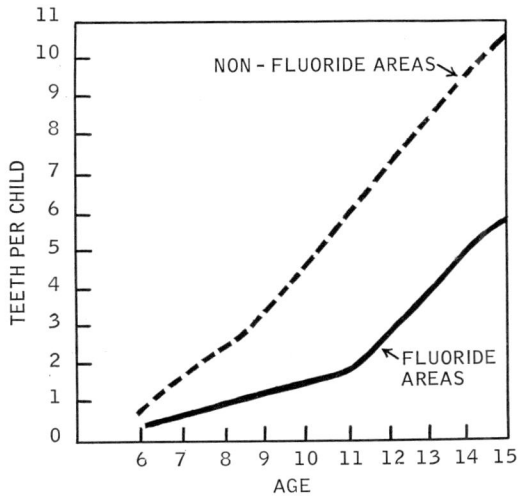

Figure 4. Number of permanent teeth per child affected with decay.

United States Public Health Service, the program has been rejected in many communities. Certain groups have consistently opposed the program, and one major deterrent has been the lack of planning and organization by the community health educators and leaders. They must plan a long-range program that is strongly supported by active participation from community members. Confidence and support must be voiced by local dentists, physicians, educators, and government officials. A strong community education program must reach all the people. The facts must be presented and the people made to realize the benefits of fluoridation and urged to secure fluorine for their community water supply.

It is interesting to note that a similar problem existed in 1910 when communities were urged to chlorinate public water supplies. Health officials were confronted with the same kinds of opposition. One has only to compare the 1910 death rate with that of today to see the results of chlorination. The psychological bases for objecting to chlorination, pasteurization, immunization, and fluoridation by certain groups are similar and include: (1) physiological fear of the chemical, (2) invasion of human rights, (3) conflicts with entrenched beliefs, and (4) resistance to change. *Education, cooperation,* and *coordination* are the key words in this area.

CAUSES OF CHILD DEATHS

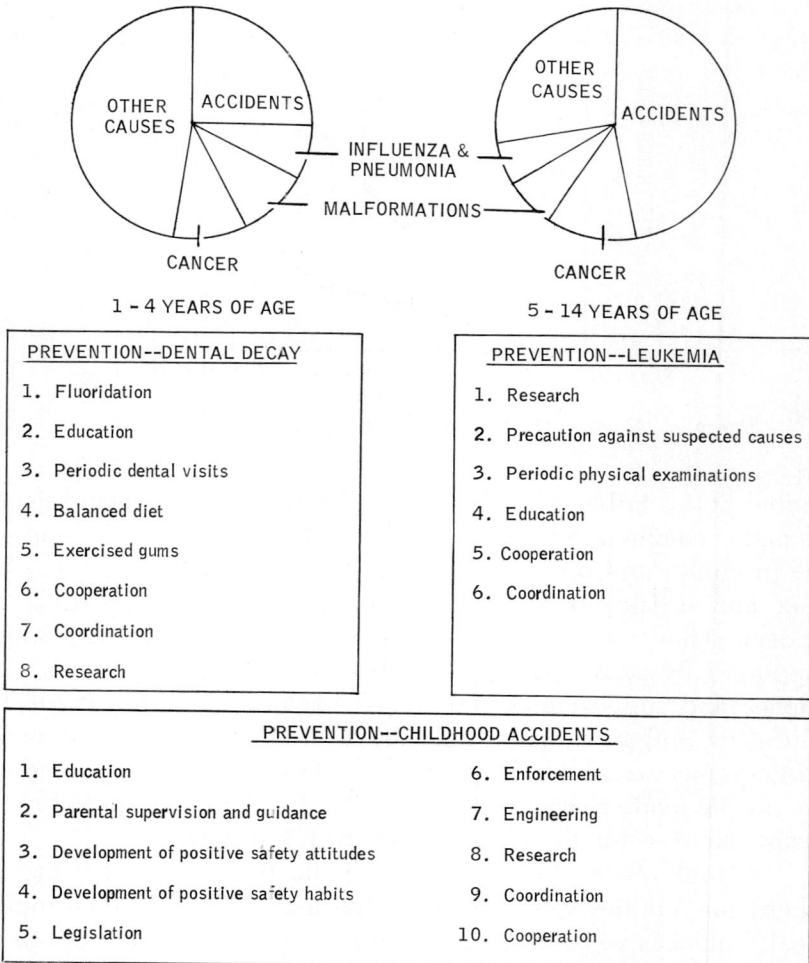

Figure 5. Causes and prevention of death among children one to 14 years of age.

COMMUNITY HEALTH PROBLEMS OF ADULTS AND THE AGED

Suicide

Suicide is an important community health problem in the United States. Deaths by suicide number over 16,000 and rank fifth as the leading cause of death in persons from 15 to 45 years of age. These figures, however, are probably conservative; many suicides are concealed, and many deaths from suicide are recorded as accidental.

The act of suicide is as old as man, and the social attitudes toward suicide have varied through the ages. Ancient laws of India permitted suicide for the diseased, and Eskimos demanded it of their aged. Suicide flourished during the days of the Roman Empire; arsenic was sold publicly in the Egyptian markets for purposes of suicide. With the rise in influence of the Catholic Church, the attitude of society toward suicide gradually changed, and the act was considered a crime against church and state.

In English common law, suicide is a crime against society. This view, which originated in Roman law, was supported by Christianity. The crime of suicide was punishable in common law by denial of a Christian burial; the corpse was buried in the highway with a stake driven through the body; and the property of the miscreant was confiscated. At present, sanctions against the body and property of the suicide have been removed. The attempt at suicide is no longer considered an attempt to commit murder; rather, it is regarded as an attempt to commit a felony, for which the maximum penalty is two years' imprisonment. In the United States, *attempted suicide* is regarded as a crime in only a few areas, but the crime of *suicide* has been repudiated by statute in the majority of states. The New York statute calls suicide "a grave public wrong."

The increasing number of suicides is causing many city and state health officials to reappraise the situation. Suicide, for example, was the sixth leading cause of death in San Francisco in 1958, with approximately 200 suicides. The city's 45 square miles represent an unusual concentration of those elements that may be responsible for suicide. More people are concentrated in less space in San Francisco than in any other metropolitan city in the nation except Manhattan. There are 17,000 San Franciscans per square mile. Many of these people are newcomers, and for them it can be a city of anonymity, isolation, and loneliness. But why is the suicide rate in San Francisco four times higher than in New York City?

Many theories have been advanced regarding the high suicide rate in San Francisco. Many investigators believe that people who pull up old roots and "go West" are more susceptible to the general tensions and anxieties of life. They must prove to themselves and the others they left behind that they can make good. Furthermore, many are faced by sudden financial loss and are less emotionally prepared for the adjustment. Many of these people have no meaningful interaction with others. Other theories include the influence of the bridges, climate, and the hectic pace in a leading financial center. For example, the Golden Gate Bridge has been a diving board for approximately 200 suicide victims since its construction in 1937. One authority suggests that people desire "togetherness" even in death.

San Francisco health authorities, however, are quick to point out that these figures may be misleading. Reasons include a high percentage of autopsies performed in San Francisco, more accurate and better reporting of suicide cases, a high percentage of older persons living in the city, mass migration to the city, and a high percentage of visitors. One other factor involves the city's China-town, where the suicide rate is twice as high as in any other section of the city.

PREVENTION. Epidemiological studies of suicide are limited because of the inadequacies of medicolegal records. Coroners, of necessity, gather information to establish the cause of death rather than to understand the suicide. If more significant insight and knowledge are to be developed about suicide, systematic information should be gathered at the time of death and more autopsies should be performed. Also, the important finding of a study of suicide in Philadelphia revealed that the majority of the suicides had been under medical supervision prior to their death, usually by the family doctor. This suggests that the family doctor is in a key position to recognize psychiatric problems in his patients at the earliest possible time and to refer them to appropriate psychiatric resources for special care and treatment. It would be helpful if

Table 4. *Average Annual Male and Female Suicides**

INSTRUMENTS OF SUICIDE	AVERAGE ANNUAL NUMBER†	
	Males	*Females*
Poisoning	2,166	1,158
Barbiturates and other soporifics	339	484
Other solids and liquids	391	336
Gases in domestic use	207	140
Motor-vehicle exhaust and other gases	1,229	196
Hanging and strangulation	2,508	822
Drowning	333	257
Firearms and explosives	6,393	808
Cutting and piercing instruments	373	97
Jumping from high place	319	161
Other means	186	103

* *An Age-Old Moral Problem Poses a Modern Medical Challenge, Suicide.* Therapeutic Notes, *65*:115, 1958.
† White persons, United States, 1953–55.

material on the problem of suicide with emphasis on prevention, and methods of detecting individuals with suicidal tendencies were introduced in college health education, medical school, and public health school curriculums.

SUICIDE FACTS

1. There are about 16,000 deaths by suicide each year in the United States.
2. Suicide is the fifth leading cause of death in persons 15 to 45 years of age.
3. The largest number of suicides occurs in spring, during the morning, on Monday or Tuesday.
4. Although twice as many women attempt suicide, men are more successful by a ratio of three to one.
5. Men are more violent and use instruments such as a rifle or rope; women most often swallow an overdose of barbiturates.
6. All occupations are represented; the incidence is higher among professional groups.
7. The suicide rate goes up at the start of an economic depression and goes down during war years.
8. The suicide rate is higher than average among Orientals, city dwellers, single persons, army officers, and Protestants; it is lower than average among Negroes, farmers, married persons, army enlisted men, Catholics, and Jews.
9. If a person attempts suicide once, he will usually try again.
10. The median age of a suicide victim is 36.2 years; over one-half of the victims are over 45 years of age. There has been a marked increase in suicides among younger age groups.
11. About 40 per cent of the men and 20 per cent of the women kill themselves because of ill health.
12. A person contemplating suicide may feel imaginary pain.
13. Suicidal threats or attempts must always be taken seriously.
14. Almost one-half of the suicides occur within three months of an emotional crisis or shortly after leaving a psychiatric hospital or sanitarium.

Alcoholism

Whether *alcoholism* is considered a mental illness, a physical illness, or both, it constitutes a serious and increasing public health problem. It is estimated that about 2,000,000 problem drinkers

Table 5.   *Mortality Rates from Suicide**
(*all ages, per 100,000, 1954*)

		BOTH SEXES	MALE	FEMALE
Countries with	Japan	23.4	29.2	17.8
Highest Rates	Denmark	23.3	31.4	15.4
	Austria	23.1	33.1	14.4
	Switzerland	22.6	33.9	12.0
U.S.A.	All races	10.1	16.1	4.3
	White	10.8	17.2	4.6
	Nonwhite	3.8	6.4	1.3
Countries with	Spain	5.9	9.1	2.9
Lowest Rates	Scotland	5.9	8.3	3.7
	Chile	4.6	7.3	2.1
	Northern Ireland	3.5	5.3	1.7
	Ireland	2.0	3.2	0.81

* An Age-Old Moral Problem Poses a Modern Medical Challenge, *Suicide Therapeutic Notes*, 65:116, 1958.

lose on the average of 22 to 25 work days per year each, in the United States; the total direct cost to industry is about $1,000,000,000 per year. The drain alcoholism places on human resources cannot be measured in dollars. An estimated 60,000,000 persons use alcohol moderately; these are the "social drinkers." They take one or two drinks a day. The major problem, however, concerns the 5,000,000 chronic alcoholics—the "compulsive drinkers." These people lack control and are seemingly driven to take one drink after the other, which usually results in interference with their work, health, and social activities. Scientists are still debating whether or not a person's dependence on alcohol is caused by physical, mental, or emotional needs.

The alcohol problem increases in importance when we realize that cirrhosis of the liver is the tenth leading cause of death in the United States and accounts for about 18,000 deaths each year. Cirrhosis or hardening of the liver is commonly associated with alcoholism. In San Francisco, for instance, cirrhosis was the fifth leading cause of death in 1958 and accounted for approximately 350 deaths. However, not all of these deaths were due to alcohol.

The apparent rise in the incidence of alcoholism in recent years is attributable in part to better reporting of deaths due to cirrhosis of the liver. Most of the diseases associated with alcoholism are the result of alcohol's interfering with diet and the way the body uses food. However, nutritional deficiency and neuritis probably constitute a relatively small proportion of the total disease picture of the alcoholic.

Alcoholism is a major problem in many states throughout the

THE UNFORTUNATE ALCOHOLIC

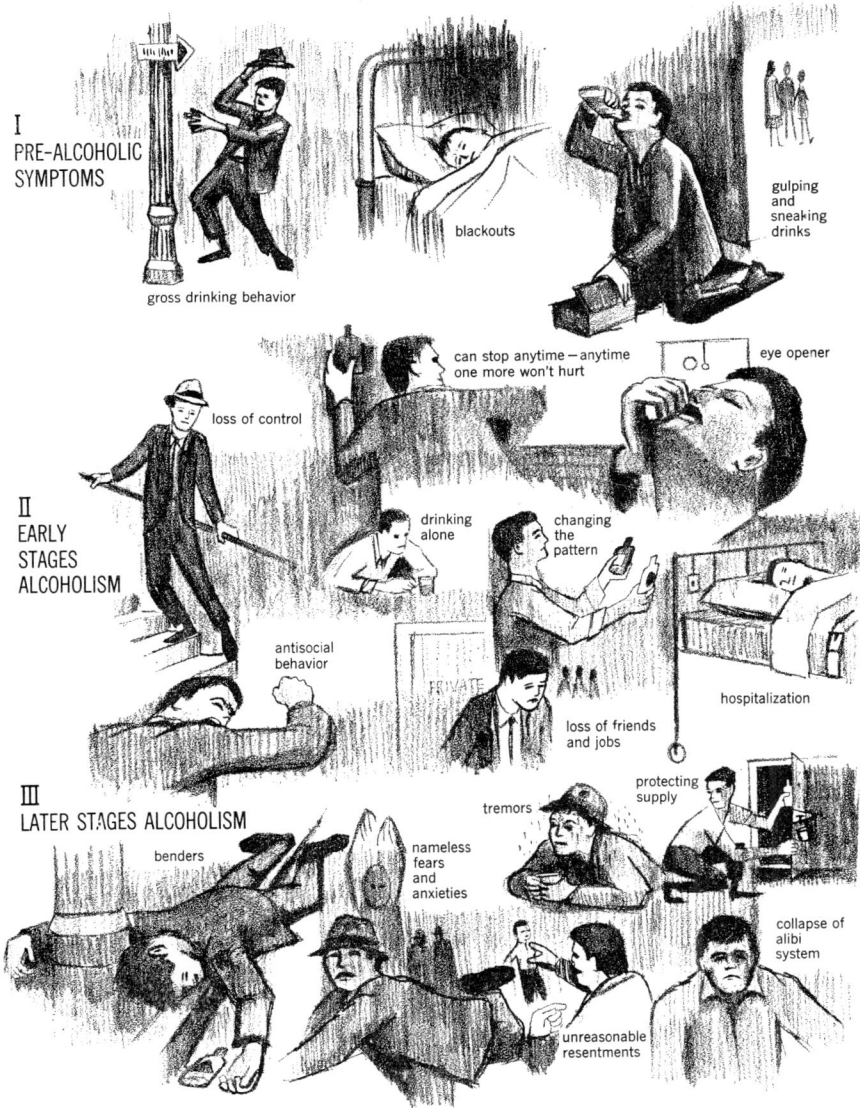

Figure 6. (From Schifferes, Justus J.: Essentials of Healthier Living, John Wiley & Sons, Inc., New York, 1960.)

country. California, for example, is estimated to rank higher in alcoholism than any other state in the Union.[6] For United States cities with more than 100,000 population, San Francisco is estimated to rank first in the nation in the number of problem drinkers and is closely followed by Sacramento.[7, 8] Correspondingly, cirrhosis of the liver is a major cause of death in these areas. Furthermore, the rate of total alcoholic admissions (of persons under alcoholic commitments) to California state mental hygiene hospitals increased from 8.9 per 100,000 population in 1945 to 25.0 per 100,000 population in 1954.[9, 10] In addition, alcohol is involved in many suicides, homicides, and fatal accidents throughout the country.

Public health authorities in cities estimated to rank high in alcoholism, such as San Francisco, for example, are quick to point out that these figures may be misleading. Reasons include a higher percentage of autopsies performed, more accurate and better reporting of cases, a higher percentage of older persons living there, mass migration to these cities, and the fact that the prevalence of alcoholism is based on a formula that has never been adequately tested for validity.[11]

It is important to note that the excise taxes and license fees collected by the state and federal government from the sale of alcoholic beverages amount to a great sum of money each year. This money, plus the great number of persons employed by the industry, plays an important part in the economy of many states.

PREVENTION. Two new and interesting research projects may open new roads to alcohol prevention. One is being directed by Stanford University sociologists.[12] Their studies reveal that it may be possible to predict 85 per cent correctly that a child from a certain type family will become an alcoholic in adult life. Research has been based thus far upon investigation of 510 children traced to adulthood. Those who became alcoholics had very similar family structures: the parents were antagonistic; fathers were escapists; and mothers showed little affection or love for their families. If this study is repeated and investigated by other researchers and proves valid, it may be possible either to change the problem family structure, or to remove the child from this type of environment.

The other research project involves laboratory work being done at the California State Department of Public Health. It has been observed that alcoholics excrete more zinc into their urine than normal. It may thus be feasible and economical to conduct large-scale screening or routine physical examinations in an effort to detect the potential alcoholic before his health is affected.

Alcoholism affects the public in phenomenal ways and involves the entire community. The alcoholism problem requires community recognition, community planning, and community action to control and prevent it. Researchers must determine the nature and extent of the problem, the role of alcohol in society, the prevailing attitudes toward its use, and the available facilities and resources needed to prevent alcoholism. Meanwhile, rehabilitation services and facilities must be made available, and community education enforced by active participation and cooperation to combat this growing community health menace.

ALCOHOLISM FACTS.

1. There are an estimated 5,000,000 chronic alcoholics in the United States today; 4,250,000 are men and 750,000 are women.
2. Only cardiovascular disease and mental illness outrank alcoholism in incidence.
3. One of every 13 men 20 years of age or more is an alcoholic.
4. About 2,000,000 workers, or 3 per cent of the entire indus-

What are physicians doing to help the alcoholic?

Between 40 and 70% treat one or more alcoholics a year.*
Of these:

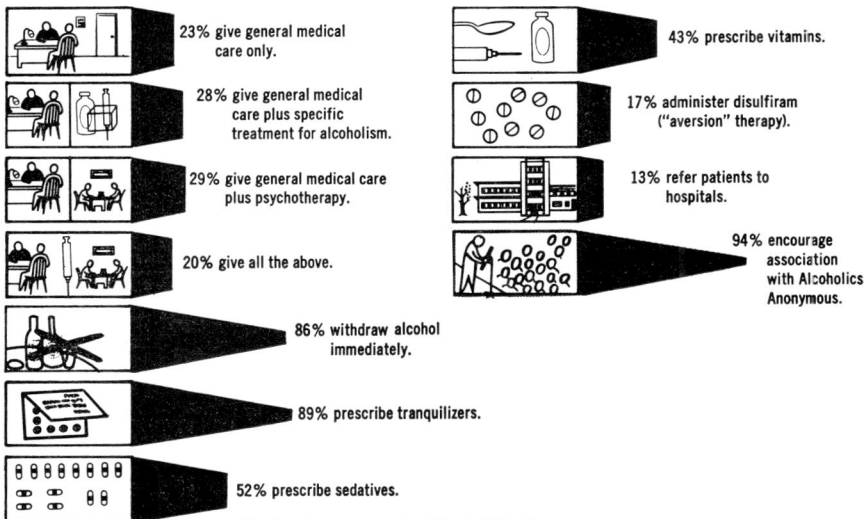

23% give general medical care only.

28% give general medical care plus specific treatment for alcoholism.

29% give general medical care plus psychotherapy.

20% give all the above.

86% withdraw alcohol immediately.

89% prescribe tranquilizers.

52% prescribe sedatives.

43% prescribe vitamins.

17% administer disulfiram ("aversion" therapy).

13% refer patients to hospitals.

94% encourage association with Alcoholics Anonymous.

*Based on 4 surveys covering 3,300 physicians in Kansas, Iowa, New York, and New Jersey.

Figure 7. The general practitioner is the key man in the treatment of alcoholics. (From Patterns of Disease. Parke, Davis and Co., June, 1959.)

trial force, are alcoholics; about 200,000 new cases arise annually.

5. Today's alcoholic is probably a man in his mid-forties, married, employed, and a resident of his community for the past five years.

6. Cirrhosis of the liver is the tenth leading cause of death in the United States and the fifth leading cause of death in persons 45 to 64 years of age.

7. About 20,000 alcoholics are admitted to mental hospitals annually.

8. Inebriety accounts for at least 70 per cent of the occupants of local jails.

9. The first large-scale federal effort against alcoholism was launched in July, 1958, by the National Institute of Mental Health.

Table 6.   Cost of Alcoholism Each Year in the United States*

$1,000,000,000	Direct cost to industry
432,000,000	Lost wages due to absenteeism
125,000,000	Accident losses
40,000,000	Aid to families of alcoholics
30,000,000	General hospital costs
25,000,000	Cost of custodial care in institutions
$1,652,000,000	Total cost

* Block, M. A.: Journal of American Association of Industrial Nurses 7:24, 1959.

ALCOHOLIC REHABILITATION. State legislatures have regulated the production, distribution, and sale of alcoholic beverages in many ways. Government activities at state and local levels were originally organized to deal with the socially unacceptable effects of intemperate drinking, including drunk driving, public intoxication, and mental disturbances. Presently many states have created an agency to engage in the treatment and rehabilitation of alcoholics, to investigate and study all phases of the rehabilitation of alcoholics, and to study all factors necessary to reduce and prevent chronic alcoholism. For example, the Division of Alcoholic Rehabilitation of the California State Department of Public Health, which was organized in 1957, has a program that emphasizes financial support to local pilot rehabilitation clinics, offers consultation and advice to communities in developing alcoholic rehabilitation facilities, investigates factors which may contribute to alcoholism, and conducts a continuous, intensive health education program.

GOALS OF COMMUNITY ACTION ON ALCOHOLISM[13]

1. *Physicians* who are ready, willing and able to treat the acute phases of alcoholism and to use their skills to join with the community team that offers help for the chronic aspects of the illness.
2. *General hospitals* whose beds are as available to acutely intoxicated patients as they are to diabetics, and nursing staffs that recognize that there is more to alcoholism than intoxication.
3. *Clergymen* who are aware of the spiritual problems faced by alcoholics and their families, and are ready to use their counseling skills to help rather than condemn.
4. *Social agencies* that offer help to families where alcoholism has intensified normal social problems, and that utilize their skills to help the individual alcoholic.
5. *Health departments* that feel as much responsibility toward alcoholism as they do toward any other public health problems.
6. *Employers* who recognize the early symptoms of alcoholism in employees, and who protect the investment that they have made in these people by getting help for them before they jeopardize their jobs.
7. *Union officials* who recognize the importance of educating people and promoting early treatment for problem drinkers.
8. *Educators* who are up-to-date on the modern concepts of alcohol education for youth.
9. *Police officers* who have some knowledge of alcoholism and who see their job as one of helping alcoholics, and at the same time, protecting the rights of others.
10. *Courts and laws* that recognize that help for the alcoholic is far more effective than is punishment.
11. *Citizens* who recognize that some people cannot drink in moderation and that these people cannot be blamed for the conditions that made them alcoholic, but can be helped and restored to normal living—in other words, an *informed public.*

Diabetes

Diabetes is the eighth leading cause of death in the United States today. About 50,000 new cases of this disease occur each year; three-fifths of these cases occur among females. Although it is estimated that there are over 2,000,000 persons suffering from diabetes, the major community health problem concerns the 1,000,000 of these persons who do not yet know that they have diabetes. It is also estimated that more than 50,000 children under

15 years of age are victims of this chronic disease. Diabetes is most common among overweight persons between the ages of 40 and 60; more women than men have the disorder.

Diabetes is definitely inheritable and follows the same inheritance path as baldness and color blindness and may skip a generation. The incidence of diabetes may seem to be increasing today because we are living longer. The diabetic is more susceptible to arteriosclerosis, or hardening of the arteries. Since this con-

CAUSES OF ADULT DEATHS

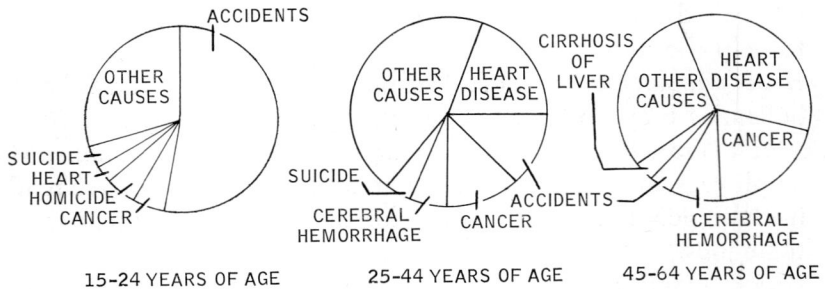

15-24 YEARS OF AGE   25-44 YEARS OF AGE   45-64 YEARS OF AGE

PREVENTION--ALCOHOLISM

1. Education
2. Coordination
3. Cooperation
4. Rehabilitation
5. Research
6. Medical and psychological treatment

PREVENTION--DIABETES

1. Weight control
2. Recognition and awareness of danger signals
3. Education
4. Research
5. Periodic blood-sugar test

PREVENTION--SUICIDE

1. Awareness and referral by family physician and others
2. Adequate medico-legal records
3. Education
4. Cooperation
5. Research
6. Coordination

Figure 8. Causes and prevention of death among adults 15 to 64 years of age.

dition leads to poor circulation in affected areas, circulation may be impaired in the hands or feet, and this in turn may lead to gangrene. Furthermore, damage to retinal vessels of the eye may lead to blindness.

Diabetes mellitus is a disease characterized by the presence of excessive quantities of sugar in the blood and by its excretion into the urine. The basic cause of diabetes is a deficiency of insulin, a hormone secreted by the pancreas. Insulin is used not as a cure, but as a replacement. Fortunately, diabetes is easy to discover, and the test, a simple urinalysis to determine whether or not sugar is present, takes only a few minutes. If the urinalysis shows suspicious signs, it is followed by a more conclusive test to learn if there is an excess of sugar in the blood.

PREVENTION. Prevention in this area stresses education. The public must learn and recognize the diabetes danger signals that include excessive thirst, constant hunger, frequent urination, and sudden loss of weight. Other preventive measures include periodic physical examinations, periodic blood-sugar tests, and maintenance of normal weight. Engaged couples and parents should be aware of the hereditary factor.

Geriatrics

The aged are the 17,000,000 men and women in America who are more than 65 years of age. By 1975, they will total 22,000,000. Since 1900, their number has quadrupled, while the population as a whole has merely doubled. With the increase in number of older persons, the problems associated with aging have increased in an even greater proportion.

Aging is a complex, continuous process that proceeds throughout life; it is a psychological as well as a biological process. The problem of old age comes almost overnight—when a man retires, or a husband dies. The aged may find themselves victims of isolation and segregation. Their fears include the loss of their precious independence, the loneliness of a furnished room, or the illness that can leave them in a nursing home or state hospital. These factors may have an adverse effect upon their personalities.

Major health problems of the aged include deteriorating diseases of the heart and blood vessels, cancer, accidents, mental illness, and rheumatism and arthritis. Diseases of the heart and blood vessels include stroke or cerebral hemorrhage, high blood pressure, and hardening of the arteries (arteriosclerosis). Cancer is the third leading cause of death in this age group. Accidents, particularly falls in the home, are the sixth leading cause of death for persons 65 years of age and over. Rheumatism and arthritis cripple and further discourage at least one-half the persons 65 years of age and over. Mental illness in the aged is caused either by degenerative body processes or by increased psychological stresses and strains placed on these persons. Large numbers of our older people are in institutions of some kind. To an alarming extent many are in mental hospitals, but their condition does not warrant that type of care. The beds they occupy are needed for others with more serious mental problems. The average rate of admission to mental hospitals of patients with a diagnosis of senile psychosis has more than doubled in the past 25 years. Nearly 30 per cent of

Table 7. Frequency of Major Disorders in New Admissions to Mental Hospitals: 1953*

AGE		PER CENT
15 to 44	Schizophrenia	24.0
	Manic-depressive psychoses	3.4
40 to 50	Involutional psychoses	4.4
	Alcoholic intoxication	3.3
60 and over	Cerebral arteriosclerosis and senile psychoses	27.0
All Ages	Personality disorders	11.6
	Psychoneurotic reactions	4.7
	Acute brain syndromes	3.4
	Mental deficiency	2.8
	Miscellaneous disorders, each of low incidence	15.4

* *Mental Health, a Paramount Problem.* Therapeutic Notes, *64*:288, 1957.

present admissions to mental hospitals is recorded as psychosis with cerebral arteriosclerosis or senile psychosis. (See Table 7, page 24.) It can be anticipated that as present trends are extended this percentage will increase. This increase in hospitalization of the aged is a social trend and does not represent an actual increase in mental disease. For example, whenever an elderly patient cannot care for himself and has no family or friends who are willing to care for him, he is usually sent to the state mental hospital.

In recent years, physicians have developed a dynamic concept of treating the ailments of old age. They have demonstrated that intensive, complete therapy, including proper nutrition and environment, can give older persons additional years of fruitful life. Doctors are developing a new understanding of dietary requirements and the effects of stress. Preventive medicine may help to eliminate many problems now confronting the aged. Advances in anesthetics are making operations safer for older people; new drugs and antibiotics are as effective for the old as for the young.

A major problem of the aged revolves around the fact that at a time when their medical needs are the greatest their earning power is at its lowest. Many older persons discover also that because of age limitations in some insurance policies they are deprived of necessary medical care, hospitalization, and accident insurance coverage. The older person does not have the means or the capacity for meeting this crisis alone. Old age thus becomes a national problem and is a growing economic factor involving great sums of money. Old age is a problem that concerns each of us and its economic and social aspects can be dealt with both by the government and personally. In relation to the latter level, President Eisenhower's personal physician, Major General Howard McC. Snyder, gave ten rules for living longer and liking it:

1. Be happy in what you are doing.
2. Overcome extremist tendencies.
3. Live on a reasonably well-regulated diet.
4. Relax and rest now and then during the day.
5. Get a good night's sleep.
6. Don't overindulge in smoking or drinking.
7. Exercise, but in moderation.

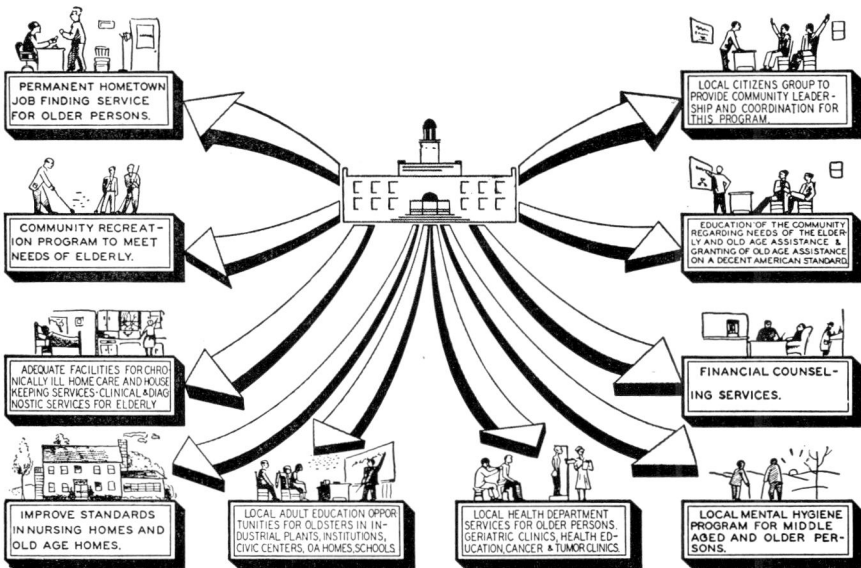

Figure 9. (From Smiley and Gould, *Your Community's Health,* The Macmillan Co., 1952.)

CAUSES OF DEATH AMONG THE AGED

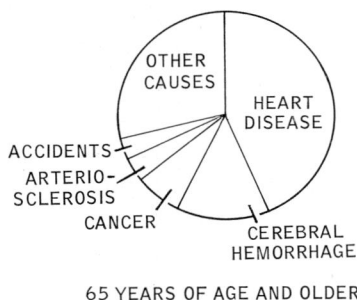

65 YEARS OF AGE AND OLDER

POSSIBLE COMMUNITY GERIATRIC AIDS

1. Modify our compulsory retirement practices

2. Modify our health insurance plans

3. Improve our housing for the aged

4. Provide new kinds of jobs and services for the aged

5. Coordinate efforts of community agencies

6. Develop new home and recreation materials and facilities specifically for the aged

7. Help the aged help themselves

8. Help prepare for old age physically, mentally, socially, and emotionally

9. Help the aged dispel fears of sickness and infirmity

10. Provide health education programs leading to increased knowledge and positive attitudes concerning the aged

Figure 10.   Causes of death and aid to the aged, 65 years of age and older.

8. Older people should shun fats if their cholesterol count is high.

9. Avoid stress and strain.

10. Be philosophical about things.[14]

PREVENTIVE AIDS.   Five types of community care now under consideration for the aged include: (1) a geriatric unit in the general hospital, (2) rehabilitation programs, (3) senior centers, (4) old age guidance centers, and (5) infirmaries for the aged. Many state and local health departments are also doing research and disseminating information on heart disease, cancer, diabetes, accidents, and cerebral hemorrhage, which are all great killers of the aged. Many health departments conduct chronic disease detection programs, cancer and mental health research centers, clinics, and other facilities designed to prevent illness and prolong life. In some areas special funds are made available to school districts in order to provide education and recreation services for the aging.

These problems must be attacked in the same way as communicable diseases. Public health has developed specialized personnel and techniques that can be used in attacking the noncommunicable diseases of later life. Many local programs are being designed to meet the needs of this older segment of the population, to prevent disease among them, and to extend and maintain healthful life, thus making a longer life more enjoyable. Governor Nelson Rockefeller of New York aptly summarized the situation:

. . . . The greatest pitfall is to think of old age as simply a government problem. It is a human problem—and also a great human opportunity. Elderly people are rich in years and potentials, each desiring to fill a useful place. They are all of us—tomorrow or the next day. . . . Any proper program for the aged must show a vigorous concern for their welfare. It is not easy for a state to find the money—and even with limitless money it would not have limitless staff or limitless knowledge. But an experimental program can often blaze new trails and can even save money in the long run as well as greatly increased human happiness. . . .[15]

QUESTIONS FOR REVIEW

1. Are the major community problems in California *similar* to those in Arkansas? Different? Explain.
2. Name and briefly discuss five methods or ways of determining the health of a community or nation.
3. (a) List in order the ten leading causes of death today in the United States.
   (b) Compare the leading causes of death among college students with the leading causes of death among elementary and high school students.
4. "We added chlorine to the community water supply without voting—let's add fluorine to the water without a vote." Discuss the merits of this statement.
5. What are some new childhood accident dangers that have risen with scientific and technological advances?
6. How can we prevent prematurity and congenital malformations?
7. How can we detect a possible suicide victim?
8. Why is alcoholism a community problem?
9. What danger signals indicate diabetes?
10. List eight possible community geriatric aids.

REFERENCES

1. Eliot, Martha M.: *The National Score, The Challenge of Fetal Loss, Prematurity, and Infant Mortality.* Association for the Aid of Crippled Children, New York, 1956, Page 10.
2. Ibid. Page 11.
3. West, Jessie Stevenson: *Congenital Malformations and Birth Injuries,* A

Handbook of Nursing. Association for the Aid of Crippled Children, 1954, Pages 2–10.

4. *Prematurity, Congenital Malformation and Birth Injury.* Proceedings of a Conference sponsored by the Association for the Aid of Crippled Children, Association for the Aid of Crippled Children, New York, 1953, Pages 176, 184.

5. Eliot, Martha M.: *The National Score, The Challenge of Fetal Loss, Prematurity, and Infant Mortality.* Association for the Aid of Crippled Children, New York, 1956, Page 12.

6. *Alcoholism and California Related Statistics, 1900–1956,* State of California, Dept. of Public Health. California State Printing Office, 1956, Page 7.

7. *California's Health, Biennial Report Edition, July 1, 1954–July 30, 1956,* Vol. 14, No. 10, Nov. 15, 1956. California State Printing Office, 1956, Page 101.

8. The Big Headache. *The California State Employee,* February, 1959, Page 14, 16.

9. *California's Health, Biennial Report Edition, July 1, 1954–July 30, 1956,* Vol. 14, No. 10, Nov. 15, 1956. California State Printing office, 1956, Page 101.

10. *Alcoholism and California Related Statistics, 1900–1956,* State of California, Dept. of Public Health. California State Printing Office, 1956, Page 46.

11. Popham, Robert E.: *The Jellinek Estimation Formula and Its Application to Canadian Data.* Quart. J. Studies on Alcohol, 17:559–593, 1960.

12. McCord, W., and McCord, J.: *Origins of Alcoholism.* Stanford University Press, 1960.

13. *Alcoholism—Society's Responsibility.* Proceedings of a Statewide Workshop on Alcoholism, Alcoholic Rehabilitation, California State Department of Public Health, 1958, Page 31.

14. *Do You Want To Live Longer?* U.S. News and World Report, February 14, 1958, Page 82.

15. *Unnecessary Fate of the Old and Sick.* Life, August 3, 1959, Page 17.

SUGGESTED READING

American Public Health Association: *Present Day Health Problems.* Am. J. Pub. Health, 50:1, 1960.

A Report of the Subcommittee on Paramedical Personnel in Rehabilitation and Care of the Chronically Ill: *Mobilization and Health Manpower II.* Washington, D. C., U. S. Government Printing Office, 1956.

Ast, D. B., and Schlesinger, E. R.: *Conclusion of a Ten-Year Study of Water Fluoridation.* Am. J. Pub. Health, 46:3, 1956.

Bachman, George W.: *Health Resources in the United States.* Washington, D. C., Brookings Institution, 1952.

Baird, Janet: *These Harvest Years.* New York, Doubleday and Co., Inc. 1951.

Bond, Floyd A., et al.: *Our Needy Aged, a California Study of a National Problem.* New York, Henry Holt and Co., 1954.

Bouton, M. A.: *A Diabetes Case-Finding Program.* Am. J. Pub. Health. 50: 524–530, 1960.

Boyington, Gregory (Pappy): *Baa Baa Black Sheep.* New York, G. P. Putnam's Sons, 1958.

Crocetti, G. M.: *Suicide and Public Health—An Attempt at Reconceptualization.* Am. J. Pub. Health, 49:881–888, 1959.

Dunham, M. C.: *Premature Birth as a World Health Problem.* Pediatrics, 7: 262, 1951.

Gordon, J. E.: *Dental Problems, an Epidemiologic Perspective.* Am. J. Pub. Health, 49:1041–1049, 1959.

Greenberg, Leon A., M.D.: *Alcoholism, A Basic Approach to Treatment.* Yale Center of Alcohol Studies, 1957.

Gruenberg, H. M.: *Public Health and the People's Health.* Pub. Health Rep., 72:1, 1957.

Health Bulletin for Teachers: *Recent Advances in Medicine and Public Health,* Vol. 25, New York, Metropolitan Life Insurance Company, 1954.

Hilleboe, Herman E., and Larimore, Granville W.: *Preventive Medicine, Principles of Prevention in the Occurrence and Progression of Disease.* Philadelphia, W. B. Saunders Company, 1959.

Lawton, George: *Aging Successfully.* New York, Columbia University Press, 1946.

Lipscomb, W. R.: *Epidemiological Methods in the Study of Alcoholism.* Am. J. Pub. Health, 49:327–333, 1959.

Mann, Marty: *New Primer on Alcohol.* New York, Rinehart and Co., 1958.

Menninger, Karl: *Man Against Himself.* New York, Harcourt, Brace and Co., 1938.

Mountin, Joseph W.: *Selected Papers of Community Services for an Aging Population.* Pub. Health Rep. 1952.

Pfeffer, Arnold Z., M.D.: *Alcoholism.* New York, Grune & Stratton, Inc., 1958.

Philip, J. R.: *Alcoholism in California—The Experience of the California State Department of Public Health.* Am. J. Pub. Health, 49:322–326, 1959.

Proceedings of Conference Sponsored by Association for Aid of Crippled Children: *Prematurity, Congenital Malformation, and Birth Injury.* New York, Association for Aid of Crippled Children, 1953.

Proceedings of Second Conference of the Association for Aid of Crippled Children: *Mechanisms of Congenital Malformations.* New York, Association for Aid of Crippled Children, 1954.

Robins, E., et al.: *Some Clinical Considerations in the Prevention of Suicide Based on a Study of 134 Successful Suicides.* Am. J. Pub. Health, 49:888–899, 1959.

Roth, Lillian: *I'll Cry Tomorrow.* New York, Fell and Co., 1954.

Simpson, Winea J.: *A Preliminary Report on Cigarette Smoking and the Incidence of Prematurity.* Am. J. Obst. & Gynec., 73:4, 1957.

Smillie, Wilson G.: *Preventive Medicine and Public Health.* New York, The Macmillan Co., 1955.

Steiglitz, Edward J.: *Geriatrics Medicine. Philadelphia,* J. B. Lippincott and Co., 1954.

The Alcoholic Foundation, Inc.: *Alcoholics Anonymous.* New York, The Alcoholic Foundation, Inc.,

The Committee for the White House Conference on Education: *A Report to the President.* Washington, D. C., U. S. Printing Office, 1956.

The National Council on Alcoholism: *Alcoholism Information Kit.* New York, The National Council on Alcoholism,

Wallace, Helen M., Baumgartner, Leona, and Rich, Herbert: *Congenital Malformation and Birth Injuries in New York City.* Pediatrics, 12:525, 1953.

West, Jessie Stevenson: *Congenital Malformations and Birth Injuries, A Handbook on Nursing.* New York, Association for Aid of Crippled Children, 1954.

Chapter II

Historical
Aspects of Community
Health in the United States

THE MAJOR health problems that confronted the citizens of such states as Massachusetts, New York and Oregon during the middle of the nineteenth century also confronted citizens of other growing states and cities throughout the country. Many health problems, such as water pollution and smallpox epidemics, were prevalent at approximately the same time throughout the entire United States. With the discovery of the causes of certain diseases; the production of vaccines, serums, and antibiotics; the organization and cooperation of official, voluntary and community health agencies; and the application of the principles of sanitation and health education, the number of communicable disease cases and deaths declined.

This decline was slow, but it appeared uniformly throughout the country. As one epidemic subsided, however, there was usually another of a different nature to take its place.

Early Health Legislation

Health measures in towns and communities were slow to develop; early settlers were primarily interested in building their homes and developing land. Woods Hutchinson, M.D., Secretary of the first Oregon State Board of Health, reflected the situation when he stated:

> . . . it was rather hard to stir up popular interest in public hygiene or to secure adequate appropriations for its promotion. . . . This of course was only natural, both because our people were so closely engaged in building the railroads, clearing the forests, breaking the prairies and providing housing and shelter in a wild, new country, that there seemed to be no time for consideration of "doctors' fussiness" about sewage and ventilation and food-inspection and quarantine. . . .[1]

The population of cities and states was small, and regulations concerning public health were not demanding at that time. For example, the original city charter of Portland, Oregon, adopted in 1851, made no provisions regarding public health except to empower the city council to enact ordinances and bylaws concerning the "good government of said corporation, and the health, morals, and safety of its citizens."[2] In 1853 the council was given additional authority "to make regulations to prevent the introduction of contagious and other diseases into the city; to establish hospitals and make regulations for the government of the same; and to secure the general health of the inhabitants."[3] Furthermore, citizens were reluctant to accept public health reforms, and public health legislation was difficult to establish.

The first state health department was organized in Louisiana in 1855. Massachusetts organized the second state health department in 1869.[4] Shortly after, other state health departments were established in rapid succession. It is interesting to note that the fear of importation of specific diseases was directly responsible for the creation of many state and local health departments. For example, the Louisiana State Board of Health was founded to prevent the further inroads of yellow fever. An epidemic of the same disease in the Southern States prompted Congress to create a National Board of Health in 1878 in order to combat the disease. The Board was unorganized and ineffective, however, and was discontinued in 1888. Fear of the importation of cholera from Europe

was directly responsible for the National Quarantine Act of 1893.[5]
Importation of diseases by steamers arriving from Europe and the
Orient constantly threatened the coastal states, especially during
the periods of heavy immigration from 1880 to 1910. In addition,
a new manner of disease importation occurred in 1883 when cross-
country rail communication was completed.

Communicable Disease Control

The major activities of local and state health departments
from 1850 to 1920 involved communicable disease control and sanitation.[6] The chief methods of controlling communicable diseases
included escorting diseased persons to the town pesthouse (isolation), quarantine, and fumigation to destroy bacteria. However,
quarantine failed as the major measure of communicable disease
protection because health officials and others did not understand the epidemiological principles of the disease carrier in relation to the spread of infection. Furthermore, the modes of transmission, and periods of incubation and communicability of infection
were not well understood. Because pride and business interests
were involved, citizens in most communities falsely denied that diseases existed in their midst.

Although tuberculosis and typhoid fever claimed many lives,
smallpox was the most dreaded disease ever to invade the country.
Smallpox instilled fear and terror in the public mind because of its
loathsome appearance and disfiguring consequences, its extreme
communicability, and its high fatality rate. Smallpox vaccine had
been introduced as early as 1796, but mass vaccination programs
were not conducted in the United States until the 1920's because
many individuals were slow to accept the preventive measure. With
the application of measures for community sanitation and health
education and with an increasing proportion of the population protected by immunization against typhoid fever, diphtheria and smallpox, the number of cases and deaths from these communicable diseases gradually decreased. (See Figure 11.)

Population Changes

The rapid change of population from a rural to an urban economy was a major factor in molding the pattern of public health organization, administration and services in the United States. From
1880 to 1910, many cities grew rapidly as a result of heavy immigra-

tion and a high birth rate. Urbanization of cities without proper understanding of the problems and hazards of crowded community life was one of the most important problems at that time. Hygienic measures that were quite adequate in sparsely settled areas were completely unsuited to the city dweller. Thus, sickness and communicable disease death rate increased to such a degree that specific sanitary problems were eventually recognized, faced, and finally solved. Another key to the high communicable disease fatality rate in the United States from 1880 to 1910 related to the age distribution of population. At that time epidemics were most fatal to children and young adults, and over 40 per cent of the nation's population was under 20 years of age.[7]

Milk and Water Control

Impure milk and water accounted for a large number of communicable disease cases and deaths from 1850 to 1915. Epidemics of typhoid fever, diphtheria, scarlet fever, diarrhea and enteritis,

Victory over disease requires constant vigilance.

Vaccination controls smallpox; incomplete vaccination keeps polio a threat.

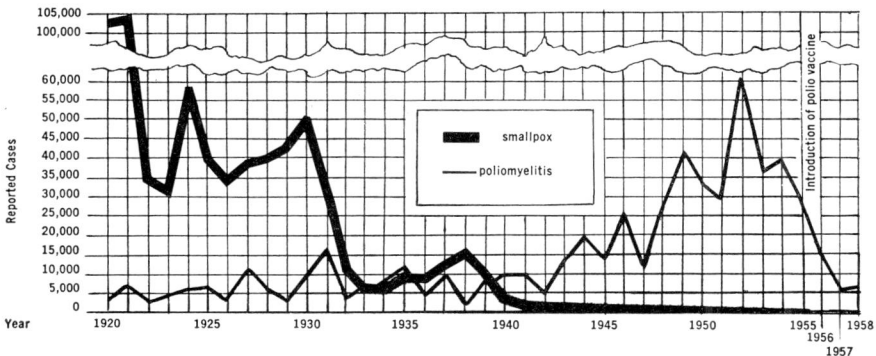

Figure 11. Widespread immunization was practiced first against smallpox, a disease well-controlled in the United States although no uniform national law exists for vaccination. In 1955, 13 states required vaccination for school enrollment, 17 states provided for "local option in face of threat," 11 states had no immunization laws covering smallpox, and 7 (Washington, California, Arizona, Utah, North Dakota, South Dakota, Minnesota) prohibited compulsory vaccination. Smallpox is still endemic in some parts of the world, and travelers from foreign countries pose a threat to the United States. In 1946, a soldier returning from Japan was responsible for an outbreak of 28 cases in Seattle; a man traveling from Mexico to New York spread infection to 8 persons in 1947. In the 1958 Detroit polio epidemic, outbreak of paralytic type was located in a downtown area of low socioeconomic level where less than 5% of the paralytic cases had received 3 doses of polio vaccine. None of the 22 fatal cases had received 3 doses. (From Patterns of Disease, Parke, Davis and Co., November, 1959.)

City of Albany, N.Y.

Average 89.4

Filters Installed

Supply Chlorinated

City of Binghamton, N.Y.

Average 56.6

Filters Installed

Supply Chlorinated

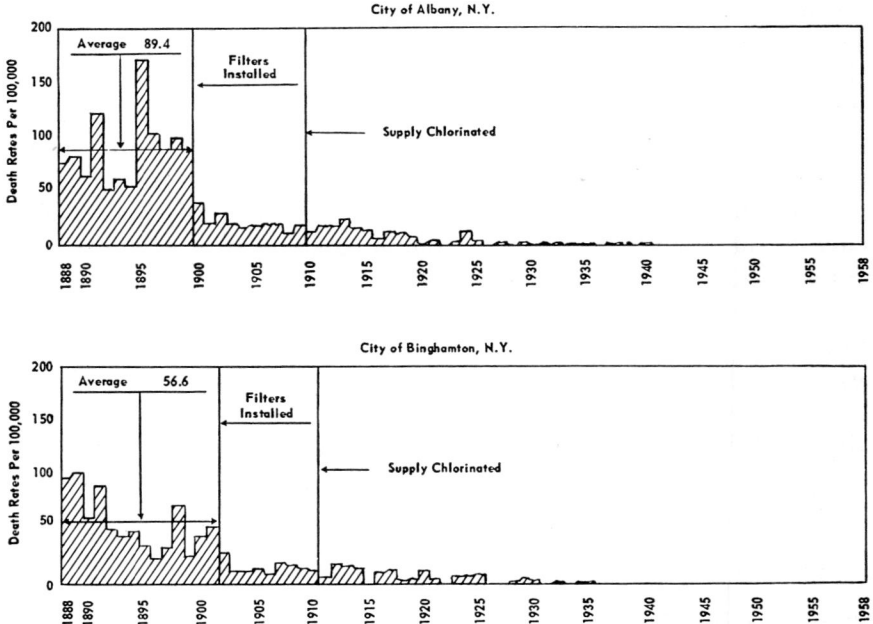

Figure 12. The effect of water purification on the typhoid fever death rate of two typical cities. (Prepared by the New York State Department of Health, 1958.)

tuberculosis and other diseases were traced directly to impure milk or water supplies. Although state and city health officials devoted a great deal of time to those major public health problems, it was not until the period from 1910 to 1915 that legislation was enacted and organized campaigns were conducted to remedy this situation. Education, scientific advances, chlorination, pasteurization, and sanitary improvements also contributed to pure milk and water supplies. A sharp decrease in the number of communicable disease cases and deaths resulted. (See Figure 12.)

Expansion of State and Local Health Departments

Although the States as sovereign powers had the responsibility and authority to guard the health of their citizens, they granted permission to separate local communities to establish local public health laws, and each community solved its own public health problems. In 1797, for instance, Massachusetts granted state-wide authority to towns and cities to establish local health services, but the state itself assumed no responsibility for public health affairs. Even such matters as maritime quarantine were carried out by the local community.[8] The creation of state boards of health, however, brought about a great improvement of public health within the state. The boards, originally designed to control communicable diseases by interstate and intrastate quarantine methods, rapidly expanded their services and personnel in an effort to prevent disease and prolong life. Bacteriology laboratories were established to aid in the diagnosis of communicable diseases. More efficient systems of reporting and recording vital statistics were introduced. In addition, county health boards were organized, health officers were appointed, and each county was required to meet certain minimum public health standards and regulations. Funds granted by private health foundations and the United States Government enabled the state boards of health to expand their services, activities and programs. Through the years, prevention of disease and prolonging of life were stressed.

Public Health and Medical Advances

An infant born in 1900 had a life expectancy of 50 years. Today, because of tremendous strides made in public health and medicine, an infant has before him a life span of more than 69 years. (See Figure 13.) When the early state boards of health were created, epidemics of typhoid fever, smallpox, diphtheria, and bubonic plague threatened the country. Tuberculosis and typhoid fever were leading causes of death at that time. Today, smallpox has almost disappeared from the country, plague is an extremely rare disease, and significant reductions have been made in the incidence of and deaths from typhoid fever, diphtheria, whooping cough, measles, scarlet fever, tuberculosis, the dysenteries, and the tick-borne diseases. The period from 1900 to 1960 has revealed a steady decline in the communicable disease morbidity and mortality rates. Maternal mortality has been reduced to a great extent, and infant deaths have been cut from 99.9 per thousand in 1915 to 26.0 per thousand in 1960.

The success of official and voluntary health agencies throughout the first half of the twentieth century is largely attributed to public health laboratory services, statistical services, environmental sanitation services, immunizations, antibiotics, public health nursing services, and health education. Although communicable diseases have decreased, tuberculosis, pneumonia, venereal diseases, poliomyelitis, and infectious hepatitis are among those still prevalent in 1960. Therefore, health officials emphasize that continued success in the control of communicable diseases cannot be maintained

THE INCREASING LIFE SPAN IN AMERICA

	IN 1900 AVERAGE LIFE EXPECTANCY	NOW* AVERAGE LIFE EXPECTANCY	INCREASE IN LIFE EXPECTANCY SINCE 1900
AT BIRTH	49.2 YEARS	69.5 YEARS	20.3 YEARS
AT AGE 10	51.1 YEARS	61.9 YEARS	10.8 YEARS
AT AGE 20	42.7 YEARS	52.3 YEARS	9.6 YEARS
AT AGE 30	35.5 YEARS	42.9 YEARS	7.4 YEARS
AT AGE 40	28.3 YEARS	33.7 YEARS	5.4 YEARS
AT AGE 50	21.2 YEARS	25.1 YEARS	3.9 YEARS
AT AGE 60	14.7 YEARS	17.5 YEARS	2.8 YEARS
AT AGE 70	9.3 YEARS	11.3 YEARS	2.0 YEARS
AT AGE 80	5.3 YEARS	6.6 YEARS	1.3 YEARS

For youths under 20, life expectancy is much higher than when the twentieth century began — 10 to 20 years longer, on the average.

For people over 60, the gain in life expectancy has been much smaller — about two to three years have been added on the average, since 1900, to the lives of those who reach 60 and over.

*1955, latest available

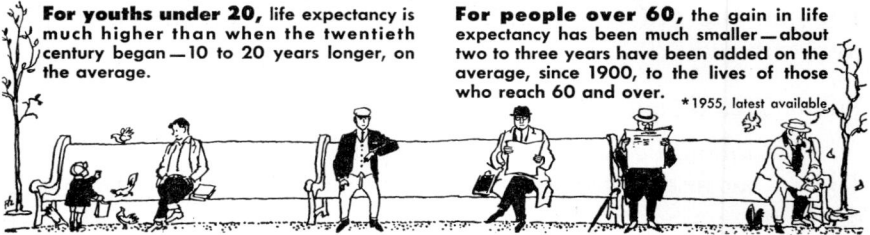

Figure 13. (From Stieglitz, Edward J., *Do You Want To Live Longer?* U. S. News and World Report, February 14, 1958.)

without continued effort and evaluation of the effectiveness of control measures.

Medical advances in recent years have been rapid and remarkable. Physicians are trying to solve the mysterious interrelation between the mind and the body. New and ingenious devices and instruments have been developed to probe the secrets of the body's cells, tissues, organs, and glands. For example, we can now study the nature of genes and chromosomes with the aid of an electron microscope. Reflecting and recording tapes attached to the head, neck, shoulder, arms, and legs of a walking man reveal the precise pattern of muscular movement.

Other devices probe more hidden body activities. Modern electronics can measure minute variations in the beating of the heart, which makes early diagnosis of many heart ailments possible. Electrodes attached to the head can reduce fluctuations in the brain's electrical activity and thus detect certain brain tumors or lesions. Radioactive isotopes reveal tumors and abnormal chemical changes taking place within the body. High voltage x-ray machines can destroy these malignant tumors. Ultrasonic waves, radium, and electric currents can also destroy unwanted cells or tissues. Devices like the heart-lung machine can take over a patient's entire circulation while the heart is immobilized. During the operation, accessory devices monitor the patient's pulse and blood volume, add coagulants or anticoagulants as needed, and maintain a complex state of anesthesia that can be altered instantly. Slender blade-like rods can scrape diseased or clogged blood vessels and thereby add years to the life of the patient with atherosclerosis.

Discovery of new antibiotics and drugs has also aided in preventing disease and prolonging life. New drugs have helped many persons defeat and prevent such previously noted killers as pernicious anemia, subacute bacterial endocarditis, tuberculosis, rheumatic fever, syphilis, and high blood pressure. Chemotherapy has given a ray of hope to many mentally ill patients, needle-plagued diabetics, and certain cancer and heart patients. Rheumatism and arthritis may be cured or at least alleviated to allow our aged to enjoy a fuller and happier life.

As longevity increases, people require more and more body replacement parts. Today there are blood banks, bone banks, eye cornea banks, cartilage banks, and artery banks, to name only a few. These replacement parts are taken during autopsy, frozen, and then stored as replacements for diseased or damaged parts of future patients. Surgeons believe that they will be able to transplant most types of tissue and even entire organs eventually.

New Problems

Despite major public health gains in the United States, new health problems have appeared. The interest in longevity has led to the boast that Americans enjoy the finest medical care in the world. Since increased longevity is achieved as a result of medical advances, the assumption is a natural one. But the fact is that there are many nations which surpass the United States in life expectancy. The Netherlands leads the world with a life expectancy of 72 years, followed in close order by New Zealand and the Scandinavian countries. (See Figure 14.)

A more realistic picture of life expectancy is obtained when comparing the decline in death rates in different age groups. Such comparison shows which segments of our population have benefited most from medical advances. (See Figure 15.) Significant differences can also be noted when the life expectancy rates are compiled according to sex, race, and social factors. The female death rate, for

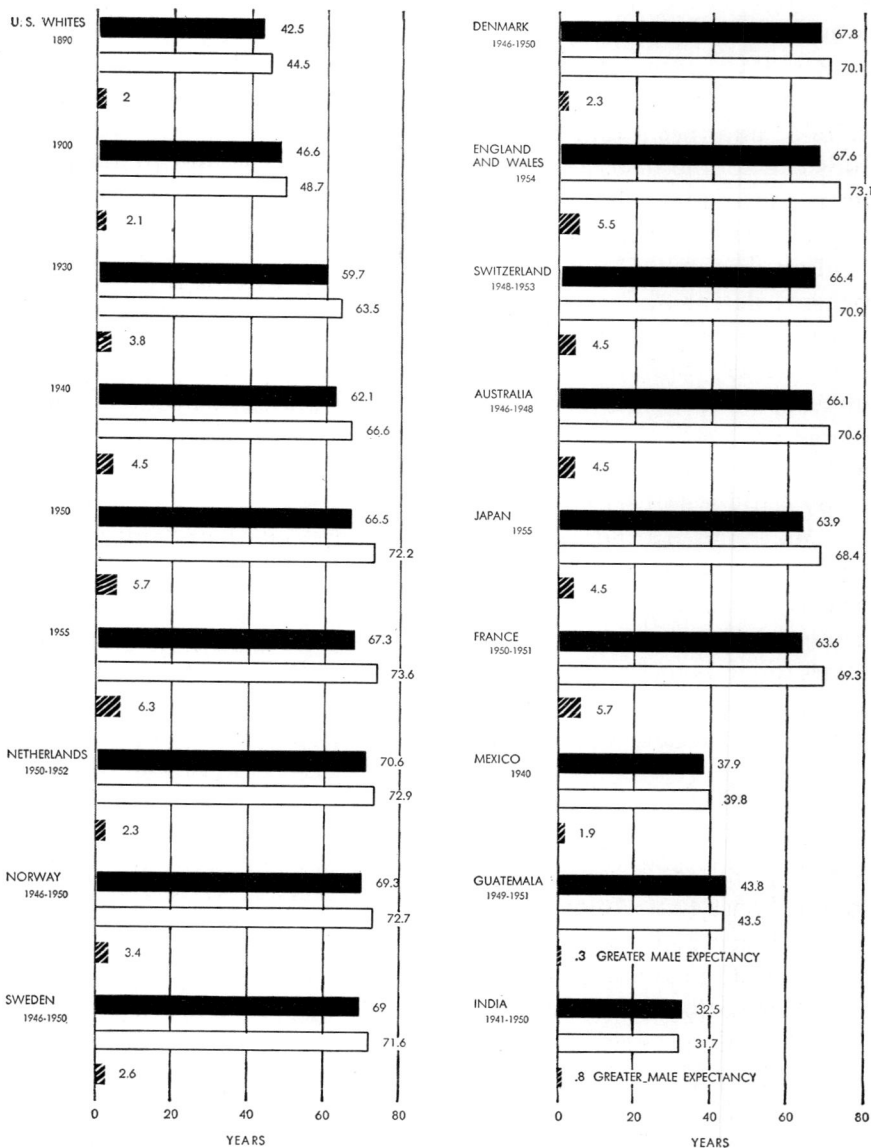

Figure 14. Life expectancies at birth of white men and women in the U. S. over a period of 65 years, and of men and women in 12 other countries over various periods, are compared. The black bars represent men; the white bars, women; the diagonal (stripes) bars, the difference between the two. (From Scientific American, *198*:26, February, 1958.)

example, has declined nearly two-thirds since 1900, while the male death rate has dropped one-half. It is interesting to note that the average life expectancy of the United States female has always exceeded the average life expectancy of the United States male. If we use mortality rate as the sole criterion of a people's health, we must not overlook the fact that certain disabling illnesses impair the victim's mental, physical, and social well-being, and may be as destructive to a nation's health as the sudden killer. Our nation is faced with many health problems in this category.

Whether the United States can materially better its present life expectancy in the near future seems doubtful to the experts. Death rates from acute diseases, they point out, are already so low that even an additional reduction would have little effect in reducing the overall rate. More important, death rates from chronic diseases have been steadily rising. Increased life expectancy has given the entire nation a population with a greater proportion of aged persons. This has caused health agencies to shift emphasis from communicable disease programs to chronic and degenerative disease programs. Mental health, industrial hygiene, air pollution, radiological health, fluoridation, hospital construction, geriatrics, safety education, school health, and recreation programs have also increased in importance. Each program is supported by research and education.

However, it is not sufficient merely to shift the attention of

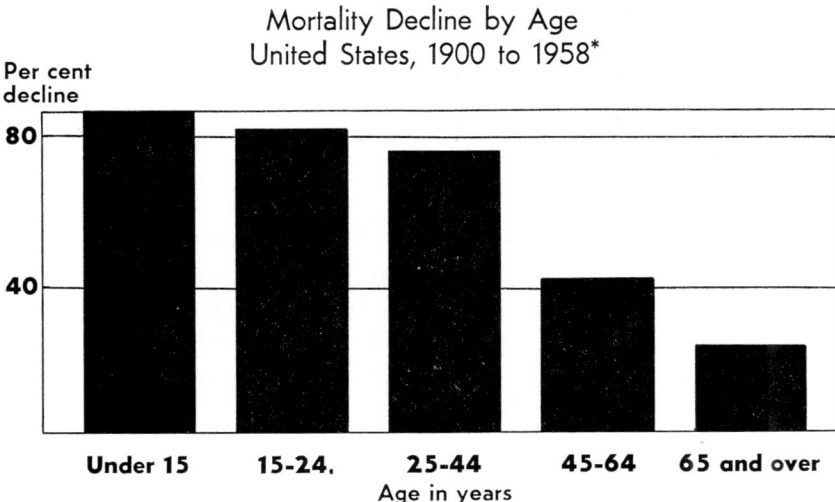

Mortality Decline by Age
United States, 1900 to 1958*

*Death Registration States only, 1900. 1958 data are provisional.

Figure 15. (From the National Office of Vital Statistics, modified from Research Series Eleven, Health Information Foundation.)

medical and public health men from acute to chronic diseases. Physicians have been concentrating on chronic diseases for some time; their intentions are excellent, but they lack weapons. Nor is it sufficient to provide additional funds for research in new drugs for cancer, heart disease, and other chronic problems, worthy as these projects are. The great need is increased emphasis on the development of fundamental knowledge in the basic sciences of physiology, biology, chemistry, genetics, and physics. A greater appreciation for basic research must be developed and encouraged as a long-term investment in knowledge, rather than for the immediate conquest of a particular disease. A disease cannot be vanquished merely because unlimited amounts of money and scientists are available; new vaccines and miracle drugs cannot be purchased with money alone. They are developed only when research in the basic sciences has yielded enough knowledge to make them possible. For example, the Salk polio vaccine resulted from 16 years of tedious work by hundreds of scientists in a dozen fields of endeavor. The information gained by these various investigations may prove vital in the control of other diseases.

The success of a dynamic attack on the chronic killers depends on the support of basic research, and there is much medical knowledge available that is not being used for the benefit of all. There is too great a lag between the development of medical knowledge and its application. The fault is threefold: insufficient health and medical personnel, inadequate training, and faulty distribution of services. A leading medical director, Dean Willard C. Rappleye of Columbia University's College of Physicians and Surgeons warns that attention should first be given to insuring that physicians, nurses, dentists, and other health personnel are adequately trained and competent to provide modern, up-to-date health services for individual patients and the community. He joins other authorities in calling for greater support of medical education. The nation's 96 medical schools, which produce nearly 7,000 new doctors each year, are in need of money. To attract and keep the needed high quality teachers, they must pay salaries that compete with high earning potentials outside medical school. The costs of operating a medical school are extremely high. Small group instruction is essential; most schools maintain an average of one teacher to four students. Nor can medical students be taught with books alone; every school must have an affiliated teaching hospital where the first-hand diagnosis and treatment of disease can be learned. Such hospitals are expensive to maintain and usually show large deficits. Also necessary are numerous medical-research studies requiring costly laboratory equipment. Although the average medical student spends about $1,000 per year for tuition, actual expense to the school for each student is about $4,000. The National Fund for Medical Education, an organization dedicated to helping medical schools survive, estimates that at least $10,000,000 a year is required to cover their basic needs. The source of financial aid has become a major problem; shall it be gifts from individuals, donations from industry or subsidies from the federal goverment? Some medical leaders fear government aid; they believe it may lead to political interference with the operation of the schools. Many advocate that government money be used only for buildings. But if support does not come from some source, many schools may be seriously weakened; if this happens, the foundations of medical care will be threatened.

There is no disagreement with the fact that this country lacks sufficient nurses to meet the growing health needs of the nation. In addition to the recruitment of more girls to enter the nursing profession, the shortage is being met by the special instruction of thousands of women as nurses' aides and practical nurses. There is, however, loud disagreement when the shortage of physicians is discussed; the American Medical Association disclaims any lack of physicians, admitting only to poor distribution in certain rural areas. Physicians, it holds, tend to concentrate in well-populated regions because of the many advantages. The President's Commission on the Health Needs of the Nation believes there is a shortage and estimates that by 1965, considering the population increase, we will have a shortage of 55,000 physicians. If medical schools were able to increase their facilities for training larger numbers of medical students, there apparently would be no lack of qualified candidates. Medical schools report that each year at least 20,000 students apply for admission. Many are well-qualified but are rejected because of lack of space and facilities. Because it takes many years to train a physician, observers believe it is imperative to settle the shortage controversy without delay.

QUESTIONS FOR REVIEW

1. (a) Name five leading causes of death in the United States in 1900.
   (b) Name in order four leading causes of death in the United States today.
   (c) Give five reasons for this change, if any.
   (d) What effect does this change have upon community health programs?
2. What major factors led to the establishment of local and state health departments?

3. (a) What were the two major activities of local and state health departments from 1850 to 1920?

(b) What are the major activities of local and state health departments today?

4. "Despite major public health gains in the United States, new health problems have appeared." Discuss this statement.

5. Name four leading causes of death in your community today.

6. Name four leading causes of death in your state today.

REFERENCES

1. Oregon State Board of Health: *Fourteenth Biennial Report to the Governor,* 1931 . . . (Salem) Pages 5, 6.

2. Oregon Laws, 1851, Page 18.

3. Oregon Laws, 1853, Page 9.

4. Smillie, Wilson G.: *Public Health: Its Promise for the Future.* New York, The Macmillan Co., 1955, Page 319.

5. Mountin, Joseph W.: *The History and Function of the United States Public Health Service.* In Simmons, James Stevens, Editor, Public Health in the World Today. Massachusetts, Harvard University Press, 1949.

6. Chapin, Charles V.: *A Report on State Public Health Work Based on a Survey of State Boards of Health.* Chicago, American Medical Association, 1916.

7. Dublin, Louis I.: *The Facts of Life From Birth to Death.* New York, The Macmillan Co., 1951.

8. Blake, John B.: *Public Health in the Town of Boston, 1630–1822.* Unpublished Ph.D. dissertation, Harvard University, 1953.

SUGGESTED READING

American Public Health Association: *A Century of Progress Through Sanitation.* Am. J. Pub. Health, *43*:6, 1953.

Budd, W.: *Typhoid Fever, Its Nature, Mode of Spread and Prevention.* New York, George Grady Press, 1931.

Chapin, C. V.: *Papers of.* New York, Commonwealth Fund, 1934.

Hanlon, J. J., Rogers, F. B., Rosen, G.: *A Bookshelf on the History and Philosophy of Public Health.* Am. J. Pub. Health, *50*:445–458, 1960.

Larsell, O.: *The Doctor in Oregon.* Portland, Binfords and Mort, 1947.

Panum, P. L.: *Observations Made During the Epidemic of Measles in the Faroe Islands in the Year 1846.* New York, American Public Health Association, 1940.

Rosen, George: *A History of Public Health.* New York, MD Publications, Inc., 1958.

Smillie, Wilson G.: *Public Health: Its Promise for the Future.* New York, The Macmillan Co., 1955.

Smolensky, Jack: *A History of Public Health in Oregon.* Doctoral Dissertation, Oregon, University of Oregon Press, 1956. (microcard)

Snow, J.: *On Cholera.* New York, Commonwealth Fund, 1936.

The Crisis in American Medicine. Harper's Magazine, October 1960, Pages 123–168.

Where Are Tomorrow's Doctors? U.S. Medical Education Is Lagging. Time, June 20, 1960, Pages 52, 53.

Winslow, C. E. A.: *The Conquest of Epidemic Diseases.* New Jersey, Princeton University Press, 1944.

Zinsser, H.: *Rats, Lice and History.* Boston, Little, Brown and Co., 1945.

Chapter III

Sociological
Aspects of Community Health

THE PHRASE *community health* is composed of two words: community and health. In order to conduct a successful community health program, health workers must consider the significance and implication of both words. We are dealing with a product, *health,* and a recipient, *the community.* Complete knowledge and understanding of both are necessary. We must understand and deal with the health problem; we must also understand and treat the social or public phase of the situation.

Health is a social responsibility in and of the community. In order to formulate ways of meeting and solving health needs by the democratic process, a community must have groups of interrelating and interacting individuals functioning for a common purpose. This demands recognition of differing groups in the community and appreciation for the fact that their goals or values may not be totally in accord with our own. We cannot have adequate motivation for health, or develop adequate participation by these groups unless we are willing to accept people, whoever they are and wherever they may live, and work with them toward sharing goals, aspirations, and tasks.[1]

Concepts and Obstacles

There are many obstacles to be overcome and certain concepts to be understood before a community can organize and successfully solve its health problems. As a result of urbanization, relationships among individuals in the community have become less effective. Some authorities believe that there has been a corresponding decrease in the effectiveness of channels of communication.[1] Another obstacle presents itself when "modern" children and "old-fashioned" parents disagree upon the objectives and philosophies behind certain health programs. In each community the family represents the most powerful example of social cohesion. Therefore, if conflicting opinions, objectives, and philosophies cause families throughout the community to become separated, community health programs are weakened and often defeated. On the other hand, certain members of the family may disseminate factual health information that, in turn, may lead to strengthened family support for certain controversial health programs. For example, many parents may be undecided concerning fluoridation of water supplies. Their high school or college boy or girl, however, may have learned that fluoridation is beneficial, and he or she may have an opportunity to discuss the problem with other members of the family. As a result, more of these informed parents may join the campaign for fluoridation. However, we must remember that in many families the parents' attitudes and prejudices are instilled in the children from early childhood, and although the child is exposed to new ideas and concepts in school, more concentrated effort and education is needed to erase unfavorable prejudices and attitudes.[2]

Present economic, sociologic, and technologic conditions have caused the family to be less closely knit than in the past, and this must be considered when organizing and planning health programs. Members of the family have barely enough time to speak to each other, and certainly haven't time to discuss community health problems. Often the young adult members of the family marry or leave for college; in addition, many families do not stay in one community long enough to learn or to concern themselves with the health problems and needs of the community. Because Americans are migrating from state to state at such a rapid pace, many new health problems are being created every day. An insecure and fast pace of living; pressure and interest groups; racial integration in schools and communities; increased chronic disease and accident fatalities; longer life expectancy; population explosion; increased mental illness; and swift methods of travel that bring cities, states, and countries closer together are other factors to consider when a community attempts to organize and promote health programs today.

Community organization involves recognition of the fact that there are definite separations among upper, middle, and lower classes and these separations are on the increase.[3] Communities are also divided into racial, religious, and national minority groups, age groups, and occupational groups to mention but a few. The college graduate is separated from the high school graduate, the factory worker from the store owner, and the owner of a Rolls-Royce is separated from the owner of a simple four-door sedan. Correspondingly, poor housing projects develop in one section of a town, and larger, more modern homes are found in another section. As a result small nucleated groups develop; these groups have little in common and in some ways may be antagonistic. A strong and united community is composed of groups of cooperative individuals who are functionally related in meeting common needs. Although each group may have different values, the health priority rating of each group and of the total community must be determined and understood. How high does health really rank in the value systems of the people? Each community must ask this question.

Often a community is divided into many different kinds of areas or tracts resulting in many and varied neighborhoods. These neighborhoods or zones gradually overlap, and sometimes social problems follow such changes. A master plan formulated by an official city planning board can greatly alleviate the results of these changes in land-use patterns. Furthermore, artificial city and county boundaries that are arbitrarily set at a certain road or creek weaken the entire community organization. Any boundary line lessens active cooperation and participation for better health and vitiates the appeal for popular support.

Interest in many community health programs often wanes because only 10 to 20 per cent of the people in any community are members of organized health groups. In rural communities the percentage is even smaller. Active participation by a cross section of all the people in the community is not accomplished if representatives are chosen only from the various agencies and groups. Instead, *all* members of the community should be considered when representatives are being chosen. Certain members within a group or community are assumed to be leaders and are therefore assigned leadership positions; community programs would be much more effective if the real or natural leaders were elected by their respective groups. Many times majority groups choose leaders or representatives from certain minority groups without consulting minority members. If members of the minority groups were asked they would readily confess that the real or natural leaders had not been chosen.

Although there are 25 to 100 organized health groups and established health agencies operating in many communities in the United States, there is usually a lack of cooperation, coordination, and planning. Health workers and other professional personnel often forget that health interests are only one aspect among many in the community. Some agencies are interested in organizing the community for their own ends, and those ends are determined in the national headquarters, not in the community. Pressure and interest groups may hinder or halt certain health programs; vested interests, ignorance, or lack of the facts are a few contributing factors. The cooperative efforts of many agencies enable communities to produce citizens with complete physical, mental, and social well-being. An effective program includes group defined philosophy, objectives, fact finding, education, decision making, community action, and evaluation. This democratic process is of the community, for the community, and by the community.

Effect of Cultural Patterns on Health

A society is any community of individuals drawn together by a common bond of nearness and interaction—a group of people who act together for the achievement of certain common goals. A person's culture determines how he thinks, feels, acts, speaks, worships, dresses, marries, eats, prepares food, treats the sick, and disposes of the dead.[3] There are usually a great many cultures in each community. Each culture respects and accepts certain values, attitudes, and beliefs. Public health programs necessarily involve the introduction of new practices and changes in values and beliefs into the culture of the society. If such programs are to be constructive rather than destructive forces, the social structure and the traditional cultural way of life of the community must be taken into account and utilized. The accepted value systems of a culture are deeply ingrained, and people adhere strongly to their attitudes and beliefs. Crowded living conditions, low economic status, and discrimination have made certain cultures look upon change or suggested change with misgivings and suspicion. Community health programs involve time, patience, sincerity, planning and understanding.

Public health programs must demonstrate to people that continuing improvement in their health, welfare, and level of living is its main purpose. A sincere and genuine interest in the people, individually and collectively, is a necessity. For example, residents of a Mexican settlement in San Bernardino County, California, were uncooperative and suspicious when asked to cooperate in a mass chest x-ray survey of that area. Fear, ignorance, and language barrier barred all attempts toward success. However, in time a Mexican public health nurse gained the people's confidence and acceptance. She helped them organize a community health council, which was composed of leading lay and professional citizens. Upon the satisfactory completion of a few successful health projects, the group decided to conduct the mass x-ray survey. Spanish literature was disseminated and films were shown. The successful x-ray survey program enabled health authorities to find and treat many early tuberculosis cases and precipitated a slum clearance project. The tuberculosis mortality and morbidity rates decreased accordingly in that area. It is interesting to note that certain groups have accepted many modern American health practices such as immunization and x-ray, but often revert to traditional cultural patterns in relation to nutrition, home remedies, and family and marriage problems.

There are many examples of the effect of cultural and social patterns on health. A few include:

SOCIAL FACTORS	DISEASE OR CONDITION
Ignorance or Lack of Knowledge	
Drinking unpasteurized milk	Brucellosis*
Drinking water from polluted stream	Dysentary, hepatitis
Visit to a "quack"	Cancer
Poor personal hygiene	Typhoid fever
Home canning, improper methods	Botulism

* The incidence of *brucellosis* is highest among farmers and packing plant workers. (See Figure 16.)

SOCIAL FACTORS	DISEASE OR CONDITION

Economic Status

Rich, fatty foods	Diabetes, atherosclerosis
Lack of balanced diet	Rickets, scurvy
Lack of shoes	Hookworm
Inadequate sanitary facilities	Typhoid fever
Inadequate prenatal care	Prematurity
Slum areas	Tuberculosis

Religious Beliefs

Eating raw pork	Trichinosis
Worship of cows	Malnutrition
Medicine man or faith healer	Cancer
Stream rituals	Schistosomiasis

Heredity

Race	Susceptible tendencies vary with certain diseases
Passed from parent to child	Diabetes, color blindness, feeblemindedness

Environment

Mineral content: lack of	
(a) Iodine	Goiter
(b) Fluorine	Dental decay
Living in the tropics	Malaria
Living at South or North Pole	Freedom from and inactivity of certain germs

Activity

Stress and strain	Cerebral hemorrhage, heart condition, mental illness
Lack of exercise	Heart condition

Occupation

Atomic or radioactive plants	Radiation sickness, sterility
Sheep, goat herder	Anthrax
Paint sprayer	Encephalitis
Dairyman	Brucellosis*
Rabbit farmer	Tularemia
Working with parakeets or turkeys	Psittacosis
Hunter	Rocky Mountain spotted fever
Miner	Silicosis
Physician	Shorter life expectancy

Faulty or Negative Attitude

"Good enough for my father"	Tuberculosis (unpasteurized milk)
"Why not overeat? Cancer or accidents will get me anyhow"	Heart disease
"Nothing hurts me yet"	Dental decay
"An apple a day keeps the doctor away"	Cancer
"Let him learn by experience"	Childhood accident
"One more fast handball game, Son"	Heart disease

SOCIAL FACTORS	DISEASE OR CONDITION
"Have to work late"	Mental illness
"It always happens to the other fellow"	Auto accident
"I can't watch him every minute"	Childhood accident
"One for the road"	Alcoholism
"He likes me slim and trim"	Malnutrition

Factors Responsible for Group Actions and Reactions

There are certain factors that determine the reactions of each community group to its health needs. One important factor involves the group's conception and meaning of the word *health*. There are many meanings of this particular word. For example, some may conceive the word health as meaning pain, abnormal, or "tired blood"; others may visualize health as a social, mental, physical, or emotional concept. Similarly, the phrase *community health* has about as many meanings as the number of people in each community. To some, community health means solving immediate, noticeable health problems, an adequate sewage treatment plant, or a pure water supply; to others, community health involves organization, long-range planning, leadership, needs, cooperation, coordination, and active involvement.

Another consideration revolves around the fact that different

Brucellosis is not just a rural problem.

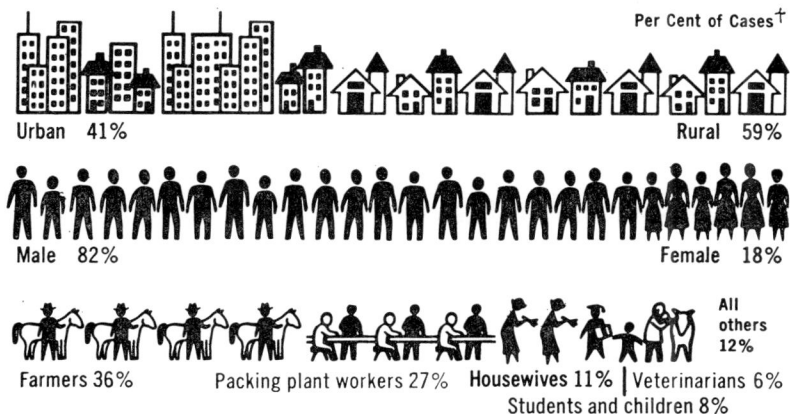

Per Cent of Cases[†]

Urban 41%   Rural 59%

Male 82%   Female 18%

Farmers 36%   Packing plant workers 27%   Housewives 11% | Veterinarians 6%
                                                Students and children 8%
All others 12%

†Based on a study of 637 cases reported in 1957. Data on residence cover 581 cases; sex, 618 cases; occupation, 570 cases.

Figure 16. Of 236 cases of brucellosis occurring among city residents in 1957, 20 were in veterinarians. Incidence of this disease is higher among veterinarians than among any other occupational group: about 283 per 100,000 practitioners. (From Patterns of Disease. Park, Davis and Co., July, 1959.)

groups attach different values to their health needs. Alcoholic beverages and tobacco are much more important than periodic physical examinations to some groups; to others luxuries such as a new car or refrigerator may rank far above the value placed upon balanced diets or sanitary living conditions. A new park or highway may take precedence over needed health facilities in certain communities. Health as a value is always in competition with other values. The value system of a particular group must be recognized and understood for a community to organize and successfully solve its health problems.

A third factor determining group reaction to health needs involves past experiences and associations with health officials or agencies. Successful and rewarding experiences foster support; distasteful and negative experiences yield uncooperative, disinterested individuals and groups. Since active participation increases interest and support, the effective leadership of the natural groups in the community must be determined and utilized.

Faulty or negative attitudes account for many groups "playing the odds" on their health. To many, heavy smoking is favored over possible lung cancer; obesity is favored over possible heart disease; and heavy drinking is favored over possible accident. Members of this group rebel against health education with such remarks as, "It hasn't been proved," or "If I don't die from heart disease, I'll die from cancer," or "You have to go sometime." Positive health attitudes and practices must be instilled in individuals at an early age. Parents and educators must join in an effort to promote long life and prevent sickness through positive thinking, planning, and individual and community participation.

Barriers to Effective Community Health Programs

There are many reasons why community health organizations are difficult to maintain and community health agency or council suggestions fail to receive acceptance or adoption. Many of these reasons revolve around sociological or cultural problems. For example, the average American community, with its pioneer heritage of individualism and ever changing group action, seems to be better prepared to cope with emergencies than to maintain an organization for planning and development. This requires a continuing, relatively stable structure.

Furthermore, studies reveal that the public is indifferent to health problems, surveys, and solutions.[4, 5] People remain passive as long as no serious health problem or large-scale fatalities occur.

Although citizens are aware of health problems, they tend to view them as unpleasant conditions, but not particularly dangerous to the community. In fact, some people may regard certain health problems as a major threat to the prestige level of their community. Most local citizens feel that any existing health problems can be handled by the proper agencies, which in most cases is the health department. Some, however, still feel that health department services are limited to its historic functions: immunizations and environmental sanitation.

Devoid of interest in many areas of public health, and caught in the grip of public health laws relating to sanitation, many persons resist the aims of those devoted to the prevention of disease. Since most preventive medicine cannot be instituted through legal enforcement, there is a need for a public that is informed, educated, and sympathetic to the goals of prevention of disease and prolonging of life. Health education thus becomes a very important tool in community health work.

Even when many persons are concerned and interested enough about a certain health problem to organize and plan as a group, disagreements, rebuttals, denials, postponements, repeated duplicate meetings, and lack of leadership, common objectives, and philosophy may be noticed. Since any one health problem may be splintered into many, it is necessary for the group to define the specific area with which it is most concerned. One well-planned, well-publicized, coordinated, cooperative meeting, with well-defined objectives is sufficient for planning an action program. Each agency representative present must tell specifically what he can do, what he will do, and how his agency can work cooperatively with other agencies. Recommendations should be made by the group, a steering committee appointed and recommendations by the steering committee submitted *in writing* to the city council or county board of supervisors for action. Action results in reaction, and this is necessary to propel motivation and interest.

Many well-meaning programs in community health have failed when they have been blanketed by generalizations in education. To educate is to form or change ideas and behavior, and some people are never clear about exactly what ideas or behavior should be formed or changed. They may not see how these changes can lead to improved individual, family, and community health. Many persons view health problems in either a curative or "contribute to Community Chest" sense.

A well-informed public is exceedingly important when one considers that community health funds are sharply controlled by a public which abhors increased taxation and may feel that other current city needs have greater priority. Some departments, whose functions are more easily recognized and on which the public has placed more value, find it easier to satisfy their needs. Contributions to voluntary agencies are viewed by many with mixed emotions. There is considerable confusion about which agencies belong to the United Fund, Community Chest, United Appeal and others, and exactly how the money is apportioned. The situation is complicated by the fact that officials of certain large health agencies, such as the American Heart Association and the American Cancer Society, generally reject any suggestions for joining with the United Fund for fund-raising or any other purpose. These agencies contend that this procedure leads to administrative control, loss of identity, and elimination of the donor's choice of agency. More important, they contend that separate fund drives raise more money.

Public spirited Americans, who contribute over $1,000,000,000 a year to organizations formed to combat health problems, are growing increasingly bewildered by the proliferation of health agencies and fund appeals. Many voluntary health agencies have developed during the past few years, and all of them are competing for public loyalty and financial support; jealousy prevails and services overlap. There are over 100 national fund drives today, as compared with only 15 in 1940. Duplication of effort is illustrated, for example, by the fact that 19 agencies compete nationally for money to aid the blind; at least three national groups compete for money to fight cancer; and three mental health agencies appeal for support. Besides increasing fund raising costs, the keen competition for money sometimes appears to result in a haphazard distribution of available funds. One top official of a fund-raising group argues that allocations of funds "are decided almost entirely by such factors as which important citizens have which diseases, what agency can hire the best promoters and involve the most influential personalities, and which cause plucks hardest at the heartstrings of the public's emotions."[6]

Since the mark of success of many voluntary health agencies is determined by the success of the fund raising campaign, such basic programs as education and research are often neglected or emphasized more before fund raising begins. If employees "volunteer" to contribute a certain amount of money each year to an agency of their choice, a feeling of employee resistance is noticed, and it seems to defeat the entire principle of "giving."

Although there have been many public health advances in the past 50 years, desire for good health has not always been the motivating force in securing necessary action. We are extremely proud of the high percentage of our communities having approved water supplies. But how many of these public water supplies were demanded and supported because the public wanted a safe water supply, as compared to their desire for the comfort and convenience of an inside toilet and running water in the kitchen? Have Grade A milk programs spread from city to city because of the demands of the people for a higher quality milk or because of economic necessity and competition? Bovine tuberculosis in human beings in the United States is practically extinct. Was it the presence of bone and glandular tuberculosis in people that brought about this remarkable achievement or the economics of the dairy and cattle industries? Legislation regarding feeding only cooked garbage to swine was prohibited in Indiana until many hogs died from a disease called vesicular exanthema. Legislators enacted a bill quickly when the hogs became ill.[7]

It is interesting and important to note here that health progress depends upon local, state and federal regulation to a great degree. Since most local health officers and voluntary agency executive directors are *appointed* by city council members, by county boards of supervisors, by boards of directors, or, in the case of most state health officers, by the governor, it is necessary for these members to exchange ideas and discuss program objectives and philosophy. Officials must be well informed on community health principles and must periodically review and evaluate the health needs, interests, and problems of the people in their area.

Community Health Progress—Real or Mirage?

Most people will agree that public health activities have made this country a healthier and happier place in which to live. Life expectancy has increased, and public health advances have had a beneficial effect on the cultural patterns of people, regardless of economic status, race, or religion. Elimination of certain diseases has given health workers more time to concentrate on mental health, chronic diseases, and geriatrics. These health fields have provided new occupations, activities, buildings, and even entire communities. These new avenues have led also to the current definition of and emphasis on health as a social and emotional aspect of an individual, community, or nation.

On the other hand public health activities may produce unexpected or undesirable results, and medicine's apparent triumphs may be mixed blessings. For example, an increase in leisure time may lead to an increase in the number of alcoholics, narcotic addicts, and delinquents. Leisure time, plus high-powered automobiles and other mechanized equipment, may lead to lack of exercise and increased auto accidents. Although a man past 45 years of age has little greater life expectancy than his grandfather had, he has the world's highest living standard; but 5 to 10 per cent of his income today goes for medical care. Our greater ingenuity and inventiveness leads to a faster, less secure way of life and often results in more divorces, suicides, and mentally ill persons. Many of the new tranquilizing drugs encourage people to forget their worries. Industries release more smoke and hydrocarbons that may account for an increase in cancer and allergies. We live longer today only to wonder about obtaining a job after retirement and contemplate whether we will die from heart disease, cancer, intracranial lesions, or accidents.[3]

Although communicable diseases have decreased, they have not disappeared; disease is an aspect of man's adaptation to his environment and as his environment changes, so do his diseases. Disease has not surrendered unconditionally. The very sanitary techniques that did so much to control infections in the nineteenth century set the stage for the ravages of polio in the twentieth century. German measles, once universal in childhood, now skips many sanitized youngsters, but if a woman contracts the disease in the first three months of pregnancy, she may have a stillborn or malformed child. The effectiveness of insulin not only prolongs the diabetic's life but increases the risk of his passing on a diabetic tendency to his children. If this happens often enough, society may face medical, economic, and ethical problems for which it is not prepared.[8]

Medical Social Worker

The aspect of social work in a community health program is growing rapidly. Increasing emphasis upon the social and community aspects of health has opened many new avenues for the social worker interested in health. Positions for medical social workers are now available with many official and voluntary agencies. The medical social worker is responsible for planning, developing, and directing services within the health agency. The activities of the social worker, although varied and broad, include: (1) consultation on the social aspects of health and medical care of individuals and groups, (2) providing services through social case work, (3) consultant to the staff and community, and (4) liaison with other community agencies.[9] The demand for medical social workers led to the establishment of the Committee on Professional Education of the American Public Health Association of a Subcommittee on Educational Qualifications of Medical Social Workers in Health Agencies. This subcommittee, working with the American Association of Medical Social Workers, in addition to the establishment of personnel qualifications, has developed a summary of the functions of medical social workers in a large health agency.[10]

QUESTIONS FOR REVIEW

1. List and briefly discuss five obstacles that must be overcome before a community can organize and successfully solve its health problems.
2. What are some examples of the effect of cultural and social patterns on health? What are some examples in your community?
3. Name and briefly discuss three factors that may be responsible for group actions or reactions to community health programs.
4. "Public health activities may produce unexpected or undesirable results." Discuss this statement.
5. Briefly discuss the opportunities and possible activities of the medical social worker.
6. What are some major barriers to effective community health programs?
7. What is the purpose and function of a community health council?

REFERENCES

1. Koos, E. L.: *New Concepts in Community Organization for Health.* Am. J. Pub. Health, 43:466, 1953.
2. Paul, Benjamin D.: *Respect for Cultural Differences.* Community Development Bulletin, University of London Institute of Education, 4:42, 1953.
3. Hanlon, John J.: *Principles of Public Health Administration (2nd Edition).* St. Louis, The C. V. Mosby Co., 1955.
4. Commission on Chronic Illness: *Chronic Illness in the United States, Volume I, Prevention of Chronic Illness.* Massachusetts, Harvard University Press, 1957, Page 43.
5. Sower, Christopher, et al.: *Community Involvement.* Illinois, The Free Press, 1957, Page 252.
6. Lancaster, Paul: *Donors' Plight: Health Agencies Grow in Number with Many Offering Same Service.* Wall Street Journal, October 11, 1960, Pages 1 and 17.
7. Burney, Leroy E.: *Community Organization—An Effective Tool.* Am. J. Pub. Health, 44:2, 1954.
8. Dubos, R. J.: *Mirage of Health.* New York, Harper and Brothers, 1959.
9. Grant, M.: *Social Service in a Health Department.* Am. J. Pub. Health, 43:1545, 1953.
10. *Proposed Report on Educational Qualifications of Medical Social Workers in Public Health Programs.* Am. J. Pub. Health, 40:994, 1950.

SUGGESTED READING

Adams, R.: *On the Effective Use of Anthropology in Public Health Programs.* Human Organization, *13:*4, 1955.

An Inventory of Social and Economic Research in Health. Health Information Foundation, 1952.

Apple, Dorian: *Sociological Studies of Health and Sickness.* New York, McGraw-Hill Book Co., Inc., 1960.

Boek, W. E., and Boek, J. K.: *Society and Health.* New York, G. P. Putnam's Sons, 1956.

Dooley, Thomas A., M. D.: *The Edge of Tomorrow.* New York, Farrar, Straus, and Cudahy, 1958.

Freeman H. B., and Reader, L. B.: *Medical Sociology.* Am. Sociol. Rev., *22:* 73, 1957.

Harlow, Rex F.: *Public Relations and the Social Sciences.* New York, Harper and Brothers, 1957.

Hunter, Floyd: *Community Power Structures* (Study of a specific city). North Carolina, University of North Carolina Press, 1953.

Jefferys, M.: *Social Class and Health Promotion. Some Obstacles in Britain.* Health Education Journal, *15:*109, 1957.

Kahl, Joseph A.: *The American Class Structure.* New York, Rinehart and Co., 1957.

Koos, Earl Lomon: *Community Organization for Health.* Pub. Health Nursing, *42:*196–98, 1950.

Lewis, A.: *Health as a Social Concept.* Brit. J. Sociology. *4:*109, 1953.

Littman, R. A., Moore, R. C. A., and Pierce-Jones R.: *Social Class Differences in Child Rearing: A Third Community for Comparison with Chicago and Newton.* Am Sociol. Rev., *22:*694, 1957.

Mayo, S. C., and Marsh, C. P.: *Social Participation in the Rural Community.* Am. J. Sociol., 57:243, 1951.

Parsons, T., Editor: *Socio-Cultural Approaches to Medical Care.* J. Social Issues, 1952.

Paul, B. D., and Miller, W. B., Editors: *Health, Culture and Community: Case Studies of Public Reactions to Health Programs.* New York, Russell Sage Foundation, 1955.

Paul, B. D.: *Social Science in Public Health.* Am. J. Pub. Health, *46:*1390, 1956.

Saunders, L.: *Cultural Differences and Medical Care,* New York, Russell Sage Foundation, 1954.

Simmons, O. G.: *Implications of Social Class for Public Health.* Human Organization, *16:*7, 1957.

Sower, Christopher, et al.: *Community Involvement.* Illinois, The Free Press, 1957.

Chapter IV

Solving Community Health Problems

BEFORE we can solve community health problems, we must know a great deal about the community. A community may cluster around such things as a church, a shopping center, a school, or common interests resulting from similar racial or national backgrounds. Communities may develop because of national or geographic boundaries which set them apart from other areas. They may be separated by man-made boundaries, such as railroads, main streets, and traffic arteries. They may exist simply because a group of similar people have elected to live near each other. A community includes a group of people who have common health interests and needs which they can identify or be helped to identify. It includes people who have enough common interests and sufficiently similar backgrounds to work together toward common health goals.[1]

COMMUNITY ORGANIZATION

Community organization involves the neighborhood or other population unit in which there is common ground for action. Community organization also involves a process by which the people and health services and agencies of the community are brought together, usually through their chosen representatives, to identify their common health problems as their own, to plan the kind of action needed to solve these problems, and to act together as a unit to solve them.[1] Knowing the neighborhoods, the people that constitute them, their interests, their needs, their cultural heritage and educational backgrounds is essential to successful community organization. All groups and all areas must have leaders if the program is to reach every home. A realistic understanding requires that we recognize the community as a power structure. Somewhere it has a point of authority. There are people in the community who decide what other people may or may not do, the best living and working conditions, and many other fundamental matters. Most citizens have good will and respect for their leaders, who, by virtue of past actions, are in a position to use this good will for the good of the community as a whole. Thus the role of the community leader becomes more and more important in planning, organizing, and conducting community health programs.

Perhaps the most successfully organized communities are those undertaken by the people themselves, with or without the aid of a professional worker. But a community can be guided into organization by many categories of professionally trained persons. If health is the prime incentive for organizing, then it is likely that the health department or a voluntary health agency will provide the guidance or stimulus. Community population and area, and available health resources and facilities must also be considered in community organization. In general, the more racial and national groups, shopping districts, and areas in the community, the smaller will be the total number of people who can be brought together to work for common health goals.

The people themselves must become involved in determining and solving their health problems. They must determine their needs, set their goals, make their plans, and put those plans into action. They may accept some guidance, but they enjoy deciding for themselves what will be done about their needs. If the neighborhood health council is to have any longevity beyond the emergent need that prompts its establishment, then its members must continue to feel that it is *they* who make the decisions. Even if committee members decide to attack a health problem that may seem of little importance to health authorities, it is necessary that everyone cooperate in making the project a satisfying, successful experience for all. A successful program requires planning, and active participation by community groups and health educators.

Interested groups and individuals can study and plan together to improve the health of their community by carrying out the following six steps: recognizing health needs of the community; interesting others in community health needs; forming a community health council; conducting a community health survey to obtain the facts; educating the public, disseminating the facts; evaluating the community health program. (*Action* is the ultimate goal.) For more information, refer to Aids to Community Health Planning Kit, National Health Council, 1790 Broadway, New York 19, New York.[2] Following is a detailed discussion of each step.

Recognizing Health Needs

An organizational plan is essential to action and to the involvement of people from all parts of the community. The leaders must be identified and recruited as a first step in developing this plan. Finding leaders does not necessarily mean calling upon those who seem to be key people in a community. It means finding those persons who are acceptable to an entire group. The council must represent *all* community interests. Before a program can be developed, thorough knowledge of the community's health problems and resources is essential. This knowledge can be gained by:

1. Observation
2. Comparing health services, activities, and facilities of the community with those of similar communities
3. Ascertaining whether or not the community is served by a local health department
4. Noting the size of population served by the health department
5. Examining the health budget to see that at least $2.50 per person per year is expended
6. Comparing the health program with leading community health programs in other communities
7. Studying the vital and communicable disease statistics of the community.

Interesting Others in Community Health Needs

Any organization or any individual can initiate action concerning a health problem by discussing it with others. After a number of people have been made aware of the problem, the interested individuals and organizations may be called together to plan for cooperative effort.

Forming a Community Health Council

Such a council, mobilizing all the forces in a community willing to work for better health services, is the ideal instrument to achieve this goal. Objectives of the health council will include:

1. Bringing together medical, allied professional, and other interested groups for discussion and interchange of opinions (The local health department, medical society, dental society, and other professional organizations must not be neglected.)
2. Serving as a clearing house for health and medical care problems and programs, facilitating joint planning where it is needed to speed up approved projects and to reduce duplication of efforts
3. Encouraging, stimulating, fostering, and actively supporting the establishment of health and medical care programs designed to improve the health of the people in the community
4. Gathering and analyzing information on medical care and health needs already obtained from surveys and initiating additional studies or survey
5. Devising means for reaching all the people, with particular attention to the extension of the projects into rural areas (theoretically, towns of less than 2,500 people) and people living outside of cities and towns.[3]

The first task of the council is to prepare a constitution stating the council's objectives, membership, officers, funds, proceedings, bylaws, committees, and amendments.* The composition of the council's membership is the key to success. The council must represent *all* community interests. There is nothing rigid about the operational chart, and each health council will need to vary its plan to meet local needs. Health council work should be an educational experience for the members and for the community. Also, there should be a good public information campaign so that the people may know the complete program, members, plans, and progress of the council. Although the success of a health council depends to a great extent upon leadership, a wise selection of activities is also of great importance. Each council will have to grow in a manner

* See Appendix I and II for outline of the constitution of the Health Council of Hamilton, New York, and also for outline of bylaws in general.

that best fits the needs of its own particular community. No general pattern can be applied equally to all councils. The concept of the health council implies that most of the existing health problems are created by the people, and therefore must be solved by the people. Working and planning together to solve health problems strengthens the group and the community.

Conducting a Community Health Survey

A survey is necessary to determine health *needs* and *resources* and to obtain facts. Once a health council has the facts, it is well on the way to better health services. Experience has proved that the people and their public servants are almost never opposed to establishing or improving local health services if only they can clearly see the need. The specific needs of the community may be determined through a professional survey or through a community self-survey. The second approach is one in which the citizens themselves, with the leadership of health authorities, make the study. One of the most widely used evaluation forms utilized to help determine community health problems and needs is the *Evaluation Schedule for Use in the Study and Appraisal of Community Health Programs,* American Public Health Association, 1960.[4] Either method is useful in determining community needs. In assessing the needs of the nation, the United States Public Health Service staff, with cooperating agencies or a specially appointed commission that includes a number of staff members and field investigators, collect the data and report on their findings.

An example of the professional survey for determining health needs by a public health authority is Hiscock's study of public health in Hawaii. Illustrative selected findings from his 1950 survey are as follows:

1. Complex housing problems for both official and voluntary health agencies
2. Cumbersome civic service and budgetary requirements and operation
3. Personnel shortages
4. Gaps in services for dental health, mental health, nutrition, and community health education resources
5. Complex water supply and sewage disposal problems
6. Lack of awareness and understanding of the organization, purposes, and low cost of a modern, practical community health program by some officials and by many taxpayers.

The community self-survey enlists the citizens as members of the health team; this tends to make them supporters and boosters for public health programs. An example of this method is the survey conducted by the health council of Clinton County, Ohio.[5] The council drew up a simple one-page questionnaire.* Then sub-committees of canvassers were organized in every township and village in the county. Approximately 5,500 families, or more than 90 per cent of the entire population, were interviewed. The following facts were revealed:

1. One pregnancy in every six ended in the death of the baby.
2. A majority of preschool children had received no inoculations against diphtheria, lockjaw, whooping cough, or smallpox.
3. 40 per cent of all the school-age children had no protection against smallpox or diphtheria.
4. 70 per cent of the rural folk and 14 per cent of the town dwellers were drinking unpasteurized milk.
5. More than half the population was drawing its water from easily contaminated wells.
6. The old-fashioned surface privy, a constant invitation to disease, was still used by 45 per cent of all persons living in towns.
7. Undulant fever, usually caused by the use of infected, unpasteurized milk, had stricken more than 500 persons among the families interviewed.
8. Thousands of persons had never been reached by the free chest x-ray service of the local tuberculosis association.[4]

Educating the Public

Once the council has the facts, it is necessary to present them to *all* the people in the community; the facts will clearly reveal certain specific health needs. Council members will present definite workable plans for the solution of these needs, and action will begin. (See Figure 17 for a community action plan.) Certain individuals and groups will always be opposed to suggested health reforms. This attitude reflects fear and ignorance, which may be overcome by revealing the facts. Dairy farmers, for example, often regard the phrase *public health* as a threat to their milk businesses. Yet countless experiences have proved that health department farm inspection and pasteurization programs have had exactly the opposite effect.

In order to disseminate factual information effectively, council members should utilize all available methods of communication. This includes films, exhibits, speakers, radio, television, newspapers, pamphlets, and other media.

* See Appendix 3 for questionnaire.

Evaluating the Community Health Program

The council must periodically evaluate the program in terms of the objectives. A good program will change with the changing health needs and interests of the community. The following questions and answers may assist in evaluating the progress of a newly organized community health council:

1. Does the program enlist all groups?
   (All groups must be enlisted if the goal of reaching all people is to be attained.)
2. Do people understand the program?
   (No program can succeed until the people fully understand it, become a part of its activities, and benefit from it.)
3. Do participating organizations and council committees assume responsibility for activities assigned to them?

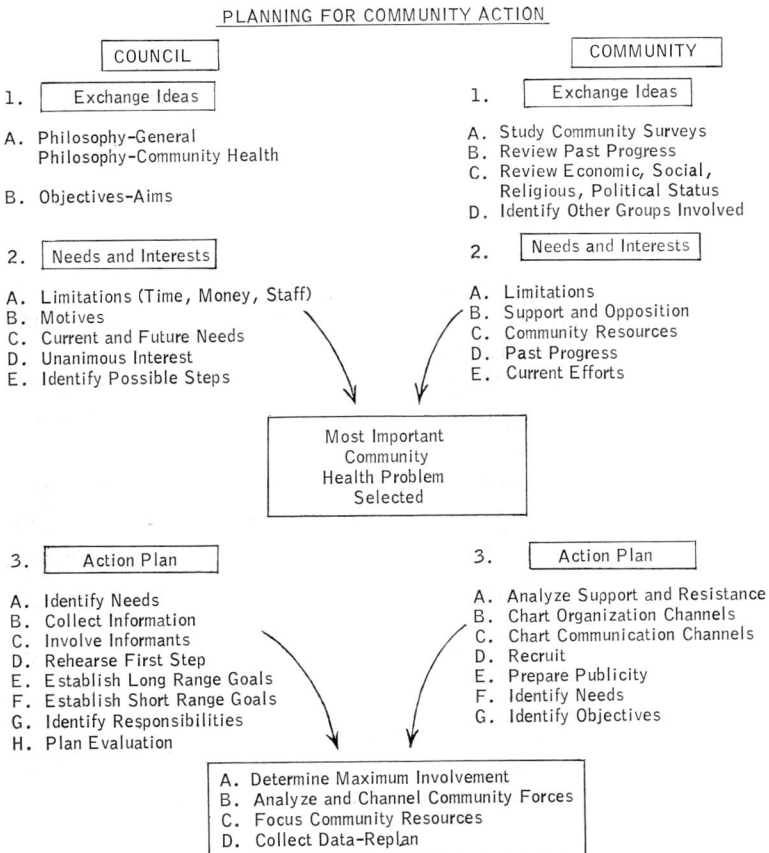

PLANNING FOR COMMUNITY ACTION

COUNCIL

1. Exchange Ideas

A. Philosophy–General
   Philosophy–Community Health

B. Objectives–Aims

2. Needs and Interests

A. Limitations (Time, Money, Staff)
B. Motives
C. Current and Future Needs
D. Unanimous Interest
E. Identify Possible Steps

COMMUNITY

1. Exchange Ideas

A. Study Community Surveys
B. Review Past Progress
C. Review Economic, Social,
   Religious, Political Status
D. Identify Other Groups Involved

2. Needs and Interests

A. Limitations
B. Support and Opposition
C. Community Resources
D. Past Progress
E. Current Efforts

Most Important
Community
Health Problem
Selected

3. Action Plan

A. Identify Needs
B. Collect Information
C. Involve Informants
D. Rehearse First Step
E. Establish Long Range Goals
F. Establish Short Range Goals
G. Identify Responsibilities
H. Plan Evaluation

3. Action Plan

A. Analyze Support and Resistance
B. Chart Organization Channels
C. Chart Communication Channels
D. Recruit
E. Prepare Publicity
F. Identify Needs
G. Identify Objectives

A. Determine Maximum Involvement
B. Analyze and Channel Community Forces
C. Focus Community Resources
D. Collect Data–Replan

Figure 17. Community health councils must continually analyze and evaluate their objectives and action in terms of their community as well as their groups.

4. Does the committee representing the professional groups properly support and provide stimulating guidance for the program?

(The experience and training of the professional groups place them in a strategic position to perform this function to the end that a sound and practical local health program will be established.)

5. Are the people willing to give time and money when needed to support the activities of the local health council?

(Greater success is assured and more lasting results can be expected when a large number of people take part in carrying out the approved program and participate in defraying its cost.)

6. Is it a genuine community effort?

(For the sake of real progress and lasting benefits, all groups should work together in harmony with intelligently directed self-interest as a motivating force. Gains for the community as a whole should take precedence over individual and special group interests.) [6]

Delayed Community Action

Although many community health councils have recognized their health needs and have all the necessary facts regarding certain major health problems, at times there seems to be little action. Health programs require a great deal of planning, organizing, and time and there are certain important influences and elements that must be considered while analyzing delays and detours.

Pressure and interest groups are always involved in any basic issue. Although issues should be aired and viewed from all sides, continued negative resistance against a statistically proven and accepted fact makes the council's work very difficult. Certain religious groups also tend to make the council's task tedious at times. However, the rights of these groups must be respected, and it is necessary to plan with representatives of these groups in an effort to reach a satisfactory agreement.

Funds are necessary to conduct any program, and many times local, state, and federal funds for certain health programs are inadequate or even deleted from the budget. Fund raising may precipitate a great deal of professional jealousy among community health agencies; other precipitation factors include salaries, rank and status in the community, and professional training and preparation. These conditions lead only to uncoordinated, uncooperative, and unsuccessful programs.

Beside the existence of these real problems in a community, there is also a definite time lag in connection with a new medical advance or discovery and a community action program utilizing this advance. For example, Edward Jenner discovered smallpox vaccine in 1798, and yet it was not until 1920 that mass vaccination took place in the United States. Another illustration confronts many of our communities at the present time. Despite the fact that 25 years of research have proved that about one part per million of fluorine in community water supplies will reduce dental decay up to 65 per cent in children and will give life-long improved dental health, communities are slow to accept fluoridation. Also, consider the Salk polio vaccine. It has proved to be 75 to 80 per cent effective during the past eight years; yet, only about 60 per cent of the most susceptible age group have received vaccine. These are only a few examples of many such discouraging facts.

The reasons for this time lag are many and varied. Marred by the tragic occurrence of disease in 79 children as a result of faulty Salk polio vaccine administered at the start of its general use, many parents now cast a suspicious eye on all vaccines. Fear of doctors and needles, lack of funds, ignorance of the facts, indifference, adopting a "what was good enough for my father" attitude, and perhaps man's suspicious nature of anything with which he is not familiar and does not fully understand are all factors contributing to the time lag. For example, most persons realize that a major prevention of disease is periodic physical examination, yet many persons neglect these examinations because they are "too busy," "too thrifty," or "too healthy." (See Figure 18.) Other persons do not recognize and accept the fact that they are either obese, alcoholic or in poor physical condition because they want to protect their ego.

Unexpected incidents sometimes motivate or initiate the public into action more than a planned or organized health council. In 1959, because of the widespread publicity of their illnesses, Secretary of State John Foster Dulles and entertainer Arthur Godfrey probably did more to advance the crusade against cancer than any organized campaign. President Eisenhower's heart attack in 1955 alerted the nation to the cause and prevention of heart disease. Community epidemics which result in many fatalities, motor vehicle accidents resulting in deaths, and prominent community leaders committing suicide or being committed to a mental institution all leave their mark upon members of a community.

Our nation's competitive spirit weighs heavily in our favor. Americans do not like to be left behind in any field, whether it is science, education, physical fitness, medicine, or public health. In our present economic situation, any weak link in a nation may lead to its destruction. Medical and public health advances of other

TOO BUSY! How could anyone expect him to give up a few hours a year for a health checkup? Every hour of his time is valuable!

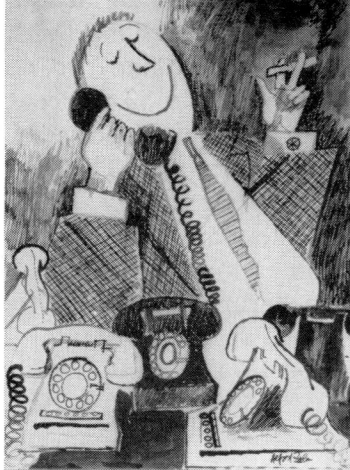

TOO THRIFTY! Why spend good money for a checkup? The doctor might not find anything wrong! How extravagant can you get?

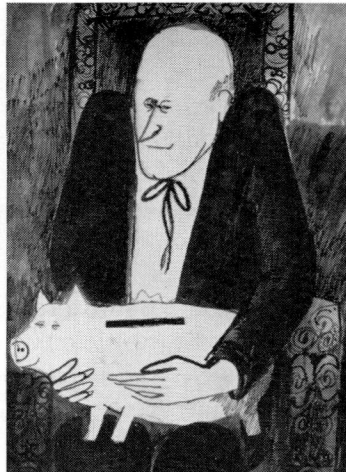

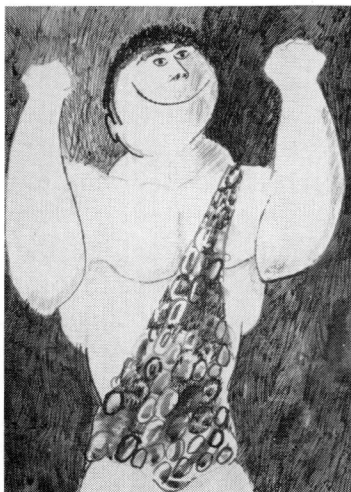

TOO HEALTHY! He's never been really sick a day in his life and he never felt better than he does right now! Why bother with a checkup?

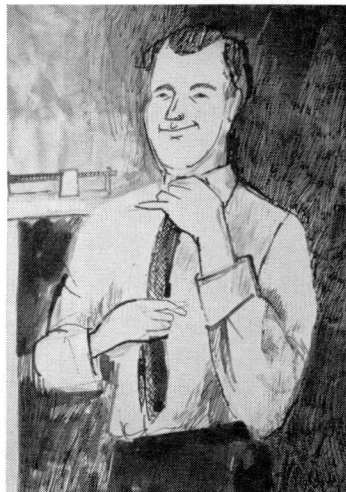

SMART ENOUGH to know that anyone can develop cancer, no matter how well he may feel...that delay in going to the doctor has caused thousands of needless cancer deaths... that his best cancer insurance is to have a thorough checkup every year and, between times, to keep on the alert for Cancer's 7 Danger Signals.

Learn how to guard yourself against cancer. Call your nearest American Cancer Society office or write to "Cancer" in care of your local post office.

Figure 18.   (From Cancer News 14:23, 1960, American Cancer Society, New York.)

nations certainly motivate many Americans to keep abreast and, if possible, ahead of them. In order to do this, community members have found that they must organize, plan, and work together in an effort to build a stronger and healthier nation.

Community Programs

Two successful and effective community programs will illustrate different methods of obtaining greater active citizen participation in understanding and solving community health problems.

The first program, the Community Education Project, was a five-year program (1953-1958) carried on through San Bernardino Valley College, California, and financed by the Fund for Adult Education established by the Ford Foundation. The project was supervised by the Board of Directors and Administration of Valley College. An advisory committee, composed of local citizens, helped establish the general policies and activities. San Bernardino, California, was one of 12 centers in the United States which cooperated with each other and shared the Fund for Adult Education in developing and testing educational programs and methods. The Community Education Project embraced the idea that if the community itself is functioning as a mature and integrated social unit, there will be an alert and informed citizenry. Within this kind of social structure, the community will desire the best health facilities and be motivated to take the necessary steps toward preventing disease and prolonging life. Health thus becomes integrated with improved community standards in all areas.

The goals of the Community Education Project were three-fold: (1) to educate the public in certain fundamental and basic American issues; (2) to make people aware of community needs and problems and (3) to guide them in their active, cooperative participation in solving them. Problems considered were not only such immediate physical matters as a shortage of water, the need for a growing and diversified industry, health problems, community planning for the future, and smog control, but also included the equally vital problems of developing an understanding of an American heritage—the free enterprise system; sound human relations practices; knowledge of world affairs; and a deepening sensitivity to good design and beauty in everyday living. The program objectives meant personal development and education for responsible citizenship.

Services offered by the Community Education Project included:
1. Discussion groups on the problems facing the people of the San Bernardino Valley
2. Training in leading and participating in group discussion and in developing sound human relations practices
3. Thought-provoking, entertaining, educational programs for radio and television.
4. Consultation services for local organizations and groups interested in more effective educational methods
5. Program and resource information of general interest for program chairmen (films, tapes, books and pamphlets, sociodramas, speakers, and others.)
6. Study materials (discussion guides, exhibit materials, facts and surveys) on San Bernardino Valley problems
7. Research into the perplexing problem of effective education for citizenship in complex, urban areas.

The following description of a program in family life and the problems of young people will illustrate the methods and materials used in promoting a community-wide educational program. A six-week educational program on family life and youth, originally sponsored by the San Bernardino Social Planning Council, the Community Education Project, San Bernardino Valley College, and the local newspaper, was offered to the people of San Bernardino Valley, California. Two hundred lay and professional community leaders were invited to a weekend Community Leadership Institute in the fall of 1953. At this meeting the Director of the Community Education Project and a representative of the Fund for Adult Education introduced the Community Education Project and outlined its objectives. The group agreed that the first project to be undertaken should be concerned with youth and family living. The omnibus program focused on young people and the difficulties they encounter in achieving a mature, responsible, effective and personally happy life. The setting revolved around the typical American family as it is affected by all the tensions and forces at work in our modern, industrial society. The core of the program was a series of six, weekly, half-hour radio dramas and an accompanying newspaper article for each program. These were directed primarily toward small discussion groups that met in private homes and in public places.

Throughout the series 150 discussion groups, averaging ten members each, met weekly. A number of related activities took place during the six-week period. These activities were designed to strengthen the program and to increase its impact on the citizens in the community. A youth and family life resource directory guide was compiled in order to aid various groups in selecting specific audio-visual aids. The guide listed qualified, available speakers and their specialties, films, sociodramas, recordings, and exhibits. Speakers and materials were readily available.

Other important aspects of the program included a youth conference of the teenagers of San Bernardino County, a workshop for program chairmen and discussion leaders, a family recreation workshop planned by the City Recreation Department, and sermons on the subject presented by local ministers. Young people were urged to participate by suggesting names for the program during a contest, volunteering as actors in radio dramas, and preparing and presenting skits.

The program was very successful. Members of the community were becoming aware of certain community problems, and they were actively cooperating in an effort to solve these problems. Various community problems were presented from time to time; each problem was analyzed, facts were obtained, action was taken, and follow-up and evaluation were continuous. Soon the people themselves brought certain health problems before the group for consideration. People realized that raising the health standards of the community was just one aspect of raising the total standards of the community; health was one important aspect of good community living. This was truely community health in action!

A second type of health program involves cooperation between school and community. For example, many schools and numerous community agencies, such as the Red Cross, have been carrying on nutrition and health programs; World War II gave impetus to these programs. A recent survey indicated, on the other hand, that there is need for additional emphasis on nutrition education, especially in elementary grades.

A nutrition program provides an opportunity for teaching good citizenship and democratic participation—an opportunity to apply, through actual experience and practical activities, the principles of sound, progressive education. Such a program can serve as a means for good public relations for any school and is a stimulant for greater participation by the community in school projects.

One such program, as entered into by General Mills, in cooperation with teachers, school administrators and community leaders

embraced four areas: (1) experimentation in cooperating schools,
(2) teacher training, (3) distribution of grade level nutrition literature, and (4) dissemination of nutrition information. The project
initiated and instituted many successful community-school nutrition
programs.[7]

QUESTIONS FOR REVIEW

1. List and briefly discuss six steps that interested groups and individuals may
   use as a guide to help them improve the health of their community.
2. List the steps you would take in promoting a community fluoridation program.
3. How would you go about *discovering* and *solving* major health problems in
   your community?
4. How can we evaluate the effectiveness of a community health program?
5. List five reasons why some community health programs are delayed.
6. In your opinion, what are the five major community health problems in your
   community? State? Why?
7. Give three different examples showing how community health programs
   failed in your community due to lack of effective communication.

REFERENCES

1. Patterson, Raymond S., and Roberts, Beryl, J.: *Community Health Education in Action.* St. Louis, The C. V. Mosby Co., 1951.
2. National Health Council: *Aids to Community Health Planning Kit.* New
   York, National Health Council, 1954.
3. American Medical Association: *The Key to Community Health.* Chicago,
   American Medical Association, 1954.
4. American Public Health Association: *Evaluation Schedule for Use in the
   Study and Appraisal of Community Health Programs.* New York, American Public Health Association, 1960.
5. *Clinton County Health Survey.* Ohio, The Clinton County Health Council,
   1950.
6. American Medical Association: *The Community Health Council.* Chicago,
   American Medical Association, 1949, Pages 14 and 15.
7. *Steps in Instituting a Community-School Nutrition and Health Program.*
   Minnesota, General Mills, Inc., 1952.

SUGGESTED READING

Abelson, Herbert I.: *Persuasion.* New York, Springer Publishing Co., 1960.
Blackwell, Gordon W.: *The Social Scientist Looks at the Health Council Move-
   ment.* Pub. Health Nursing, 42:316–21, 1950.
Cannell, C. F., et al., Editors: *Community Change: An Action Program in
   Puerto Rico.* J. Social Issues, 9:12–15, 1953.
Deasy, L. C.: *Socio-Economic Status and Participation in the Poliomyelitis
   Vaccine Trial.* Am. Sociol. Rev., 21:185–191, 1956.
Glasser, Melvin A.: *What Makes A Volunteer.* New York, Public Affairs Pam-
   phlet, 1955.
Griffiths, W.: *Health Workers' Attitudes Toward Community Development
   Programs.* Health Education Monographs No. 4, Oakland, California,
   Society of Public Health Educators, Inc., 1959.

Haldeman, Jack C., Burney, L. E., Yoho, R., and Mattison, B. F.: *Financing Local Health Services*. Am. J. Pub. Health, 45:965–83, 1955.

Hunter, F.: *Community Power Structure*. Chapel Hill, University of North Carolina Press, 1953.

Hunter, F., Schaffer, R. C., and Sheps, C. G.: *Community Organization: Action and Inaction*. Chapel Hill, University of North Carolina Press, 1956.

Kimball, S. T., and Pearsall, M.: *The Talladega Story*. Alabama, University of Alabama Press, 1954.

Koos, E. L.: *The Health of Regionville*. New York, Columbia University Press, 1954.

Leavell, Hugh R.: *Contributions of the Social Sciences to the Solution of Health Problems*. New England J. Med., 247:885–897, 1952.

Luszki, Margaret B.: *Interdisciplinary Team Research, Methods and Problems*. New York, New York University Press, 1958.

Means, Russell C.: *What's in the Health Council Idea?* Pub. Health Rep., 1952.

Miller, P. A.: *Community Health Action*. Michigan, Michigan State College Press, 1953.

Pickney, E. R.: *Public Health Cooperation Between Physicians and Local Public Health Department*. J.A.M.A., 160:1450, 1956.

Prince, J. S.: *The Health Officer and Community Power Groups*. Health Education Monographs No. 10, Oakland, California, Society of Public Health Educators, Inc., 1958, Pages 16–31.

Rosenstock, I. M., Derryberry, M., and Carriger, B. K.: *Why People Fail to Seek Poliomyelitis Vaccination*. Pub. Health Rep., 74:98–103, 1959.

Sills, David L.: *The Volunteers*. Illinois, The Free Press, 1958.

Sower, C., Holland J., Tiedke, K., and Freeman, W.: *Community Involvement*. Illinois, The Free Press, 1957.

U. S. Public Health Service: *The Chicago-Cook County Health Survey*. New York, Columbia University Press, 1951.

Wellin, Edward: *Implications of Local Culture for Public Health*. Human Organization, 16:16–18, 1958.

Chapter V

Community Health
Education—Methods and Materials

HEALTH EDUCATION has been defined as "the sum of experiences which favorably influence habits, attitudes, and knowledge relating to individual, community, and racial health."[1] In order to provide people in the community with such experiences, it is necessary to make them aware of individual and community health needs and problems, to secure the facts, to disseminate the information, and to motivate them to act. As the above definition points out, any education program must consider the habits, attitudes, and knowledge of the people. In our modern society, the senses of the average citizen are constantly bombarded by publicity, propaganda, advertising, promotional and educational forces. Some of them are subtle; others are not. The community health educator must recognize this competition and must devise and employ techniques

72

that will obtain a fair share of public attention. The community health educator must continually consider and utilize two important factors in planning and conducting his program: *motivation* and *communication*.

Motivation

In order to motivate people to use their health knowledge, they must be confronted by a basic human emotional urge to take action. The urge may be based on personal emotion such as fear, jealousy, ambition, pride, or any combination of these. However, the health educator desires to motivate people intrinsically, advancing such factors as growth, prevention, prolonging of life, social and emotional well-being of individuals. For example, a man may seek a complete physical examination because he fears he may have cancer; the same man supports the community fluoridation program because he seeks the support and acceptance of the group that is in favor of fluoridation. The health educator's task, however, is to motivate this man to seek a physical examination in order to *prevent* cancer and prolong life; the same man must be willing to support fluoridation because he knows it will help *prevent* tooth decay in his children, and because he understands that fluoridation is best for the health and well-being of the community.

The motives that are likely to be involved in public acceptance to preventive health programs include:

1. Desire to conform to group pattern
2. Desire to seek relief from fear of disease because of family history and symptomatology
3. Screening as a convenient, quick, inexpensive, and usually painless method of examination
4. Curiosity
5. Hypochondriasis
6. Desire for maintenance of optimum health and therefore to stay on the job
7. Compulsion of a legal, economic, or social nature
8. Various personal motives including the individual's desire to find a disease present and through it avoid responsibility.

Motives causing rejection of preventive health programs include:

1. Fear of a particular disease and its accompanying physical effects, as in the case of cancer (See Figure 19.)
2. Fear of the economic consequences of discovering that one

has tuberculosis (e.g., loss of job, cost or care, inability to continue supporting one's family)

3. Fear of social stigma still attached to certain diseases, such as epilepsy and syphilis
4. Religious or cultist beliefs
5. Traditions of medical practice (i.e., attachment to personal relationship with a family physician, as against the impersonality of a mass screening procedure, for example, in which examination may be by unknown physicians and technicians)
6. Misinformation or lack of information
7. Lack of confidence in the effectiveness of a particular procedure
8. Inconvenience as to time and place at which a preventive service is offered
9. Indifference (which may often be a cloak for unstated fears with respect either to a particular procedure, or to the disease or diseases to which it relates)
10. Cost of the procedure (for the individual)
11. Emphasis of a particular preventive procedure on common aspects of chronic illness rather than on specific disease entities
12. Cultural and social patterns of ethnic and other subgroups in the population.[2]

A person's motives are linked with and strongly influenced by the groups to which he belongs. An individual can and does belong to a long list of "publics" simultaneously. A person's overlapping membership in many "publics" lends stability to the powerful force of public opinion. Citizens are continually forming, disbanding, and reforming "publics" holding specific views towards specific issues. Community health educators realize the importance of these groups and communicate with the individuals in them. Appeals must be significant and relevant to a particular group interest in a particular situation. The roles people play and the value and attitudes they build around them are largely determined by the group to which they belong. A person's group relationships provide the setting for most of the health education he receives and transmits.

Communication

In order to disseminate information to increase the knowledge of others or to change their concepts, personal discussions, carried out in terms familiar to the listener and related to his personality and circumstances, are required. For example, a poster stating "Protect . . . get your D P T" may not convey the message as well as "Be wise . . . Immunize." The word *immunize* relates a common experience to most people; few people, however, are familiar with the term D P T (multiple antigen—diphtheria, pertussis, and tetanus). Health education programs depend upon effective communication. Although communication appears to be a simple process, research has successfully isolated and identified the following variables: (1) exposure and access to the message, (2) the media of communication used, (3) the content of the message, (4) the receiver's predisposition to the message, and (5) relationships within groups receiving the message.

Health educators must be able to classify community groups and organizations in order to plan an effective, well-balanced communications program. Although the public is continually growing, moving, and changing, the following groups should be considered before launching a community health education program:

1. Teachers and students—all levels
2. Government officials and agencies—local, state and federal
3. Women's groups
4. Service clubs
5. Business and professional groups
6. Industrial groups
7. Church groups
8. Veterans.

Four Typical Reactions to Life-Saving Facts About Cancer

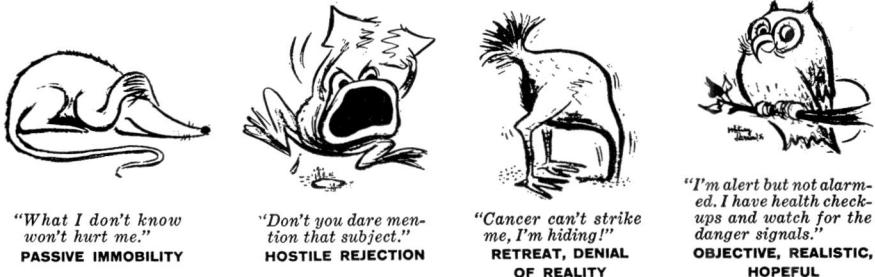

"*What I don't know won't hurt me.*"
PASSIVE IMMOBILITY

"*Don't you dare mention that subject.*"
HOSTILE REJECTION

"*Cancer can't strike me, I'm hiding!*"
RETREAT, DENIAL OF REALITY

"*I'm alert but not alarmed. I have health checkups and watch for the danger signals.*"
OBJECTIVE, REALISTIC, HOPEFUL

Figure 19. The purpose of the information program is to motivate, to persuade people to act for their own protection. To motivate, it is not enough merely to present facts or to achieve visibility for the program. Life-saving information must be presented in such a way as to overcome common anxieties and resistances. Some of the public's attitudes to be considered are illustrated above: the owl, of course, is not a problem, but an active volunteer in the American Cancer Society. (From Basic Information Guide: American Cancer Society, New York, 1960 Cancer Facts and Figures.)

Health educators must continually compare the objectives of their program with the characteristics and interests of each group in order to analyze the relationship. Understandably, certain groups are better targets than others in any given program. Names and meeting places of various groups may often be supplied by the local chamber of commerce or local health department.

The 7 C's of communication, as advanced by Cutlip and Center, are:

1. Credibility—competent source
2. Context—provides a link with reality and participation
3. Content—realistic meaning
4. Clarity—simple, clear message
5. Continuity and consistency—repetition with variation
6. Channels—established channels of communication should be used
7. Capability—require little effort on part of the recipients.[3]

One important principle in effective communication is to keep the message simple and direct with a minimum number of choices. For example, to offer an individual his choice of the tuberculin test, patch test, or chest x-ray may deter, confuse, and even repel the person from the original objective. Another principle involves the positive clear message. It seems doubtful that we can change behavior or attitudes with weak and misleading messages as "If you must smoke, smoke less than one pack per day." A third principle involves timing and group or individual readiness. For example, public or individual acceptance toward immunization is more favorable just before or during the polio season. Also, individuals are more concerned about the prevention of disease, promotion of fluoridation, or old-age health insurance at the time when their community, friends or family are directly involved. The fourth principle relates to the necessity of determining the most effective message and the most effective methods of communicating this message. Health education programs must continually strive to influence and change attitudes and behavior as well as to present information. Considerations should include such factors as age group intended, individual or group problems, availability of services, and socioeconomic factors.

In order to motivate and communicate with groups, health educators must select and plan program methods; study leadership principles; choose effective tools of communication; and discover major sources of community health education materials. These important areas are discussed on the following pages.

PROGRAM METHODS AND LEADERSHIP

Program Planning

A good program can be planned by interested group members who consider the needs and interests of all members. Needs and interests may be obtained by various methods including interviews, informal conversations, meeting census, registration cards, suggestion or question boxes, and questionnaires. (See page 78 for sample questionnaire.) Other considerations in program planning include choosing a topic that is capable of solution and limited in scope. A good program should:

1. Start with the interest of members
2. Have a variety of subjects and methods
3. Start and end on time
4. Have a good speaker, film, reading or other needed resource
5. Make provision for fellowship
6. Get members doing things
7. Provide for physical comfort
8. Add something to each person's life.[4]

Program Methods

A good community health program involves group discussions or an exchange and critical examination of ideas between individuals. Through such participation, the individual adds to his information and has his own contribution evaluated by others. Thus discussion is an important part of the learning process. There are also emotional values that accrue to the individual through his participation in discussion. Discussion, therefore, aids in the personal and social development of individuals. Tensions are relieved through the airing of beliefs and opinions; talking through a problem may have emotional value for all who participate. Suppressed biases and prejudices are brought into the open for examination. Group discussion is a cooperative effort to use facts in the solution of a problem, to test facts proposed in the solution of a problem, to propose alternatives for the solution to a problem, and to present divergent points of view on a problem. Desired outcomes of effective discussion include:

1. Increased knowledge or information
2. Increased ability to use knowledge in new situations
3. Increased skill and precision in thinking and in communicating thoughts to others

COMMUNITY HEALTH COUNCIL—SAMPLE QUESTIONNAIRE

FROM: Program Committee
TO: All Members
SUBJECT: The kind of program you want to have next year. If you would like to help us plan next year's program, please fill out this questionnaire and return it today.

I. *I am most interested in:*   *Specific service, speaker or area.*
  A. Services of voluntary health agencies
  B. Services of local health department
  C. Chronic or communicable disease
  D. School health program
  E. Mental health
  F. Dental health
  G. Civil defense
  H. Safety education
  I. Environmental sanitation
  J. Maternal and child health
  K. Air pollution
  L. Geriatrics
  M. Suicides
  N. Alcoholism
  O._____

II. *Our group needs:*   *Very much   Some   Not at all*
  A. A stronger treasury
  B. More members
  C. More fellowship
  D. More active participation
  E. More significant programs
  F._____

III. The five most important health problems our community faces are:*
  1.
  2.
  3.
  4.
  5.
  * Put a circle around the number of the problem, if any, you think our group can do something about.

  4. Marked changes in individual interest
  5. More and new rational attitudes
  6. Improvement in the social and personal adjustments of individuals
  7. Increased awareness and appreciation of problems and of the source of materials used in their solution.
  8. Increased skill in reaching concensus concerning possible action
  9. Directing effective *action* to the attainment of present goals.

The group method is the basic method of democratic socialization, and the framework in which the individual can improve himself as a contributing member of society. The following types of meetings are utilized in group discussions: speaker, symposium, forum, panel, institute, working conference, workshop, group dynamics, role-playing, buzz-session, and brainstorming. (See page 80 for a handy check list of some program methods.)

Leadership in Discussion Groups

Behind every effective discussion group there is usually an able and competent leader. He considers the needs and interests of each member and guides the group toward the achievement of its goals. (See page 81 for group leader's outline.) Eventually, the leader becomes a productive group member and actually increases his contribution to the group. He fosters and propels continuous communication between group members in a climate of freedom and mutual respect.

Qualities of good leaders include:
1. They accept all contributions as something to be considered thoughtfully.
2. They are tactful and friendly.
3. They have a good knowledge of the topic being discussed.
4. They have no preconceived notions about where the discussion should go.
5. They take no particular viewpoint in the discussion.
6. They help the group recognize the main issues in the discussion.
7. They see to it that every member of the group gets an opportunity to make a contribution.
8. They prevent the development of bad feelings among members.
9. They make certain that the group knows what conclusions have been decided.

Qualities of good participants include:
1. They prepare for discussion.
2. They cooperate with the leader.
3. They think before speaking.
4. They consider the feelings of others.
5. They speak correctly.
6. They challenge ideas they cannot accept.
7. They listen.

Leadership in Community Health Programs

Community organization involves good leadership. Conviction

HANDY CHECK LIST OF SOME PROGRAM METHODS

METHOD	CHIEF CHARACTERISTIC	SPECIAL USEFULNESS	LIMITATIONS
Lecture, film, reading, recitals, etc.	Information giving	Systematic presentation of knowledge	Little opportunity for audience to participate
Forum	Information giving, followed by questions for clarification	Audience can obtain specific information on particular aspects of the subject	Formality; lack of freedom to interchange ideas
Symposium panel or debate	Presentation of different points of view	Issues, approaches, angles spotlighted; analysis stimulated	Personality of speaker may overshadow content; program can be monopolized
Discussion	High degree of group participation	Pooling of ideas, experience and knowledge; arriving at group decisions	Practical with only limited number of people
Project, field trip exhibits, etc.	Investigation of a problem cooperatively	Gives first-hand experience	Requires extra time and energy for planning
Buzz groups	100 per cent participation by large audiences through small clusters of participants	Makes individual discussion, pooling of ideas possible in large groups; develops leadership skill in members	Contributions are not likely to be very deep or well organized.
Group interview	Spontaneous giving of opinions and facts by experts in response to questions	Brings knowledge from a number of sources to bear on one problem	Becomes disorganized without careful planning of material to be covered

on the part of leaders will bring acceptance by large groups of people for any promulgated idea and will provide a basis for community-wide support and solidarity in relation to the particular program under consideration.

A recent study indicates that a person may be nominated for leadership in a community if:

1. He belonged to a recognized power clique.
2. He had the will to exercise power and leadership.
3. He had a moderate amount of wealth or property.
4. He had strong relationships with major civic associations.
5. His community residence was satisfactory.
6. He controlled a number of employees.
7. He had control of a corporate enterprise.
8. He was of prime age, or about 50 years old.
9. He was closely allied with major economic or political enterprises.

GROUP LEADER'S OUTLINE*

TOPIC: How should children be educated about sex in Midville?

TIME: Sixty-minute panel discussion followed by fifteen minutes of audience participation.

2 min.   Preliminary words of welcome to audience by group leader

6 min.   I. *The Felt Difficulty*

   A. Statement of problem and why it is important
      1. Failure of the home to impart sex education
      2. Restrictions placed upon formal education in this regard
      3. Increasing incidence of delinquency relating to sex
   B. Introduction of panel members
   C. Definition of terms
      1. Sex education
      2. What constitutes "children"
   D. Limitation of subject
      1. Sex education
      2. Of children
      3. In Midville

25 min.   II. *Analysis of the Problem*

   A. Background
      1. Is our problem part of a national one? (scope)
      2. When did sex education become a problem here?
   B. How is this problem manifested?
      1. Is this problem serious?
      2. Who is affected?
   C. Casual factors
      1. Why do we have this problem?
         a. Ignorance of psychological aspects of sex
         b. Obstacles in the path of dissemination of accurate sex
            information
            (1) Social lag
            (2) Educational lag
      2. What are the effects of this problem?
         a. Promiscuity
         b. Unwed mothers
         c. Venereal disease
         d. Neuroses and mental illness
         e. Sex crimes and perversion
         f. Divorce
         g. Research aimed at solving problem
   D. Goals
      1. It is possible to educate children in this regard?
         a. Children should have sex education commensurate with
            their mental age
         b. Information must be scientific and accurate
         c. The solution should be long range, carefully planned, and
            efficiently administered

10 min.   III. *Finding Possible Solutions*

   1. In the light of the preceding discussion, what solutions are
      suggested?
   2. What solutions have been attempted?

15 min.   IV. *Evaluation of Proposed Solutions and Choice of Best Solution*

   A. Will some offered solution meet our present need?
   B. Will it lessen or eliminate the cause of the problem?
   C. Will it work?
   D. Will its advantages outweigh its disadvantages?
   V. *Applying the Solution*   [In this discussion presentation there would be no means of evaluating the plan in action
      inasmuch as it would not have been tried.]

2 min.   Concluding summary by chairman

15 min.   Forum period

Friends, you have heard our proposed solutions. Have you any questions or can you help us with suggestions?

*Wagner, Joseph A., *Successful Leadership in Groups and Organizations* (San Francisco, California: Howard Chandler 1959—handbook), p. 28

10. He maintained good press relations.
11. His personal qualities were in conformity to standard community conduct.
12. His social clubs and church affiliations were in conformity with his station in life.
13. He had good interaction with other community leaders.

A man lost in power rating if:

1. He was known to be a follower of another person in such manner or degree that his opinions could not be considered his own.
2. He accepted responsibilities for a community project, and the project failed.
3. He made an unsuccessful bid for public office.
4. His personal qualities were objectionable to top leaders.
5. He was considered a controversial figure by top leaders.
6. He belonged to an ethnic group that did not have the praise of leadership groups.[5]

The study also indicated that a typical, strong leader in community action programs is about 50 years of age, an owner of a large corporate enterprise, a person who is willing to assume community responsibilities, a person who has prestige in the community, and one whose social position is on a high level.

Although strong leaders are necessary to organize and promote health action groups, other major influencing factors include personal motives such as desire for social prestige, personal gains, or traits of personality. But above and beyond individual concerns, people participate because they feel a sense of loyalty and obligation to the community.

It is interesting and important to note here that there is a lack of concensus among physicians as to their role in community health affairs. Dr. Louis H. Bauer, President of the American Medical Association in 1953, emphasized the lack of medical leadership in community health affairs:

The medical profession has been so long devoted to its own scientific affairs that until recently it has not been very active in civic affairs. Even now many of the profession pay little attention to what should be an important part of their lives. While physicians must always remain physicians, they are citizens first. One of the reasons why the country has experienced inflation and attempts at socialization and has wandered away from the principles and traditions of true Americanism is that so many citizens, particularly the professional groups, have neglected the duties of citizenship. Physicians ought to interest themselves in the civic affairs of their community. Their failure to do so is one reason why so many other groups have "run off with the ball" in health matters.

I have previously stated that physicians should be the leaders in community health councils and activities. We ask our fellow citizens to support us in our activities and problems and yet fail to give the leadership we should. . . .[6]

Physicians, as a group, cannot be classified as community power leaders and policy makers, but like other professional groups, they have recognized delegates who speak for the entire group. Individual practitioners are usually aware of the generalized pattern of community power and authority, even though they may not participate directly in the overall processes of decision making.[5]

THE TOOLS OF COMMUNICATION

The economical, effective avenue of contact with the general public is through the mass media: newspapers, pamphlets, radio, television, and magazines. The health educator must understand how, when, and where to utilize the media. (See Figure 20.)

Newspaper

The newspaper is perhaps the most universally available printed medium for use in a community health program. As an important social agency, the local paper ranks high as an effective ally of health groups. If health activities are to receive the desired space in the press, health officials must gain and retain the respect of both news and editorial staffs.

Advantages of the newspaper include: intimacy and confidence of local "publics"; large community circulation; possibility of descriptive pictures; favorable medium for a cumulative publicity build-up or promotional campaign; foundation for promoting television and radio programs; and the leisure and convenience with which a newspaper can be read and digested. On the other hand, the newspaper has certain limitations. Perhaps the major limitation is the fact that most people read only a portion of the daily newspaper, and that portion may have little to do with community problems. It is interesting to note, however, that one survey revealed that 66 per cent of the persons polled wanted additional coverage of public health, medicine, and other scientific information.[7] It is questionable, though, whether or not the facts and information in a newspaper lead to changes in attitude and behavior. For example, many physicians have among their patients obese women who read every column and article on reducing but continue to gain weight.

A few suggestions for health committees to keep in mind when preparing an article for the press are:

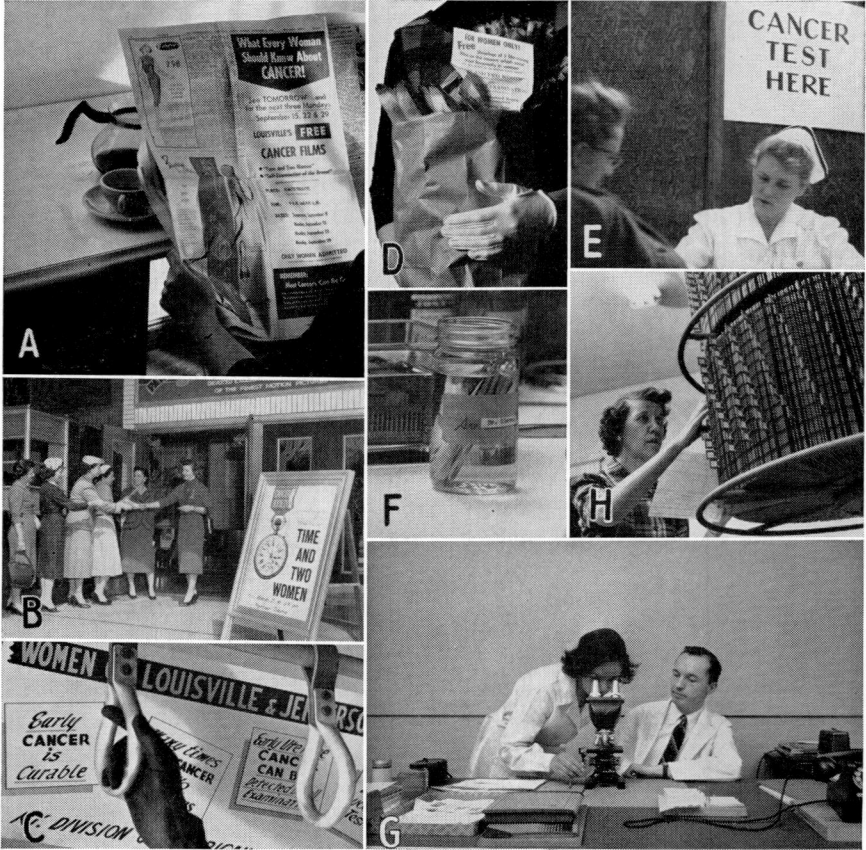

Figure 20. Community cancer cytology program embraces such educational aids as: A, newspaper ads; B, film showings; C, bus and car cards; D, handbills. Detection aspects include: E, registration and medical history; F, vaginal smear; G, microscopic examination of slide; H, record-keeping on each of the women participating. (Courtesy American Cancer Society.)

1. Write simply and use words that can be understood by the least educated reader.
2. Keep the story interesting, brief, and concise.
3. Present the *facts*—who, what, where, when, why and how.
4. Write sympathetically, especially about false notions that may be present in the community.
5. Use a positive approach and try to avoid controversial material.
6. Write about recent local events that occur near home.
7. Do not overlook the possibility of using local group and

organization publications as vehicles for messages to special audiences.

8. Keep in mind the various community groups that will read the article. (There must be reader interest.)
9. Convey the message intended.
10. Give the main points and indicate why the item is important in the first paragraph.
11. Write a story with a real reason for being written. (It must be of public interest.)
12. Submit the original draft to several interested persons and groups for suggestions.
13. Type the final copy neatly and recheck for errors in spelling, content, and meaning.
14. Place routine material in the editor's hands at least 24 hours prior to the day of publication.
15. Write articles that emphasize problems, programs, and organizations, not individuals.
16. Be impartial in distributing newsworthy stories.
17. Consider inviting reporters and editors to witness certain programs or incidents occasionally.
18. Seize the opportunity for follow-up with other articles, if practical.

To make writing more readable, there are three general rules to follow:

1. The more words there are in a sentence, the harder it is to read and understand that sentence.
2. The more parts there are in a word, the harder it is to read and understand that word.
3. The more personal references there are in a passage, the easier it is to read and understand that passage. (Personal references include pronouns, names, and words that refer to people, like *boy, friend, sister.*)

Although the press is an excellent medium, it cannot be used to the exclusion of all other media. Dissemination of information involves launching an attack via all channels of communication.

Radio

Radio has become part of our daily lives and exerts a strong influence on the public. One major advantage of the radio is the flexibility of the medium. For example, the ubiquitous radio may

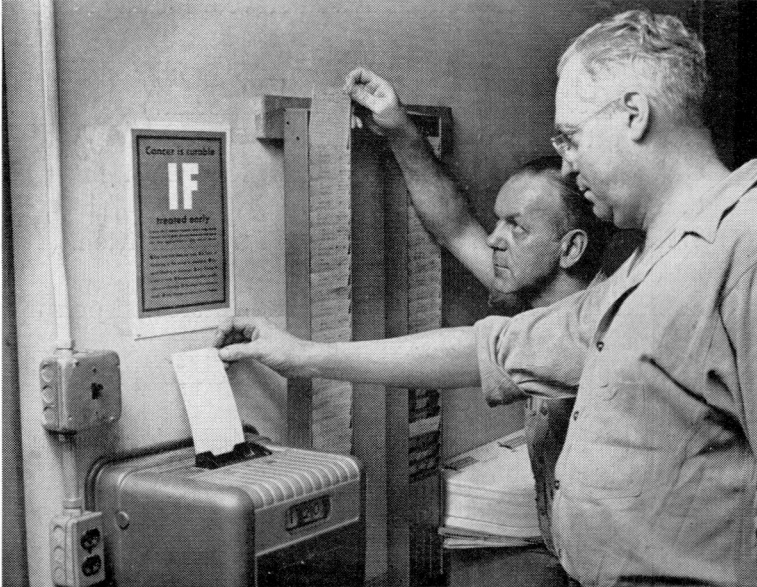

Figure 21. Two other effective methods of communication include exhibits and posters. Before preparing or displaying either medium, one should consider such factors as the purpose or objectives, eye catching colors or movement, specific groups or age levels intended, cost, ease of transporting and assemblying, participation by viewer, simplicity of message, motivation, needs and interests of intended group, and strategic locations. (From *Basic Educational Program for Business and Industry—* American Cancer Society.)

be present in two or three rooms of a home, the garage, and the automobile. The advent of the transistor and the pocket radio has made the radio more popular than ever. Other advantages include low cost of operation, ease of shifting from one station to another, large number of programs, possibility of selecting specific audiences, current news and music. There is no need for visual attention and the spoken word can be more compelling, more personal, friendler, and timelier than other media. However, ease of turning the dial, may often be a disadvantage to educators.

Most radio and television stations allot a certain amount of air time for nonprofit programs of an educational nature, among which are included public health programs and commentaries. Short spot announcements or 15 to 30 minute programs can be very effective. Quiz programs, panel discussions, or brain storming may warrant different approaches.

Television

Television has impact and realism, is welcomed in the home, and is readily available as an informational medium for the community health worker. The potential of this medium is so great that we have already witnessed its impact on presidential elections, criminal investigations, diplomatic and foreign policies and relations, education, and medical research and surgery. Television's mass appeal has been demonstrated; many families now own two television sets. However, before plunging blindly into planning a television program, community health leaders must consider that the medium requires money, people, time, facilities and materials, research, planning, and teamwork.

Commercial stations throughout the nation donate thousands of hours of free public service time to educational organizations in the interest of community culture and welfare. Since many public groups are inclined to visualize only their needs and interests in asking for time on commercial stations, it is well for community leaders to understand the considerations of station personnel in granting requests for free broadcasting in terms of value, availability of time, and quality of the public service program. For example, a half hour television program may cost as much as $2,000, and time is at a premium. The public service program must compete with programs scheduled at the same time on other channels. Station personnel want to schedule public service programs that meet high broadcasting standards and attract as wide an audience as possible. Health education possibilities are infinite. For example, a series of programs devoted to explaining and discussing the various health problems within a certain community is certainly an excellent springboard to community health organization and planning. (See Figure 22.)

Since television is becoming more significant and important as a source of health education, a few factors necessary for planning and conducting a program will be discussed. In television, as in all other media of expression, an idea must be present. The main theme may revolve around major community health problems, obstacles, objectives, needs, programs, services, and accomplishments. If these things can be shown as well as explained, the embryo of a television program is present.

The program idea must be tested or refined by asking the following questions:

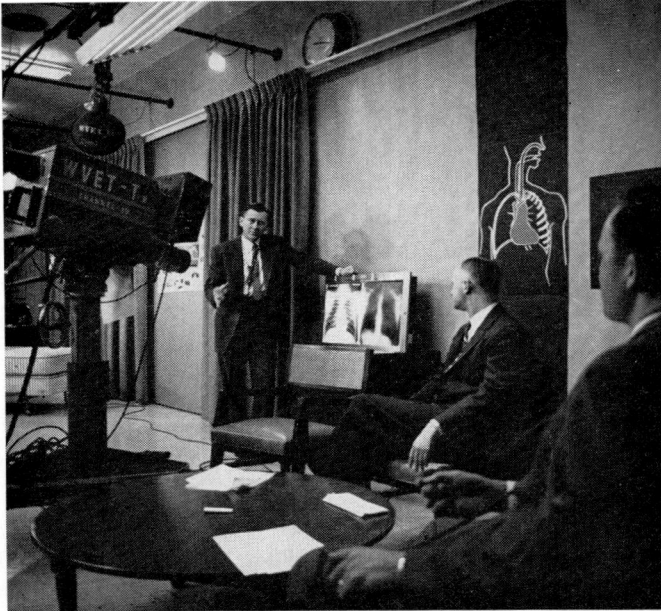

Figure 22. At rehearsal before air-time, a doctor explains the difference between a healthy and tuberculous lung in an x-ray. (From Today's Health. A.M.A. April, 1960.)

1. Is the subject of direct interest to my audience?
2. Can the importance of the subject be clearly shown to my audience?
3. Is it timely in terms of current developments, research findings, local problems, or seasons of the year.
4. Does it further community health education programs?

A good educational presentation involves research and careful planning. (For television broad planning check list, see page 88.)

BROAD PLANNING FOR TELEVISION

1. Type of Programming: Public service or instructional TV?

2. Purpose of Programming: Enrichment
General information
Teacher training
Adult education

3. Choice of Medium: Open circuit
Closed circuit

4. Course Content or Series Theme: Community health problems
College basic course in health education
Specific prevention program (safety, cancer)
Services of local health agencies

5. General Format: Demonstrations
Films and panel discussions
Illustrated lectures

6. General Participation: School personnel
Community leaders
Parent groups

7. Extent of Programming: Hours of preparation
Number of programs a month

8. Scheduling: Series or spot programming
Several stations

9. Utilization: In-school viewing
Out-of-school viewing
Viewing by community groups

10. Supplementary Materials: Work sheets, study guides
11. Evaluation: Rating sheets
Seminars
Questionnaires

12. Publicity: Channels, methods, extent
13. Sponsorship: Noncommercial

It is important that participants be given enough time to prepare a program to insure a feeling of security and excellent results. An analysis of some basic television formats includes:

FORMAT	TIME INVOLVED	SKILL INVOLVED	FACILITIES INVOLVED
1. Talk	*	**	*
(one lecturer or speaker occasional guests)	(depends upon the degree of visualization)		
2. Demonstration	**	***	***
(one performer with many materials, with or without supporting participants)			
3. Film and MC	*	*	*
4. Interview	*	*	*
(MC and guests)			
5. Discussion	*	*	*
(panel, etc.)			
6. Dramatization (completely scripted)	****	****	****
7. Dramatization (spontaneous, such as role-playing)	*	**	*

Frequently a combination format is used for education programming, involving several of the above basic formats rather than one.

    * The asterisk system indicates the relative complexity of the formats as regards (1) the amount of time involved, (2) the degree of skill required, and (3) the elaborateness of facilities, ranging from simple (*) to highly complex (****)[8]

Any format can be made interesting and meaningful if: (1) performers are carefully chosen, (2) the subject is attractive to a wide audience, and (3) audio-visual techniques are employed to provide variety and clear communication.

Pamphlets

Most health educators and health committees are often confronted with the task of preparing an educational pamphlet for distribution to the public. Authorities have recommended certain standards for use as guides in the selection and production of effective educational materials. The following outline is a brief summary of standards that apply to health education materials, and is intended for use by health educators, teachers, health council members, and other persons whose responsibility is to compose health pamphlets for distribution among people in the community:

1. Is it accurate? Is it up-to-date? Are source, author, date noted?
2. Is it impartial? For what kind of readers are you choosing the pamphlet?
3. Is the purpose of the pamphlet to arouse interest, develop attitudes, give information or stir to action?
4. Is the reader expected to read and keep the pamphlet or read and throw it away?
5. Is it attractive in format? Is it easy to read? Is it eye catching; would illustrations enhance the appeal?
6. Does it cover essential and factual information?
7. Is the material well-written, well-organized, and easy to understand?
8. Will readers remember essential points?
9. Is it personalized?
10. Does it have the positive approach?

Films

Films are valuable adjuncts to any community health education program. Free 16 mm. films, covering all aspects of community health, are available from many sources. The following sources are especially valuable: state and local health departments, county schools office or local college visual-aids department, state and local voluntary agencies, and the large insurance companies. When a group or agency has embarked upon a definite project with clear-cut objectives for which it needs public understanding, support, or participation and for which cooperating national or state agencies cannot supply suitable films, the agency may be justified in making its own films.

Nothing destroys the value of a film presentation more quickly than an antiquated film which is patently dated by outmoded wearing apparel, automobiles, buildings, and other scenery, materials, and techniques. To get the most from films, they must be previewed by the educator, introduced to the group, shown and discussed by the group. Lighting, seating, condition of the film itself, mechanical smoothness of projection equipment, environment, and room temperature are important factors to consider when presenting a film. Before a film is decided upon the following questions should be raised:

1. Is a film the best medium to accomplish the objectives set for a particular meeting, or would other materials and methods be more suitable?
2. Is a particular film best suited to the purpose you would like it to serve, e.g., to raise issues as a stimulus to discussion, to present information on a certain subject, or to arouse emotions for action to follow?
3. Has the film been previewed before use?
4. How can you get the most out of it?

After the film has been decided upon, the following questions should be raised:

1. Has the request for the film been confirmed? (Order it at least one month ahead of time.)
2. Have you arranged for an operator who knows how to run the projector efficiently?
3. Is the projector in good working order? Is the sound mechanism working correctly?
4. Is an electric outlet handy? Are there two or three pronged adapters? Will an extension cord be needed?
5. Is an extra projection lamp available? Is there an exciter bulb for sound?
6. If the film is to be used during the day, are there adequate window blinds in the room?
7. Has the screen been set up where it can remain during the whole meeting?
8. Are chairs and tables placed so that they need not be moved for showing?
9. Is the film ready to run when the time comes to use it?
10. Is the film in good condition?
11. Have you run through the entire procedure?

SOURCES OF COMMUNITY HEALTH
EDUCATION MATERIALS

The best sources of audio-visual aids in health education are the local and state health departments. Other major contributors are the local voluntary health and safety agencies. In order for community health workers to keep well informed and abreast of current local, national, and world health affairs, they may subscribe to the following list of suggested periodicals:

AREA	NAME OF PERIODICAL	WHEN PUBLISHED	COST
Local	Local city or county health newsletter, local health department.	Varies	Free
State	State health department periodical, state health department.	Varies	Free
Nation	*American Journal of Public Health*, 1790 Broadway, New York 19, New York	Monthly	$12.00 per year
Nation	*Public Health Reports*, Superintendent of Documents, Government Printing Office, Washington 25, D.C.	Monthly	$4.25 per year
World	*World Health*, World Health Organization, Pan American Sanitary Bureau, 1501 N. Hampshire Ave., N.W., Washington 6, D.C.	Bimonthly	Free
World	*WHO Chronicle*, World Health Organization, Palais Des Nations, Geneva, Switzerland	Monthly	$3.00 per year

Pamphlets

Sources of health education materials are infinite; the local health department and the local vouantary health and safety agencies will have most of the current materials available free of charge. However, they may not have the materials from the following agencies available for distribution, since there is usually a small cost involved:

Department of Health, Education and Welfare
United States Public Health Service
Washington 25, D. C.

American Dental Association
222 East Superior Street
Chicago 11, Illinois

American Medical Association
535 North Dearborn Street
Chicago 10, Illinois

National Health Council
1790 Broadway
New York 19, New York

Health Information Foundation
420 Lexington Avenue
New York 17, New York.

For a more complete list of national sources of health education material, see *How To Find What Health Education Materials You're Looking For,* American Journal of Public Health, *46:*1460–65, November, 1956.[9] Also, for a selected list of public health periodicals published in various countries throughout the world, see Rosen, George, *A History of Public Health,* New York, MD Publications, Inc., 1958, pages 516–19.[10]

Films

The best sources of community health education films are the local and state health departments. Individuals may write to these departments for a list of available films. Other major contributors include local voluntary health and safety agencies. Many industries are now producing excellent health education films; two examples include *Hemo, the Magnificent,* produced by the Bell Telephone Company, and *A Is For the Atom,* produced by General Electric.

QUESTIONS FOR REVIEW

1. In what ways can we motivate people to participate in a community health program?
2. Give three different examples showing how effective communication aided and supported successful community health programs in your community.
3. What community groups are we most concerned with in our health programs?
4. What is the nature and function of a community health council?
5. What are the major qualifications of a superior community health leader?
6. Briefly discuss the major tools of communication available to health educators in disseminating information to the public.
7. Prepare a brief health article for the press.
8. Prepare an educational pamphlet relating to a major health issue for distribution to the public.
9. List five major sources of health education materials in your community.
10. Name five periodicals in the area of community health.

REFERENCES

1. *Fourth Yearbook of the Department of the Superintendent of the National Education Association.* Washington, D. C., 1926.
2. Commission on Chronic Illness: *Chronic Illness in the United States, Volume I, Prevention of Chronic Illness.* Massachusetts, Harvard University Press, 1957, Pages 82 and 83.
3. Cutlip, Scott M., and Center, Allen H.: *Effective Public Relations.* New Jersey, Prentice-Hall, Inc., 1958, Pages 140 and 141.
4. Knowles, Malcolm S.: *Your Program Planning Tool Kit, The Leader's Digest.* Adult Leadership, *1:64,* Adult Education Association of the U.S.A., 1952.
5. Hunter, Floyd, et al.: *Community Organization: Action and Reaction.* Chapel Hill, The University of North Carolina Press, 1956.
6. Bauer, Louis H.: *The President's Page.* J.A.M.A., *151:*390, 1953.
7. Krieghbaum, H.: *Readers Crave News of Health, Science.* Published and Edited by H. Krieghbaum, 1958.
8. Kendig, K. D., and Gaither, L. M.: *The ABC'S of TV, A Handbook on Instructional and Public-Service Programming for Educators and Community Leaders.* San José, California, San José State College, 1957, Page 115.
9. *How To Find What Health Education Materials You're Looking For.* Am. J. Pub. Health, 46:1460, 1956.
10. Rosen, George: *A History of Public Health.* New York, MD Publications, Inc., 1958, Pages 516–519.

SUGGESTED READING

Albig, William: *Modern Public Opinion.* New York, McGraw-Hill, 1956.

American Public Health Association: *How to Find What Health Education Materials You're Looking For.* Am. J. Pub. Health, 46:1460–1465, 1956.

Bales, R. F., Strodtbeck, F. L., Mills, T. M., and Roseborough, M. E.: *Channels of Communication in Small Groups.* Am. Sociol. Rev., *16:*461–468, 1951.

Barnouw, Erik: *Mass Communication: Television, Radio, Film, Press.* New York, Rinehart and Co., 1956.

Bauer, W. W., et al.: *What Is Health Education?* Am. J. Pub. Health, 37:641–652, 1947.

Berelson, Bernard, and Janowitz, Morris: *Reader in Public Opinion and Communication,* Revised Edition. Illinois, The Free Press, 1953.

Bowker, Benjamin C.: *PR Helps Build a Hospital.* Pub. Relations J., 9:3–7, 1953.

Bullette, Cleve: *How Psychology Plus Promotion Built Deposits in Tulsa Blood Bank.* Pub. Relations J. 9:2–8, 1953.

Cutlip, Scott M., and Center, Allen H.: *Effective Public Relations.* New Jersey, Prentice-Hall, Inc., 1958.

Davis, Keith: *A Method of Studying Communication Patterns in Organizations.* Personnel Psychol., 6:15–22, 1953.

Festinger, Leon: *A Theory of Cognitive Dissonance.* Illinois, Row Peterson and Co., 1957.

Griffiths, W., and Knutson, A. L.: *The Role of Mass Media in Public Health.* Am. J. Pub. Health, 50:515–23, 1960.

Hare, A. P., Borgatta, E. F., and Balles, R. F., Editors: *Small Groups, Studies in Social Interaction.* New York, Alfred Knopf and Co., 1955.

Hovland, C. I., Janis, I. L., and Kelley, H. H.: *Communication and Persuasion.* Connecticut, Yale University Press, 1953.

Hovland, C. I., Lumsdaine, A. A., and Sheffield, F. D.: *Experiments on Mass Communication.* New Jersey, Princeton University Press, 1949.

Jenkin, N.: *Affective Processes in Perception.* Psychol. Bull., *54*:100–27, 1957.

Kelly, H. H., and Volkart, E. H.: *The Resistance to Change of Group-Anchored Attitudes.* Am. Sociol. Rev., *17*:453–465, 1952.

Klapper, Joseph T.: *Studying Effects of Mass Communication.* (Teachers College Record, Volume 57) New York, Columbia University Press, 1955.

Kutner, B.: *Surgeons and Their Patients: A Study in Social Perception.* Patients, Physicians, and Illness, Edited by Jaco, E. G., Illinois, The Free Press, 1958, Pages 384–397.

Lee, Alfred McClung: *How To Understand Propaganda.* New York, Reinhart and Co., 1952.

Levy, Harold P.: *Public Relations for Social Agencies.* New York, Harper and Brothers, 1956.

MacDougall, Curtis: *Understanding Public Opinion.* New York, Macmillan Co., 1952.

Martineau, Pierre: *Motivation in Advertising: Motives That Make People Buy.* New York, McGraw-Hill, 1957.

Medalia, N. Z., and Larsen, O. N.: *Diffusion and Belief in a Collective Delusion.* Am. Sociol. Rev., *23*:180–186, 1958.

Minnis, M. S.: *Cleavage in Women's Organizations: A Reflection of the Social Structure of a City.* Am. Sociol. Rev., *18*:47–53, 1953.

National Health Council: *Directory of Member Organizations:* New York, National Health Council, 1958.

Patterson, Raymond S., and Roberts, Beryl J.: *Community Health Education in Action.* St. Louis, The C. V. Mosby Co., 1952.

Patterson, Robert G.: *Foundations of Community Health Education.* New York, McGraw-Hill, 1950.

Postman, L.: *Perception, Motivation, and Behavior.* Personality, *22*:17–31, 1953.

Reissman, L.: *Class, Leisure and Social Participation.* Am. Sociol. Rev., *19*:76–84, 1954.

Scaff, A. H.: *The Effect of Commuting on Participation in Community Organizations.* Am. Sociol. Rev., *17*:215–220, 1952.

Schatzman, L., and Strauss, A.: *Social Class and Modes of Communication.* Am. J. Sociol., *60*:329–338, 1955.

Scott, J. C.: *Membership and Participation in Voluntary Associations.* Am. Sociol. Rev., *22*:315–326, 1957.

White, J. E.: *Theory and Method for Research in Community Leadership.* Am. Sociol. Rev., *15*:50–60, 1950.

Wright, C. R., and Hyman, H. H.: *Voluntary Association Memberships of American Adults: Evidence from National Sample Surveys.* Am. Sociol. Rev., *23*:284–294, 1958.

Chapter VI

Chronic Disease

CHRONIC DISEASE is a problem whose scope is as great as the total population of the country. Each member of the population is a potential victim and, to the extent that control is possible, the key to individual control lies with the individual. While all people are possible targets of chronic disease, and the largest number of victims are under 65 years of age, older persons are more likely to be disabled by chronic conditions. In the population of the United States, the proportion of older persons is growing, and chronic diseases will become an increasing problem. (See Figure 23.) The Commission on Chronic Illness adopted the following definition of chronic disease: Chronic disease comprises all impairments or deviations from normal that have one or more of the following characteristics: are permanent; leave residual disability; are caused by nonreversible pathological alteration; require special training of the patient for rehabilitation; may be expected to require a long period of supervision, observation, or care.[1]

There is wide agreement that the major medical-care problem in the country is chronic disease. One of every six persons is chronically ill; more than two-thirds of our deaths are caused by chronic illness. It is interesting to note that the chronic disease mortality trends are similar in most modern world countries. (See Figure 24.) Three of every four hospital beds are occupied by victims of long-time illnesses. Many of these patients are chronically ill because they did not seek the attention of doctors early enough. Some patients would be better off at home if professional supplementary home care were available. Others who are incapacitated could learn to take care of themselves and with proper rehabilitation could learn to lead useful lives. As a result of these conditions, the chronically ill are consuming a disproportionate amount of time of

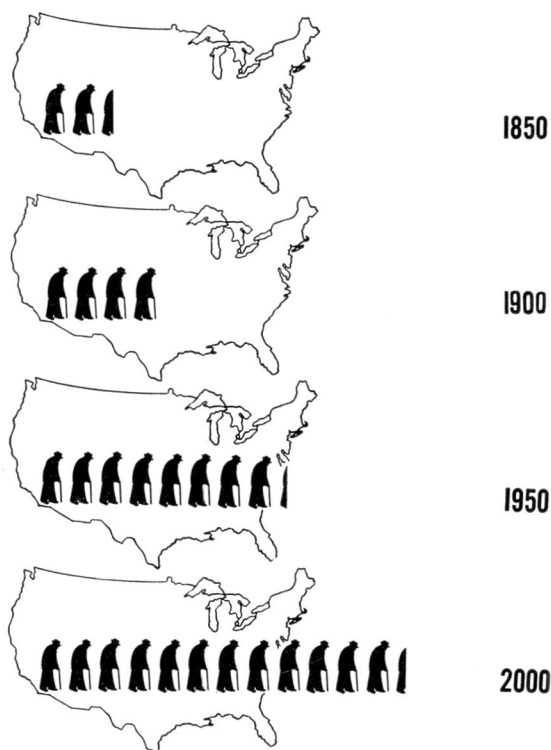

NUMBER OF PERSONS PAST THE AGE OF 65
PER 100 POP. IN THE UNITED STATES

Figure 23. Number of persons past the age of 65 per 100 population in the United States. (From Waterman, T. C., and Lang, V. F., *Chronic Illness*, St. Louis, C. V. Mosby Co., 1955.)

The Ten Principal Causes of Death in the Modern World

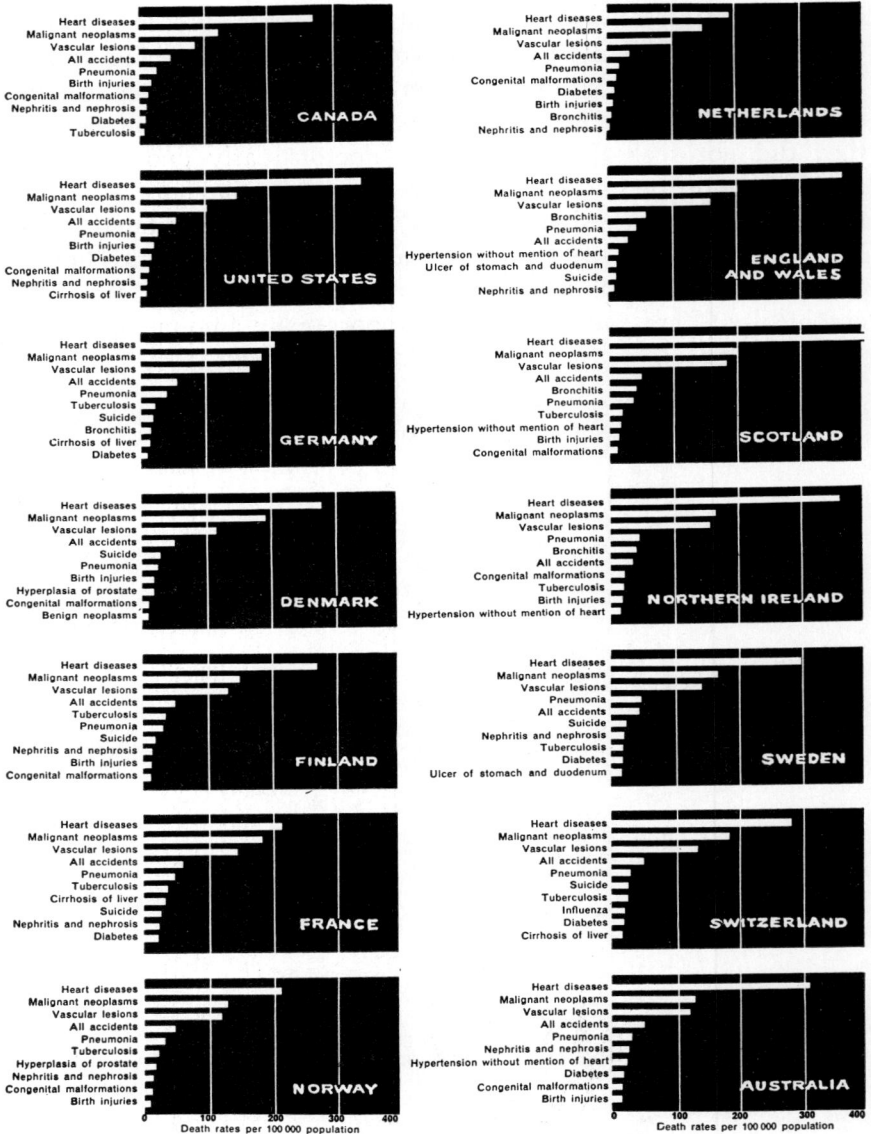

Figure 24. These graphs show ten principal causes of death in 14 countries that have reached a comparable degree of development. (From World Health. World Health Organization, Geneva, Switzerland, January-February, 1960.)

already overworked doctors, nurses, and welfare workers, and they are overloading hospitals and other medical facilities. Other problems involved in the chronic illness picture include expense and inadequacy of facilities for adequate early diagnosis and treatment, inequalities in distribution of physicians, mounting costs of medical care, and the insidious nature of the increase of chronic illnesses.

Prevention and treatment of chronic illness are community problems and affect each member of a community. Although two of every three deaths are caused by chronic diseases, the disability that results is of equal or greater importance. Consequences of prolonged disability from chronic diseases include medical expenses, loss in productive activity, and prolonged suffering of the patient. The major share of the financial burden for the care of the chronically disabled is usually derived from community, state, and federal taxes.

Age Group Affected

As an individual ages, his tissues undergo changes which increase his chances of becoming a victim of one or more chronic diseases. However, chronic diseases are not a problem confined to the older segment of the population. Chronic or degenerative conditions of cardiovascular disease and cancer cause more deaths among school age children than do all the infectious and parasitic diseases combined.[2] The degree to which individuals in the various age groups are affected by disability is illustrated partially by the following statement:

It is true that the highest rate of prevalence of chronic disease and disability occurs among the olders persons in the population, but, as the National Health Survey discovered, more than three-quarters of those with chronic illness and two-thirds of the invalids are between the ages of fifteen and sixty-four and more than half the chronic invalids are under the age of forty-five.[3]

One chronic disease case of every six involves a person under 25 years of age, and one chronic disease case of every two involves a person under 45 years of age. Cerebral palsy, which affects more than 500,000 persons, occurs most often before, during, or soon after birth. For example, it is estimated that there were approximately 570,000 cerebral palsy cases in 1957, and 280,000 of those cases were persons under 21 years of age.[4] Rheumatic fever, which has crippled at least 750,000 Americans with rheumatic heart disease, almost always strikes for the first time during childhood. Rheumatoid arthritis most often strikes between the ages of 35 and 40.

Diabetes and cancer are primarily diseases of middle and old age, but often strike earlier. Multiple sclerosis, a remissively progressive disorder of the central nervous system, characteristically affects persons betwen the ages of 20 and 40; onset is rare below the age of 12 or after 50 years of age. Muscular dystrophy, a disease that gradually wastes away all the voluntary muscles of the body, is a scourge of childhood and youth. Diseases of the heart or arteries, though concentrated in the years after 40, are distributed to some extent in every age group.[5]

Members of the United States Public Health Service estimate that about 3,000,000 persons under 20 years of age suffer from chronic illness or physical impairment. Some of these young people can be treated successfully but often at considerable expense. Others require special educational programs and placement services if they are to lead adjusted, useful lives. Each time the community allows one of these young people to spend his entire life in inactivity, it sacrifices nearly 50 man-years of productive effort and contented living.

Prevention

Prevention of chronic illness and disability requires mobilization of individual and public resources. Freedom from chronic illness can be achieved through united efforts toward individual health promotion, toward averting the occurrence of illness, and toward early detection of disease through health examinations and mass screening programs. At present, the prevention of severe forms of many chronic diseases depends largely upon early detection. Usually this implies the discovery of cases by means of screening procedures, examination, and diagnosis. There is evidence for the fact that severe forms of chronic disease and complications can be averted by early treatment. However, the majority of cases are already in severe or advanced forms when detected. Clinical and public health practices lag in utilizing the existing knowledge and measures for the prevention of chronic disease.

Chronic disease experts agree that there is no certain method of primary prevention at the present time for the following diseases or conditions: alcoholism, arteriosclerosis, degenerative joint disease, diabetes, epilepsy, essential or primary hypertension, multiple sclerosis, glaucoma, and rheumatoid arthritis. However, prompt and continuing application of known measures of primary prevention will result in a substantial reduction in the amount of and impairment by the following chronic diseases.

CHRONIC DISEASE	PREVENTION
1. Blindness	
retrolental fibroplasia	Control of oxygen administered to premature babies
congenital cataracts	Expectant mothers avoid contact with German measles or be exposed to the disease earlier
cataracts	Protective goggles—safety equipment
glaucoma	Early detection and treatment
ophthalmia neonatorum	Silver nitrate drops in new-born babies' eyes
2. Paralytic poliomyelitis	Immunization
3. Cardiovascular diseases	
rheumatic fever	Early detection and penicillin
atherosclerosis	Dietary control
syphilitic heart disease	Early treatment
4. Cancer	Avoiding certain pollutants, excessive radiation, chemicals and other irritants; early detection and treatment
5. Deafness	Expectant mothers avoid contact with German measles, syphilis, and other diseases
6. Dental caries	Fluoridated water supply, periodic visits to dentist

PERIODIC HEALTH EXAMINATIONS. Secondary prevention means halting the progression of a disease from its early unrecognized stage to a more severe one and preventing complications or sequalae of disease.[6] One of the best methods for detecting chronic disease is a periodic physical examination. A good periodic health examination should have four main sections: (1) a complete medical history, (2) a thorough and comprehensive medical examination, (3) appropriate laboratory, x-ray and other diagnostic procedures, and (4) health guidance and follow-up. The periodic health examination represents only a partial solution to the problem of early detection of chronic disease. The weaknesses and limitations of the health examination are time, cost, personnel limitations, cursory nature of some examinations, poor public acceptance, inability to detect all incipient disease, and limited facilities for diagnosis and treatment.

SCREENING EXAMINATIONS. Screening is another method of secondary prevention. Finding chronic diseases in their early, treatable stages would be no problem if everyone in the United States could and would go to his physician for a complete health appraisal once or twice a year. For this reason, medical and health authorities have urged regular health checkups in order to detect early signs of disease. Since time, costs, personnel shortages, and other factors already mentioned preclude the possibility of regular comprehensive health examinations for the majority of the population, relatively simple and inexpensive procedures of other types are needed to sort out persons with probable evidence of chronic disease in order to refer them for diagnosis and medical care. To help solve this problem, a fresh and interesting idea is the multi-test clinic. This clinic screens persons for two, six, or twelve diseases at a time. One blood sample can be tested for signs of diabetes, anemia, and venereal diseases; the same chest x-ray can be inspected for signs of tuberculosis, lung cancer, and heart defects; the urine sample can be examined for diabetes and kidney disorders. Multiple screening is not intended to diagnose diseases, but to discover persons who have need of consulting their physicians for diagnosis and treatment. The results of the screening tests are sent to the individual's physician or to the doctor named by him. The process is inexpensive, flexible, fast, and can be done by nonmedical personnel. Surgeon General Burney[7] stressed the value of screening as a measure to prevent blindness from glaucoma:

> It is estimated that 2 per cent of all persons over 40 years of age suffer from glaucoma and, with the increasing proportion of aged persons in our population, the number of persons included in that 2 per cent is constantly growing. With early detection and treatment, glaucoma seldom progresses to blindness; yet at present, 12 per cent of all blind people are blind as a result of glaucoma. Obviously, we are not detecting and treating cases in time.
>
> Encouraging progress has been made in the development of tonometry and other detection techniques. However, there are 59 million Americans over 40 years of age who, ideally, should be examined annually for glaucoma. The task is formidable, but a promising start is being made in a few communities through the use of mass screening, comparable to the mass casefinding programs that have proved so successful in the control of tuberculosis and venereal disease.*

A screening program will be most effective when it has the support of the medical association and voluntary and official agencies. A few effective screening tests include:

TEST	DISEASE DETECTED
1. X-ray	Tuberculosis
	Heart defects
	Cancer

* Address by L. E. Burney, M.D., Surgeon General, U. S. Public Health Service, Department of Health, Education, and Welfare, before the House of Delegates, Indiana State Medical Association.

2. Visual field and tonometry   Cataracts
Glaucoma

3. Audiometer   Hearing loss

4. Blood and urine tests   Diabetes
Anemia
Syphilis
Kidney disorders

5. Cytology (especially uterine cervix)   Cancer

The great advantage of screening is that it affords a means of bringing the benefits of early detection to large groups of the population. Selection of population groups for screening programs should include hospital patients, prisoners, members of industrial and labor groups, students, recipients of social and welfare services, members of group health plans, federal, state and local government employees, and members of the Armed Forces. Multiple screening is one way of detecting early signs of disease and of assuring speed, efficiency, and economy. Screening provides an excellent opportunity for health education, but, it is not a panacea. Its ultimate value in the community will be achieved when it becomes an integral part of a well-rounded chronic disease program.

OTHER PREVENTIVE MEASURES. Other suggested preventive measures are:

Prompt treatment. Many chronic diseases can be minimized and even cured if detected early. If parents and teachers are able to observe the signs and symptoms of certain diseases, they should refer children to physicians quickly and therefore prevent chronic or disabling consequences. For example, a hemolytic streptococcal infection usually precedes rheumatic heart disease. If detected early enough, however, the streptococcal infection can be treated with penicillin to prevent the disease. Protective hormones such as cortisone and ACTH are often used to soften the effect of the infection.

Adequate nutrition. "Lengthen the belt line and shorten the life line" can certainly be applied to specific chronic diseases. For instance, diabetes and heart disease are more prevalent in obese persons. Nutritional diseases and lowered resistance occur more often among those individuals who are unaware of the necessity of a wholesome and healthful diet.

Industrial hygiene. Industrial hazards such as dust, chemicals, and radiation can lead to a variety of occupational diseases which are chronic in nature. These air pollutants are increasing at a dangerous rate; management and medicine working together have shown that the worker can be protected from these hazards. More and more industries have come to realize that promotion of the health of workers represents a sound investment, and there are many ways in which industry can play an important role. An increasing number of businesses and industries are establishing policies requiring the preemployment and periodic medical examinations of workers; many plants engage in superior health education programs; rehabilitation programs also benefit business and industry.

Accident prevention.   Accidents kill more persons between the ages of one and 35 than any disease and rank fourth among the causes of death for all ages. Motor vehicle accidents and falls cause over 60 per cent of all accidental deaths yearly. Every year many more accident cases are added to the list of chronically disabled individuals. Developing safe behavior habits and attitudes in children and adults; initiating community safety education programs; creating community health and safety councils; and developing more and better safety equipment and regulations for industry are a few suggested preventive measures. Also important are the following: employment of trained safety engineers; adoption and enforcement of more stringent traffic laws; and the addition of safety education in the school curriculum.

Education.   Public education is of prime importance in conducting a chronic disease prevention program. The facts must be presented to all the people, and the people must be motivated to act accordingly.

Rehabilitation

Each of the 50 states, the District of Columbia, and Puerto Rico operate a rehabilitation program in cooperation with the Office of Vocational Rehabilitation of the Federal Security Agency. Under this federal-state plan, a handicapped person may apply for whatever help he may need to become self-supporting. About 60,000 men and women a year are being rehabilitated by this system. In most cases their disabilities are a result of illness. The Office of Vocational Rehabilitation estimates that between 1,500,000 to 2,000,000 Americans of working age are so severely disabled that they cannot support themselves, and that another 250,000 are disabled each year, primarily by chronic disease. The Office of Vocational Rehabilitation believes that most of these individuals could become self-supporting if Congress or the state legislatures, or both, voted enough money for rehabilitation. With present funds, the number of rehabilitants probably cannot exceed 60,000 a year. Once rehabilitated and working again, the handicapped person no longer needs support from community, state, and federal taxes. In fact, the person begins paying taxes again. Individual and family happiness contribute to the success of the rehabilitation program.

Community rehabilitation centers serving several hospitals, or established as part of one or more existing hospitals, have been very successful. The personnel required varies with the size of the community. A city of 100,000 population, for example, requires the services of a psychologist, a social service worker, a vocational counselor, as well as occupational and physical therapists. All programs and activities are supervised and directed by medical authorities.

Community Programs

Many successful chronic disease programs have been developed in communities throughout the country. Home-care programs, for example, have been very successful in caring for the patients and making more hospital beds available for others. It has been estimated that 70 per cent of chronically ill individuals would be better cared for in their own homes, providing the homes maintained satisfactory facilities for nursing care. Chronically ill patients may also be cared for in privately operated nursing homes. Operators of these homes are encouraged to maintain high standards, and to foster a close relationship between doctors, hospitals, and nursing homes. Also important is the willingness and ability of welfare agencies to pay adequate fees for impoverished invalids.

There is a need for more chronic hospitals, qualified privately-owned nursing homes, and other similar facilities. Many communities or counties have established central services for their chronically ill. The first central service was established in Chicago in 1944 by the Institute of Medicine, the Welfare Council, and the Community Fund. Others have since been established in Milwaukee, Essex County, New Jersey, and in San Francisco. Each program conducts some or all of the following activities:

1. Surveying the problem of chronic disease. In Chicago the central service knows the approximate number of persons affected, their ages, sex, financial status, diagnosis, degree of disability, and the amount and type of care needed. It also knows what facilities

are available for various types of treatment and care at what cost, and what additional facilities are needed.

2. Referring disabled persons and their families to the institutions and agencies best able to serve them. A Milwaukee hospital was ready to discharge a 60 year old woman who had been admitted for a fractured hip. But where could she go to convalesce? Besides her hip trouble she had such a severe case of arthritis that she hadn't walked in five years. The Central Agency for the Chronically Ill referred the patient to a nursing home where Milwaukee's Curative Workshop helped with her rehabilitation at the request of her physician. Today she is back in her own home, not only taking complete care of herself, but also doing some of the housework.

3. Working to expand facilities for the chronically ill. Both the Milwaukee and the Chicago agencies have encouraged qualified persons to open nursing homes and have given practical advice on how to run them. The Essex County group in New Jersey has started a homemaker service to aid the chronically ill person at home.

4. Acting to stimulate community interest in every phase of the problem.[8]

Federal, state, and local health agencies have stepped up their chronic disease programs. The key word, *prevention,* is stressed by all agencies. Their tools include legislation, education, research, and treatment, supported by coordination and cooperation. Chronic diseases warrant the current emphasis placed upon them.

CANCER

Cancer is uncontrolled, abnormal cell growth. Mankind has been afflicted with cancer for a long time; tumors have been found in prehistoric animal skeletons and in human remains from very early civilizations. Today, no race, creed, nor nationality appears to be free from cancer. The warning signs may be trivial or minor, and thus are ignored or forgotten.

There has been a marked increase in the number of cancer cases and deaths since 1900. However, certain factors, such as increase in average life expectancy, increase in population, more accurate diagnoses, increased use of radioactive elements, and other possible cancer-producing materials may partially account for this increased cancer rate.

One of every four persons now alive will develop cancer at some time in his life unless new preventive measures are found. About 700,000 men, women, and children are under treatment for the disease at this time. Approximately 700 Americans die of cancer every day; cancer kills one man, woman, or child every two minutes in the United States; over 250,000 Americans die of cancer each year. There are about 500,000 new cancer cases each year.

The cancer fatality rate could be decreased by 33 per cent if proper treatment were begun in time. In other words, we are losing about 85,000 Americans each year who could have been saved if they had received early diagnosis and prompt treatment. Many thousands more could be saved if men and women would have a complete medical examination once a year. Although more than $30,000,000 was voluntarily contributed by the public to the cancer research fund in 1960, 390 times as much, or $10,000,000,000 was spent on alcoholic beverages. Furthermore, 210 times as much money was spent on tobacco products and smokers' accessories during the same year. Experts testify that 30 million dollars is only a fraction of the amount needed for cancer research. A more concentrated education program is necessary in order to present the facts to all the people and motivate them to act.

Causes

Scientists have found many causes of cancer. However, each case seems to vary, and no conclusive facts can be presented at this time. Cancer has been attributed to chronic irritations, virus, acid substances within the cell nuclei, radioactive elements, ultraviolet to cosmic rays (sunburn), tobacco, inherited susceptibility, chemicals, congenital origin, precancerous conditions (moles), diet, hormones, proteins, enzymes, atmospheric pollution, and specific occupations. Research on each of these causes is still in progress. The leading causes of cancer deaths in men are lung cancer and cancer of the prostate gland. The leading causes of cancer deaths in women are breast cancer and cancer of the uterus.

Lung Cancer and Tobacco

Since interest in the correlation between lung cancer and smoking is high, the latest findings in this area will be discussed. (See Figure 25.) Lung cancer is the leading cause of cancer death among men, and is rapidly increasing as a cause of death among women. The disease, which is common among heavy cigarette smokers, is cured in less than 5 per cent of the cases. A few facts, as advanced by the American Cancer Society follow.

    1. If you smoke cigarettes *you may not live as long* as one who does not smoke.

Table 8. Cancer Status Chart: Leading Sites

SITE	ESTIMATED CASES, 1960	ESTIMATED DEATHS, 1960	DANGER SIGNAL (when lasting longer than two weeks see your physician)	SAFEGUARDS	COMMENT
Breast	63,000	24,000	Lump or thickening in the breast.	Annual checkup. Monthly breast self-examination.	The leading cause of cancer death in women.
Colon and Rectum	69,000	39,000	Change in bowel or bladder habits; bleeding.	Annual checkup. Routine proctoscopy.	Considered a highly curable disease when digital and proctoscopic examinations are included in routine checkups.
Kidney and Bladder	24,000	13,000	Bleeding or urinary difficulty.	Annual checkup with urinalysis.	Protective measures for workers in high-risk industries are helping to eliminate one of the important causes of these cancers.
Lung	43,000	36,000	Persistent cough or lingering respiratory ailment.	Annual checkup. Chest x-ray.	Evidence indicates cigarette smoking to be the chief cause of lung cancer, now the leading cause of cancer death among men.
Mouth, Larynx and Pharynx	19,000	8,000	Sore that does not heal. Difficulty in swallowing. Hoarseness.	Annual checkup including larynx.	Many more lives should be saved because the mouth is easily accessible to visual examination by physicians and dentists.
Prostate	32,000	15,000	Urinary difficulty.	Annual checkup. Routine palpation.	Occurs mainly in men over 60. The disease can be detected by palpation and urinalysis at annual checkup.
Skin	60,000	4,000	Sore that does not heal, or change in wart or mole.	Annual checkup. Avoidance of overexposure to sun.	Skin cancer is readily detected by observation, and diagnosed by simple biopsy.
Stomach	28,000	20,000	Indigestion.	Annual checkup.	A 40% decline in mortality in 20 years, for reasons yet unknown.
Uterus	40,000	14,000	Unusual bleeding or discharge.	Annual checkup including pelvic examination and Papanicolaou smear.	Uterine cancer mortality has declined 40% during the last 20 years. Now with the "Pap" smear, it can be virtually eliminated as a cause of death.
Leukemia	15,000	13,000	Leukemia is a cancer of blood-forming tissues and is characterized by the abnormal production of immature white blood cells. Acute leukemia strikes mainly children and is treated by drugs which have extended life from a few months to as much as three years. Chronic leukemia strikes usually after age 25 and progresses less rapidly.		Cancer experts believe that if drugs or vaccines are found which can cure or prevent any cancers they will be successful first for leukemia and the lymphomas.
Lymphomas	17,000	13,000	These diseases arise in the lymph system and include Hodgkin's disease and lymphosarcoma. Some patients with lymphatic cancers can lead normal lives for many years.		

From Cole, W. H.: Medical Progress. The New York Times, March 27, 1960, Section 10, page 7.

WHAT ARE YOUR

CHANCES

OF

DEVELOPING

LUNG

CANCER?

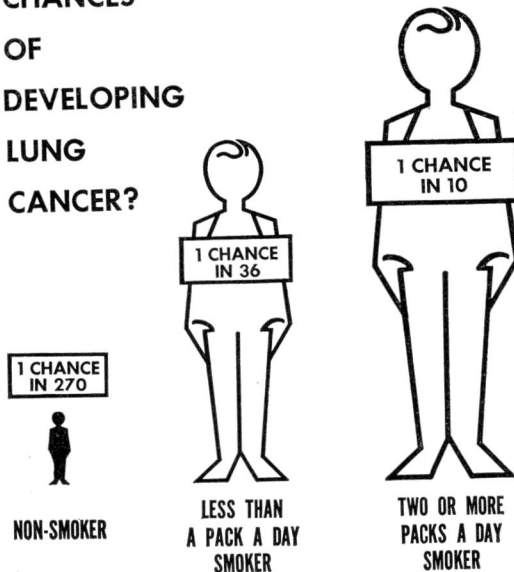

1 CHANCE
IN 10

1 CHANCE
IN 36

1 CHANCE
IN 270

NON-SMOKER

LESS THAN
A PACK A DAY
SMOKER

TWO OR MORE
PACKS A DAY
SMOKER

Figure 25. (Courtesy American Cancer Society.)

2. If you smoke two packs or more of cigarettes a day your chances of dying of lung cancer are *20 times greater* than those of a nonsmoker!
3. If you *give up* smoking, you have a *lower risk of death* than if you keep on smoking. It is not too late!
4. Persons with heart trouble *die much sooner* if they smoke.
5. Cigarette smokers are *more susceptible* than nonsmokers to cancer of the esophagus, larynx, mouth, tongue and back of the throat.
6. *Inhaling* cigarette smoke causes changes in lung tissue—the more smoking the worse the changes.[9]

A study of teen-age smoking in Portland, Oregon, revealed that of 21,980 high school students, about one-fourth the boys and more than one-eighth the girls smoke regularly every week, and most of them smoke every day. Other findings of the study include:[10]

1. The percentage of smokers is highest among children of families in which both parents smoke cigarettes; lowest in families in which neither parent has been a smoker, and

intermediate in families in which only one parent smokes cigarettes.

2. The smoking behavior of boys tends to conform more closely to that of the father, while smoking behavior of girls follows more closely that of the mother.

3. The percentage of smokers among children of families in which one or both parents continue to smoke is significantly higher than the percentage in which one or both parents gave up cigarette smoking.

4. Each successive school grade has a higher percentage of smokers.

5. The percentage of smokers is higher among students in Catholic parochial schools than among students in the city public schools. It is lowest among students in the suburban public high schools.

6. The percentage of smokers among boys who do not participate in athletics is substantially higher than those who do and have a coach. The percentage of smokers is higher among students who do not participate in any school activities.

Many scientists are convinced that cigarette smoking is the major cause, although not the only cause, of lung cancer. This opinion is not unanimous. Most of the evidence, however, makes it clear that cigarette smoking is largely responsible for the tenfold increase in lung cancer since 1930.

Prevention

Each year 85,000 lives can be saved from cancer. These people can be saved if they follow three simple but basic rules:

1. *Learn the seven danger signals of cancer.*
   Any sore that does not heal
   A lump or thickening in the breast or elsewhere
   Unusual bleeding or discharge
   Any change in a wart or mole
   Persistent indigestion or difficulty in swallowing
   Persistent hoarseness or coughing
   Any change in normal bowel habits.

2. *Have regular physical examinations.* The seven danger signals do not *necessarily* appear early in the course of cancer's growth. Some cancers can be detected by the medical doctor's thorough examination before they have had a

chance to sound the alarm and signal their presence to you. (See Figure 26.) Sometimes it is possible to find cancer in persons who seem to be perfectly well. Therefore, it is necessary to form the habit of having routine physical examination periodically—not less often than once a year. All men over 45 should have regular x-ray examinations of the chest; and all women over 35 should have regular vaginal smears taken. These examinations will check on the most common areas of cancer growth. Fortunately these examinations are simple and effective. The personal responsibility for seeking out possible cancer through periodic physical checkups is one of the more important responsibilities in your life.[11]

3. *Examine Yourself.* This important cancer detection method is a personal responsibility. Its usefulness is restricted to a few organs, and even where it is practical it does not replace the periodic survey by a doctor. The skin, a frequent location of cancer, lends itself readily to self-inspection. We can

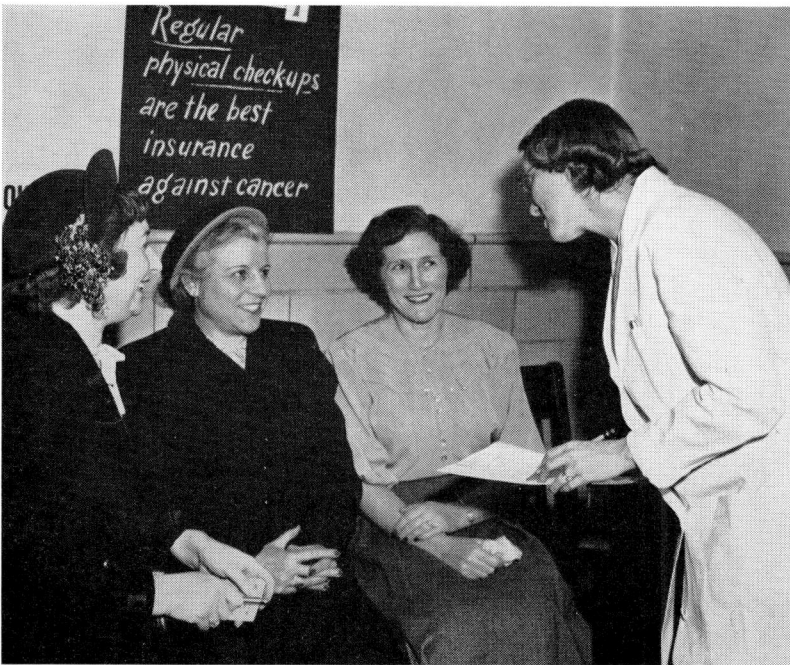

Figure 26. Women reporting to their doctor for yearly physical examinations. (Courtesy American Cancer Society.)

hardly fail to recognize and be conscious of moles, lumps, or sores that occur on the face. But it is astonishing to find that so many people are wholly unaware of similar lesions on their backs, arms, or legs. Why? Because they have simply not troubled to look for them. The same is true of the mouth, into which most people seem disinclined to look. We have already seen that self-examination of the breasts, if universally practiced, could double the curability of cancer arising there. And that small cancers of the rectum, which are highly curable, give an early warning signal in blood in the stool. Yet if we do not look for these signals, they will go by unnoticed.[11]

A simple smear test developed by Dr. George N. Papanicolaou has saved thousands of women with early cancer of the uterus. The test is easily administered, painless, and about 90 per cent accurate. It consists of drawing off a portion of the vaginal fluid, placing it on a slide, fixing it with a dye, and then examining the slide under a microscope. The trained technician can tell with a great degree of accuracy whether or not there are cancer cells present in the specimen.

The Papanicolaou smear was tested on a mass basis in 1950 and in 1955 in Tennessee and Georgia and showed that about five cases of such cancer are detected for each 1000 women examined. The test is slowly gaining in popularity among physicians, but must be supported by education programs designed for both the doctor and the public.

A new approach to early diagnosis of cancer involves the development of ways to identify groups of persons with high risk or susceptibility to particular kinds of cancer. Such persons would then become the focus of special programs aimed at earlier detection in specific sites of cancer. The Society's Cancer Prevention Study under way among 500,000 families will undoubtedly yield valuable clues to such patterns of cancer incidence and frequency.

Present methods of cancer diagnosis, although generally accurate, are too slow and cumbersome in view of the magnitude of the problem. If a simple detection test is developed, there are not enough physicians or clinics available to accommodate the public. Thus, the number of approved cancer clinics and general hospital clinics are being increased. An additional step has been taken to increase the number of physicians trained in cancer diagnosis and treatment.

Most health departments have an active cancer-control program consisting of educating the public to the need for early detection; the training of laboratory technicians in techniques for early detection, such as the microscopic examination of cervical smears; conducting epidemiological studies of cancer; and the development and evaluation of cancer control services within the various states.

A basic element of many cancer-control programs involves the tumor registry, in which is filed various information about cancer cases. These reports give the essential information about diagnosis and treatment of the cases, as well as some of the important characteristics of the patient. These registries provide a tremendous reservoir of information that is useful in evaluating the progress of cancer-control measures. The follow-up mechanism, by which reports are made on each case every year until time of death, helps keep patients under continuous medical supervision. This is as important in cancer as it is in tuberculosis and other chronic diseases. The registry supplies data for research and contributes to a better understanding of the epidemiology of cancer.

Education must be promoted and state laws enacted in a continuing effort to protect citizens from fraudulent drugs and curative devices. The "cancer quacks" are particularly vicious because they kill hundreds of cancer victims by keeping them from early detection and competent treatment. State and local health departments, in conjunction with the United States Food and Drug Administration, have investigated many "cancer quacks" and have been successful in bringing about court convictions.

The biggest and best known private organization in the cancer field is the American Cancer Society, organized in 1913 by a group of doctors and laymen as the American Society for the Control of Cancer. The Society's original and early contribution to the nation's fight against cancer was its educational campaign to convince the public and the medical profession that cancer could be cured if found early enough. Congress finally recognized the need for basic and fundamental research in this field, and in 1937, established the National Cancer Institute within the United States Public Health Service.

Funds to combat cancer have increased slowly but steadily. From an income of less than a million dollars in 1945, the Society's annual income has grown to over 30 million dollars in 1960. Congressional appropriations have increased from $561,000 in 1945 to

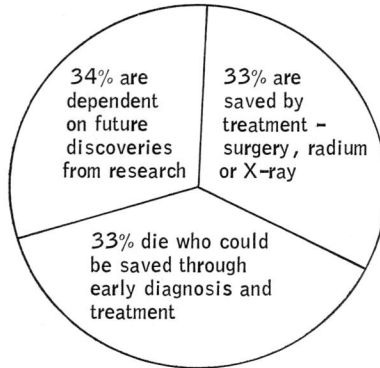

Figure 27. What is happening to those who get cancer?

$91,000,000 in 1960. The National Cancer Institute utilizes this money for research and grants to institutions, medical schools, and researchers.

Treatment

Surgery, x-ray, and radium are the standard treatments, but promising results are being obtained with hormones, radioactive isotopes, and growthblocking chemicals.

However, cancer differs widely in it symptoms, behavior, and response to treatment. For example, certain cancers of the breast grow rapidly and spread quickly to other parts of the body. Others grow slowly and remain localized for many years. Many cancers are aggressive, but one of the most common of all, basal cell cancer of the skin, is indolent and slow-growing.

Cancers also differ in their response to treatment. Most skin

CURABILITY OF CANCER				
Kind of Cancer	Present Cure Percentages	Possible Cure Percentages	Lives Lost Last Year	Lives Lost Which Could Have Been Saved through Earlier Detection
Uterine cancer	30%	70%	16,000	9,100
Breast cancer	35%	70%	21,000	11,300
Rectal cancer	25%	70%	11,000	6,600
Mouth cancer	35%	65%	3,000	1,400
Skin cancer	85%	95%	4,000	2,700
Lung cancer	5%	50%	27,000	12,800

Figure 28. (From Schifferes, J. J., *Essentials of Healthier Living,* John Wiley and Sons, 1960.)

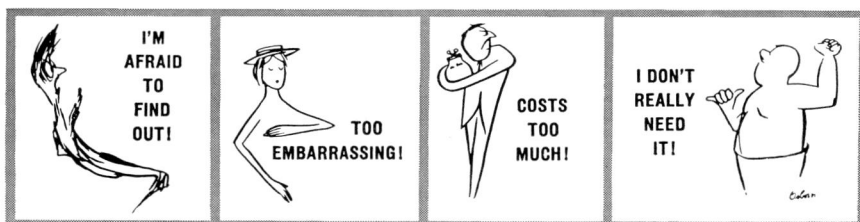

Figure 29. Why people delay examination and avoid cancer check-ups. These are rationalizations, not reasons. Early detection is the best protection against death from cancer. (From Schifferes, J. J., *Essentials of Healthier Living,* John Wiley and Sons, 1960.)

cancers are readily destroyed by x-rays or radium, but one form of cancer, melanoma, that usually originates in the skin is highly resistant to these agents. Cancer of the uterus is often cured by radiation, but cancer of the stomach is not approached in this manner. Some of this variation is due to the location of the diseased area, since some areas are more accessible than others to the cancer-destroying rays. However, there are also significant differences that seem to be inherent in the various cancer cells.

The Future

Techniques of diagnosis and treatment have been greatly improved. Drugs, radioactive isotopes, anti-cancer chemicals, hormones, surgery, and radiation are helping save one cancer patient in every three; 15 years ago only one in four cancer patients was saved. New high-voltage radiation equipment permits more effective treatment of certain cancers; x-ray dosages can be more skillfully calculated and aimed to provide maximum destruction of cancer tissue with minimum harm to healthy cells. Better understanding of the body's chemical balances and needs, techniques of rapid blood transfusion, and the use of new drugs controlling infection have made remarkable new surgical procedures possible. A more significant development has been the increased activity of medical schools in cancer teaching and research and in the training of young surgeons, radiologists, and internists through American Cancer Society fellowships.

Some of the goals researchers and scientists hope to achieve in the near future include:

1. Discovery of cellular trigger mechanisms which start malignant cell growth
2. A means of checking metastasis—the spreading of cancer

3. Chemicals to selectively kill or halt division in cancer cells
4. Understanding of possible immune defense mechanisms that may work against cancer
5. Proof that viruses are a cause of some forms of cancer in humans
6. A simple and practical blood test to disclose early cancer.[12]

CARDIOVASCULAR DISEASE

The leading cause of death in the United States today is diseases of the heart and blood vessels. Each year heart disease is responsible for one of every two recorded deaths, or nearly one million Americans. For each patient who dies, 11 others are chronically ill, and many of them are afflicted in their most productive years. Cardiovascular disease is an important cause of disability for all ages above 15, and about four billion dollars is lost annually due to employee absenteeism.

Causes

Basic causes of the major cardiovascular diseases are unknown. Many possibilities are being explored including obesity, hormones, diet, exercise, over-work, occupation, cigarette smoking, emotional tension, environment, and social characteristics.

The death rate of men from heart diseases exceeds that of women at all ages, but the greatest variation between the sexes is caused by the soaring rate among men aged 45 to 64. Furthermore, a man's chance of dying from a heart attack if he lives in New York State is more than twice as high as that of a resident of New Mexico.

Some defects may be present in a child's heart or great vessels at birth. For example, the pulmonary artery and aorta may be transposed and cause death soon after birth. Scarring and narrowing of the valves may be acquired later in life as the result of rheumatic fever. However, 90 per cent of all heart disease in the United States is due to arteriosclerosis and hypertension or high blood pressure.

Cerebral Hemorrhage or Stroke

Cerebral hemorrhage is one form of cardiovascular disease and is listed as the third leading cause of death in the United States. Among physicians, disorders of the blood vessels in the brain are called "C.V.A.," or cerebral vascular accident. To the layman, however, any C.V.A. is known as a stroke or apoplexy. The term encompasses all kinds of C.V.A.'s and all degrees of severity, with or without paralysis. Four causes of strokes are:

1. Hemorrhage in the brain caused by the bursting of a blood vessel. (This type is usually severe and causes paralysis.)
2. Thrombosis or clotting in the artery affected.
3. Embolism or traveling clot.
4. Spasm of an artery.

In any case, a stroke may or may not irreparably damage that part of the brain where nerve centers controlling sight, hearing, speech, memory, and skilled acts are located.

Prevention

The local health department and the local branch of the American Heart Association joined forces long ago to combat heart disease by providing research, professional and public education, and community service. At the national level, the American Heart Association and the National Heart Institute of the United States Public Health Service have cooperated in the development of a single-focused attack on cardiovascular diseases.

Research grants include studies concerned with such problems as the movement of metals across cell walls, the effects of stress on bodily absorption of fats, the electrical forces of heart muscle, the pattern of life that leads to heart disease, and the role of diet, physical exercise, occupation, cigarette-smoking, stress, obesity, and cholesterol levels in heart disease. Epidemiologic studies of various kinds are necessary to help find the causes of this disease.

Emphasis is placed upon health education in the fight against heart disease. Although diet and exercise are stressed, six suggestions for the prevention and treatment of arteriosclerosis are:

1. Reduce weight if obese.
2. Follow your doctor's advice and if blood cholesterol is high, try to reduce the level by change in dietary habits.
3. Reduce the proportion of solid animal fats to the liquid vegetable fats and also reduce the total quantity of both.
4. Get more regular exercise.
5. Avoid excesses of all kinds.
6. Reduce blood pressure, if elevated.[13]

Since it is known today that rheumatic fever is preceded by a streptococcal infection, teachers, parents and others are being alerted to this fact; prevention is possible if antibiotics are administered early. An estimated two million persons in the United States have had, or will develop, an attack of rheumatic fever during their lifetime. Rheumatic fever and resultant heart disease is the fifth leading cause of death among children from five to 14 years of age.

Advances and Treatment

Advances in treatment of heart disease are given in the following list.

DEFECT OR DISEASE	ADVANCE OR TREATMENT
Syphilis	Penicillin
Diphtheria	Immunization
Subacute bacterial endocarditis	Antibiotics
Rh negative baby	New blood supply
Hypertension	Drugs
Arteriosclerosis	Surgery—drugs
Rheumatic fever	Penicillin
Heart and blood vessel defects	Surgery

As the list indicates, many new advances include surgery and antibiotics. Other advances include the heart-lung machine, replacing diseased arteries with nylon arteries, and the use of radioactivity and electronics in aiding rapid and efficient diagnosis. Individual surgeon skills and smooth cooperation of the operating team account for a great deal of success in this area. Also important is hypothermia or bathing the patient in ice water to lower the temperature as much as 20 degrees, thus reducing the need for blood and oxygen. With the body "hibernating" in this manner, for example, the aorta can be closed long enough to permit replacing the diseased section without damaging vital nerve cells.

Community services for heart patients have two major objectives:

1. To develop and improve facilities that will assist the physician in the total management of the cardiac patient.
2. To help the patient and his family, through organized community effort, cope with many personal, social and economic problems caused by cardiac disease.

One of the most important phases in the treatment of patients with coronary artery disease is rehabilitation. It is vitally important that these patients return to gainful employment as soon as feasible. Work records indicate that these patients make an excellent adjustment, are good workers, and have a low rate of absenteeism. They seem to be less prone to emotional instability if they return to work early.

QUESTIONS FOR REVIEW

1. What is the difference between chronic disease and communicable disease?
2. Which age groups are affected by chronic disease? Which chronic diseases are most prevalent in these age groups?
3. Are the number of chronic disease cases in the nation increasing or decreasing? How does this affect community health programs?
4. List five different examples of how we can prevent five specific chronic diseases.
5. Explain the difference between primary prevention and secondary prevention.
6. In what ways can we develop successful chronic disease programs in communities throughout the country?
7. Have the number of cancer cases and fatalities increased since 1900? Explain.
8. "Until there is definite proof that tobacco causes lung cancer, why not continue smoking?" Discuss this statement.
9. Discuss three new community approaches to cancer prevention.
10. (a) What part does the local health department play in cancer prevention?
    (b) State health department?
    (c) United States Public Health Service?
    (d) Local cancer society?
    (e) State cancer society?
11. List and briefly discuss five reasons why people fail to obtain periodic physical examinations.

REFERENCES

1. Commission on Chronic Illness: *Chronic Illness in the United States, Volume I, Prevention of Chronic Illness.* Massachusetts, Harvard University Press, 1957, Page 4.
2. Kahn, Harold A.: *Changing Causes of Death in Childhood.* Pub. Health Rep., 66:1246, 1951.
3. National Health Assembly: *America's Health: A Report to the Nation.* New York, Harper and Brothers, 1949, Page 85.
4. United States Public Health Service, National Office of Vital Statistics: *Summary of Health and Vital Statistics.* Washington, U.S. Government Printing Office, 1958, Page 23.
5: Yahraes, Herbert: *Something Can Be Done About Chronic Illness.* In The Commission on Chronic Illness, Public Affairs Pamphlet No. 176, Page 4, New York, 1954.
6. Commission on Chronic Illness: *Chronic Illness in the United States, Volume I, Prevention of Chronic Illness.* Massachusetts, Harvard University Press, 1957, Page 28.
7. Burney, L. E., M.D.: *Address Before the House of Delegates.* Indiana, Indiana State Medical Association, October, 1956, Pages 5 and 6.
8. Yahraes, Herbert: *Something Can Be Done About Chronic Illness.* In The Commission on Chronic Illness, Public Affairs Pamphlet No. 176, Page 26, New York, 1954.
9. American Cancer Society: *To Smoke or Not To Smoke.* New York, American Cancer Society, 1959.
10. Horn, D., Courts, F. A., Taylor, R., and Soloman, E.: *Cigarette Smoking Among High School Students.* Am. J. Pub. Health, 49:1497, 1959.
11. Cameron, Charles S.: *The Truth About Cancer.* New Jersey, Prentice-Hall, Inc., 1956, Pages 255–257.

12. Beadle, G. W.: *Research Advances.* The New York Times, March 27, 1960, Section 10, Page 6.
13. Earle, Howard: *The Last 10 Years: Giant Steps Against Disease.* Today's Health, 37:31–32, 1959.

SUGGESTED READING

Allen, E. V., M.D.: *High Blood Pressure.* New York, American Heart Association, 1958.

American Cancer Society: *Literature Available List.* American Cancer Society, New York, 1960.

American Cancer Society: *To Smoke or Not To Smoke.* New York, American Cancer Society, 1957.

American Heart Association: *Diseases of the Heart and Blood Vessels: Facts and Figures.* New York, American Heart Association, 1958.

American Heart Association: *Congenital Cardiac Defects—A Physician's Guide for Evaluation and Management.* New York, American Heart Association, 1958.

American Heart Association: *How the Doctor Examines Your Heart.* New York, American Heart Association, 1958.

American Heart Association: *Returning Cardiacs to Work: A Guide For Physicians.* American Heart Association, 1958.

Berenblum, I.: *Man Against Cancer: The Story of Cancer Research.* Baltimore, The Johns Hopkins University Press, 1952.

Blakeslee, Alton L.: *How To Live With Heart Trouble, Public Affairs Pamphlet No. 184.* New York, American Heart Association, 1958.

Cameron, Charles S., M.D.: *Cell Examination—New Hope in Cancer, Public Affairs Pamphlet No. 252.* New York, Public Affairs Committee, 1957.

Cameron, Charles S., M.D.: *The Truth About Cancer.* New Jersey, Prentice Hall, Inc., 1956.

Children's Bureau, U.S. Department of Health, Education and Welfare: *Folder No. 42.* Washington, D.C., U.S. Government Printing Office, 1956.

Hammond, E. C., and Horn, D.: *Report on Forty-Four Months of Follow-up of 187,783 Men.* J.A.M.A., 10: 1159, 1958.

Hilleboe, Herman E., and Larimore, Granville W.: *Preventive Medicine, Principles of Prevention in the Occurrence and Progression of Disease.* Philadelphia, W. B. Saunders Co., 1959.

Huxley, Julian: *Biological Aspects of Cancer.* New York, Harcourt, Brace and Co., 1958.

Keith, John D., M.D., Rowe, Richard D., M.D., and Vald, Peter, M.D.: *Heart Diseases in Infancy and Childhood.* New York, American Heart Association, 1958.

Long, N. R.: *The Decline of Chronic Infectious Disease and Its Social Implications.* Bull. Hist. Med., 28:22–24, 1954.

Marvin, H. M., M.D., Jones, T. Ducket, M.D., Page, Irvine, H., M.D., Wright, Irving S., M.D., and McCarthy, Maclyn, M.D.: *You and Your Heart.* New York, New American Library (Signet Key Book), 1957.

Miller, Lois Mattox, and Monahan, James: *The Facts Behind Filter-Tip Cigarettes.* New York, Reader's Digest, July, 1957.

Miller, Lois Mattox, and Monahan, James: *Wanted—And Available—Filter-Tips That Really Filter.* New York, Reader's Digest, August, 1957.

Mitchell, R. S.: *Cigarette Smoking, Cigarette Advertising and Health.* J. School Health, 30:251–59, 1960.

National Health Education Committee: *Facts on the Major Killing and Crippling Diseases in the United States Today.* New York, National Health Education Committee, Inc., 1957.

The Commission on Chronic Illness:
Chronic Illness in the United States, Volume I.;
Prevention of Chronic Illness, Volume II;
Care of the Long Term Patient, Volume III;
Chronic Illness in a Rural Area, and *Chronic Illness in a Large City,* Volume IV. Massachusetts, Harvard University Press, 1957.

White, Paul D., M.D.: *Heart Disease Caused by Coronary Atherosclerosis.* New York, American Heart Association, 1958.

Wright, Irving S., M.D., and Luckey, E. Hugh, M.D.: *Cerebral Vascular Diseases.* New York, Grune and Stratton, Inc., 1955.

Chapter VII

Communicable Disease

PUBLIC HEALTH officials point with pride to the decrease in incidence of communicable disease during the past 50 years; it is remarkable and encouraging. However, there are thousands of germs of many different kinds, and they are all tough, prolific, insidious, patient, and continually moving about looking for a "new home." The decline of one variety of germ usually shows an increase in a new or different type of germ such as the virus of infectious hepatitis. Thus, communicable disease continues to remain a major public health problem.

Statistics showing the leading communicable disease killers are listed in Table 9.

These figures may be misleading because the reports of many physicians are incomplete and inaccurate. Five of the eight diseases listed in Table 9 are caused by a virus; one disease, encephalitis, is transmitted by the bite of a mosquito. (See Figure 31 for other major human viral diseases.)

122

It is interesting and alarming to note that although there are known effective procedures for the prevention and control of tuberculosis, syphilis, poliomyelitis, and encephalitis, these diseases continue to take many lives. The solution to this complex problem involves reinforced mass health education; intelligent use of existing knowledge; development and improvment of techniques, methods, and materials; and continued research. The communicable disease problem is magnified when we consider the recorded absenteeisms due to disease in school and industry, and the crippling physical, mental, and economic impairment resulting from certain diseases. The economic loss is great to industries, school districts, and individuals; enormous expenditures are required for treatment and hospitalization.

Pneumonia and Influenza

Table 9 shows that the most fatal communicable diseases today are pneumonia and influenza, in spite of the virtual conquering of pneumococcal pneumonia by antibiotics. These acute respiratory conditions continue to take their toll of human lives, especially among the very young and very old. Although there have been periodic influenza epidemics in this country from time to time, e.g., the "Asian flu" epidemics in 1957 and 1960, nothing has been seen to equal the great "Spanish flu" pandemic of 1918 that was

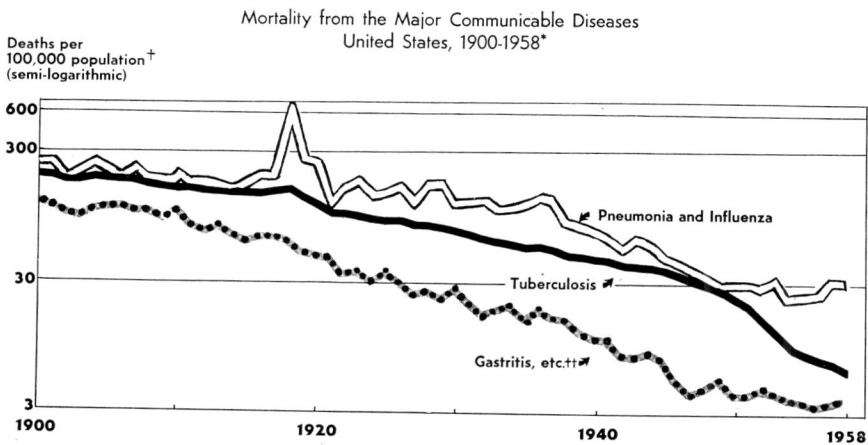

Mortality from the Major Communicable Diseases
United States, 1900-1958*

Deaths per
100,000 population†
(semi-logarithmic)

*Death Registration States only, 1900-32. 1958 data are provisional.
† Adjusted to 1940 standard.
††Gastritis, duodenitis, enteritis and colitis.

Figure 30. (From the National Office of Vital Statistics, modified from Research Series Eleven, Health Information Foundation.)

Table 9.   *Leading Communicable Disease Killers, 1956*

ETIOLOGIC AGENT	DISEASE	REGISTERED DEATHS
Virus	Pneumonia and influenza	47,103†
Bacillus	Tuberculosis	14,061
Spirochete	Syphilis	3,870
Virus	Infectious hepatitis	806
Coccus	Meningococcal infections	762
Virus	Poliomyelitis	566
Virus	Measles	530
Virus	Encephalitis, infectious	424

* *Summary of Health and Vital Statistics*, U.S. Department of Health, Education, and Welfare, Public Health Service, National Office of Vital Statistics, June, 1958.
† Over 86,000 deaths in the 1957–58 epidemic.

accompanied by a death rate exceeding the total number of American casualties in World War I. Public health agencies throughout the world are continually vigilant to prevent another such pandemic.

With the new techniques of tissue culture, much faster progress is being made in finding vaccines and drugs to combat the viral respiratory diseases such as colds, influenza, and typical pneumonia. Vaccines have already been developed for influenza, and many people are now being immunized against this disease. (See Figure 32.) The United States Public Health Service recommends routine influenza immunization for all persons 65 years of age or older, pregnant women, and patients of all ages who suffer from heart, lung, kidney, or metabolic disorders. Since the typical "flu season" begins in November, the Public Health Service advises vaccination prior to this time.

Infectious Hepatitis

Infectious hepatitis or yellow jaundice plagued Napoleon's troops and continued to plague military forces in World War I, World War II, and in the Korean War. This virus disease, which causes liver inflammation, has been noted with increasing frequency in recent years, and is considered a major health problem by many. The problem is very difficult and complex because the disease has a strange cyclical nature or wave pattern; the resistant virus is not destroyed by pasteurization or chlorination, and it is relatively insensitive to heat, cold, chemical and ultraviolet rays. Further, the

Major human viral diseases...
the epidemiologic facts.

Disease	Season of Occurrence				Age Range of Greatest Incidence	Incubation Period	Transmission
	Winter	Spring	Summer	Fall			
Common cold					0-20	1-6 days	Airborne, close contact
Influenza					5-9, 25-34	1-2 days	Airborne, close contact
Virus pneumonia					All ages	1-3 weeks	Airborne, close contact
Poliomyelitis (paralytic)					0-4 years	8-36 days	Close contact
Smallpox					All ages	12 days	Close, indirect contact
Chickenpox					0-10	14-16 days	Airborne, close contact
Measles					0-10	12-19 days	Close, indirect contact
German measles					0-15	14-21 days	Close, indirect contact
Mumps					5-15	18-21 days	Close contact, airborne
Infectious mononucleosis					15-25	4-10 days	Close contact
Infectious hepatitis					5-15	15-40 days	Parenteral, contact with contaminated waste material
Serum hepatitis					All ages	60-160 days	Parenteral
Rabies					All ages	1-3 months	Bite of rabid dogs, foxes, skunks, bats and other small, warm-blooded animals
Yellow fever					All ages	3-6 days	Mosquito
Eastern equine encephalitis					0-10 years	5-10 days	Mosquito
Western equine encephalitis					20-50, infants	5-10 days	Mosquito
St. Louis encephalitis					All ages	4-21 days	Mosquito

Figure 31. By 1948, some 60 viruses were known to be associated with infections in man. Two thirds of these parasites were transmitted by arthropods and infected other animals, involving man only as a secondary host. By 1958, more than 90 human viruses had been recognized and studied in the laboratory. New laboratory techniques have opened up a "Pandora's Box" of viral agents, and at present several hundred apparently new viruses isolated in worldwide laboratories await classification. (From Patterns of Disease, Parke, Davis and Co., November, 1959.)

virus which causes hepatitis has not been isolated and refuses to infect any organism other than man. The disease may cause many weeks or months of severe debilitating illness, and cannot be cured with antibiotics or other miracle drugs. Passive immunization through injection of large doses of gamma globulin is of proven efficiency but is of limited value since it affords only temporary protection. Personal and community sanitation will help to reduce the spread of this disease. The United States Public Health Service believes that the virus is largely transmitted by person-to-person contact and advises, "Wash your hands."

Measles

Although measles is treated lightly by most people throughout the world, the disease is often fatal or may cause brain injury. The virus is sometimes the direct cause of fatal pneumonia, but more often it is the precursor of a bacterial infection. Measles also has a tendency to attack the middle ear, which may lead to permanent deafness. The disease can also cause encephalitis or brain inflammation with a high (10 per cent) mortality rate and a higher rate of permanent damage. Most deaths occur among infants under three years of age.

In 1958, 552 deaths caused by measles were officially recorded by the United States Public Health Service, as compared with 255 deaths caused by poliomyelitis. Although measles is a reportable disease throughout the United States, fewer than a fourth of all cases are actually reported to health authorities. Since 95 per cent of the population eventually contracts measles, in reality there are probably more than 3,000,000 cases per year in the United States. It is estimated that 4,000 of these cases develop encephalitis and about 800 of these die; 2,000 measles patients survive with varying degrees of brain injury, and the remainder reveal no apparent permanent damage. It is encouraging to note, however, that dramatic progress is being made toward the development of a safe and sure vaccine against measles.

The Major Zoonoses—A Community Health Problem

Some of our nation's most serious diseases are those animal diseases transmissible to man and called the zoonoses. (See Table 10 for a listing of the major zoonoses and their human toll in 1957.) The incidence of many of these diseases appears to be greatest in children. Education and legislation are necessary adjuncts for the prevention of zoonoses. A few of the important and most common zoonoses will be discussed.

RABIES. Rabies is probably the most feared of the viral zoonoses. Once the symptoms develop, rabies is always fatal to animals and to humans. If the long, expensive, and sometimes dangerous Pasteur treatment is begun early enough, however, rabies may be prevented. The Pasteur treatment consists of 14 or 21 consecutive daily doses of rabies vaccine. The seriousness of rabies in this country cannot be measured by the small number of cases in man—only about five to ten annually. In 1959 there were five deaths from rabies in the United States. Approximately 60,000 persons receive injections of rabies vaccine each year because of bites by rabid animals. Although the cat, wolf, fox, skunk, and bat may transmit rabies, dogs seem to present the greatest problem to children and adults. It is interesting to note that children under 15 years of age accounted for over 50 per cent of all human rabies deaths from 1944 to 1954. This is attributed to higher inherent susceptibility and greater opportunities for severe exposure. The problem is magnified when we consider the tremendous loss of livestock and the time and money spent by state and local health departments to combat this problem.

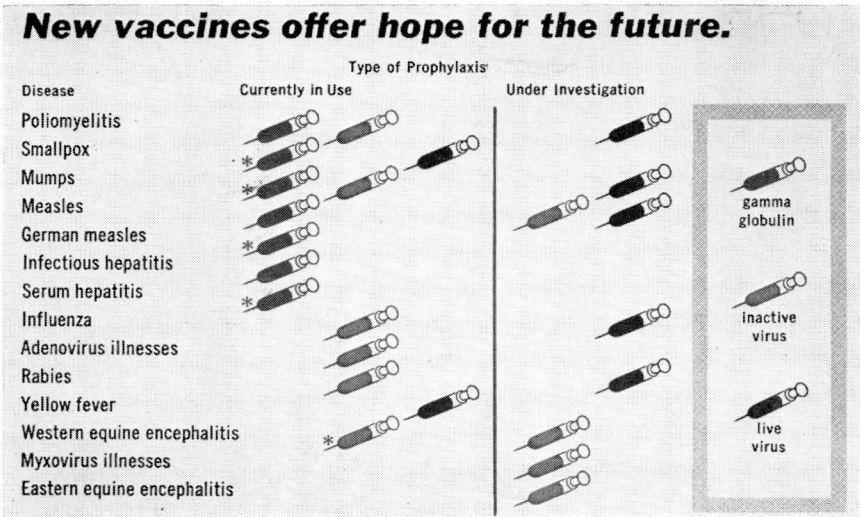

New vaccines offer hope for the future.

Figure 32. The live polio virus vaccine, which is taken by mouth, has proved effective in studies conducted abroad and in the United States. As for acute respiratory diseases of undifferentiated character, some studies indicate that an appropriate vaccine must contain 25 distinct viral antigens to protect children. Multiple immunization is the best weapon for victory over viruses. Asterisk indicates vaccines of questionable value. (From Patterns of Disease, Parke, Davis and Co., November, 1959.)

Prevention of human deaths from rabies depends upon programs of animal bite investigation; destruction of rabid animals followed by strict quarantine of the victim; prophylactic treatment of exposed persons; and control of domestic and wild animals. Control of rabies in dogs is based upon registration, vaccination, and control of stray dogs. The adoption of dog vaccination ordiances by local government officials is a major preventive measure. (The impact of control programs on brucellosis and murine typhus is illustrated by Figure 33.) Wild-life control is based upon poisoning and trapping. Poisoning is dangerous to people and domestic animals, and trapping is slow and impractical. Controlling rabies in

The impact of control programs—striking.

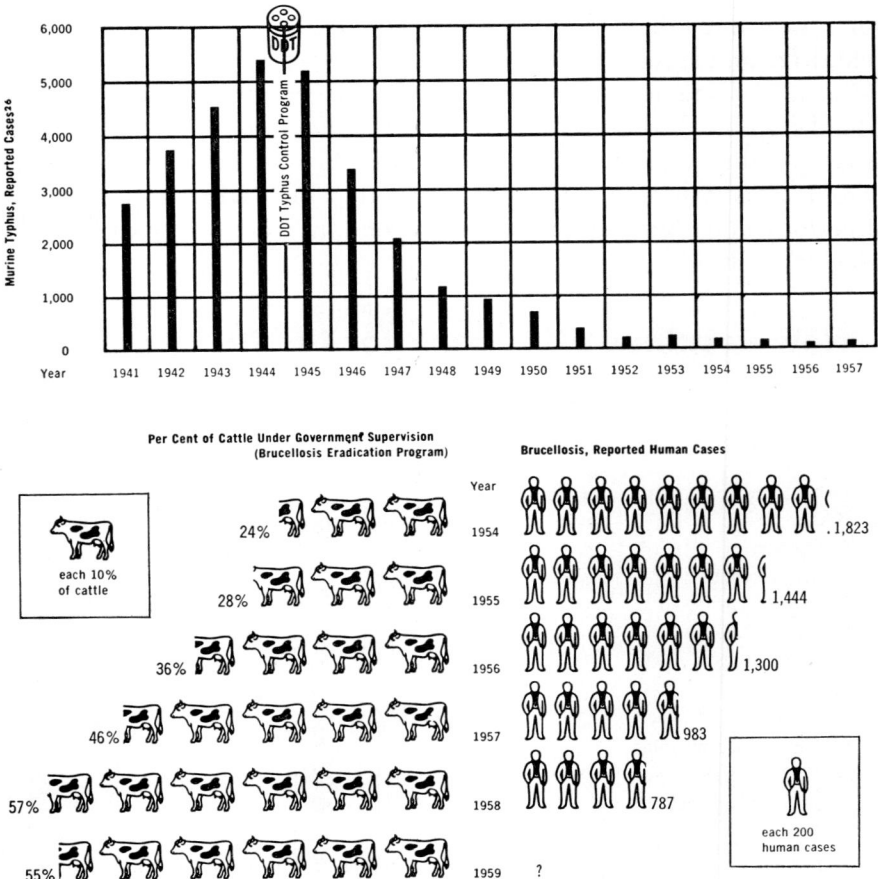

Figure 33. The Cooperative State-Federal Brucellosis Program brought about a drop in bovine brucellosis incidence from 10% in 1935 to under 2% in 1957. An accelerated eradication campaign was instituted in 1954. In Minnesota, progressive eradication of brucellosis in cattle under a state area control plan has coincided with a marked drop in human cases. Since 1940, the human case rate in areas certified brucellosis-free has been one third the rate in noncertified areas. (From Patterns of Disease, Parke, Davis and Co., July, 1959.)

Man and the horse—accidental hosts of encephalitis.

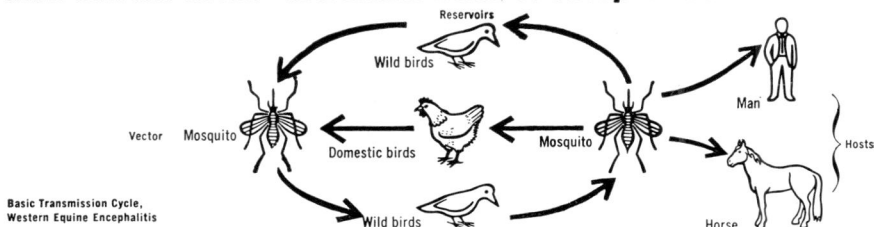

Figure 34. The 3 types of arthropod-born encephalitis—St. Louis, western, and eastern—are maintained primarily by bird-mosquito-bird infection chains. Neither man nor horse is the usual reservoir, as was once believed. Many types of mosquitoes carry the virus, and it may reside temporarily in various domesticated animals and rodents. Where the virus is maintained (unobserved) during interepidemic periods remains a mystery. (From Patterns of Disease, Parke, Davis and Co., July, 1960.)

dogs is much sounder and more feasible than wild-life control. These measures must be supported by mass and intensive health education programs.

ENCEPHALITIS. Acute encephalitis is a major problem in California, Texas, North Dakota, and many other states. The mosquito transmits the virus from infected birds to horses and to man. (See Figure 34 for the basic transmission cycle of encephalitis.) Encephalitis fatality is high, and serious and permanent neurological consequences may develop in a patient. With the development of many thousands of additional acres of irrigated land and the great increase in the volume of commercial and industrial waste waters, the mosquito problem is magnified in many states.

Preventive measures include mosquito abatement programs, new and more effective insecticides, and continued research and health education. Education programs must stress the fact that certain mosquitoes may carry disease germs and that mosquitoes lay their eggs in stagnant water.

PSITTACOSIS. Although parakeets and parrots are probably the most common source of human psittacosis, infections have been traced to pigeons, ducks, chickens, turkeys, canaries, sea gulls, egrets, and road runners. Parakeets are the usual source of human cases because of the growth in popularity of this bird. Prevention includes education and health legislation establishing a control program for banding and recording all birds that are sold commercially.

TRICHINOSIS. Trichinosis is a major public health problem even though the simple measure of thoroughly cooking pork and pork products will prevent the disease. It is estimated that every American consumes three servings of infested pork a year, and that 25,000,000 to 50,000,000 Americans carry trichina larvae in their muscles and internal organs. Between 200 and 300 human cases are reported each year despite the fact that trichinosis is not reportable in most states. The practice of feeding hogs raw garbage has kept the disease prevalent in pork.

Preventive measures include legislation requiring that hogs be fed only cooked garbage, and education programs that stress the importance of cooking pork at 140 degrees Fahrenheit for at least 30 minutes per pound.

Food Handling and Disease

Food is an excellent medium for germs, and about 30 diseases can be transmitted by insanitary food practices. (See Table 11.) For example, those germs commonly transmitted by mucus left on eating utensils include pneumonia, influenza, diphtheria, scarlet fever, colds, whooping cough, measles, and mumps. The increased number of restaurants, picnics, and banquets demand increased emphasis upon safe preparation, storage, and serving of food, and personal hygiene.

Food poisoning is a common disease recorded each year from insanitary food practices; usually great numbers of people are afflicted at one time. The cause is usually the same; the food is contaminated during preparation and allowed to stand at room temperature for one hour or more. Bacteria, usually staphylococci, multiply and produce poisons or toxins. The foods most likely to cause this form of food poisoning are the cream-filled pies, potato salads, meat and fish salads, and creamed dishes. Most outbreaks are reported from large group gatherings where the food had been prepared in advance.

A more serious form of bacterial food poisoning is salmonella food infection. The diarrhea, fever, and nausea from this form of food infection are sometimes fatal. In this case, the bacteria, not its toxins, produce the illness. The food may have been contaminated when purchased or contaminated by the food handler. Rats and mice occasionally contaminate exposed uncovered food. Dried eggs and poultry have often been the cause of salmonella food infection. Persons recovering from salmonellosis can remain carriers for various lengths of time and must be prevented from spreading the disease.

Food poisoning can be prevented. A simple but very effective precaution is to keep hot foods hot and cold foods cold until ready to serve. The health department sanitarians spend a great deal of time evaluating the sanitary aspects of food establishments and educating food handlers. Many local health departments offer food handling courses which are designed to educate the employer and employee and keep them informed of the latest methods and

Table 10. The Major Zoonoses and Their Human Toll*

DISEASE	ANIMALS INVOLVED	MODE OF HUMAN INFECTION	TOTAL HUMAN CASES, 1957
Anthrax	Cow, horse, sheep, goat, wild animals	Contaminated food, water, wool, hair, hides, air	26
Brucellosis (undulant fever)	Cow, hog, goat, sheep, horse, dog	Milk, meat or other contaminated food; occupational exposure	983
Encephalitis, (arthropod-borne)	Horse, mule, birds	Mosquito bite	144
Leptospirosis	Rat, dog, cow, hog, rodents	Skin, mucous membrane	47
Psittacosis	Parrot, parakeet, hen, duck, pigeon, turkey	Inhalation, contact	278
Q-fever	Bandicoot, rat, cow, sheep, horse, dog, goat	Tick bite, inhalation (?), milk	41
Rabies	Dog, cat, wolf, fox, bat, skunk	Animal bite	6
Rocky Mountain spotted fever	Wild rodents, other animals	Tick bite	240
Salmonellosis	Cow, hog, hen, sheep, rat, dog, cat	Contaminated food	6,693
Tularemia	Wild animals, birds	Tick bite, skin contact, water	601
Typhus fever, endemic (murine)	Rat	Flea bite	113
Trichinosis	Hog	Contaminated pork and pork products	250[1]

* Patterns of Disease, pamphlet published by Parke, Davis & Company, July, 1959.

The World Health Organization lists 87 zoonoses—diseases of lower animals transmissible to man. Of these, 49 are known to occur in the Southern United States, 46 in the state of Texas alone. Several of the zoonoses, e.g., trichinosis, are not reportable in many states, and adequate prevalence figures are not available.

Table 11.   Disease Germs in Food

GERM GROUP	ROUTE TO THE VICTIM	DISEASE
Salmonella group	Food contaminated by unwashed hands, rats, or underdone meats.	Food infections
Staphylococcus Eberthella typhi	Food contaminated by sores, boils. Water, milk, shellfish contaminated at the source. Food contaminated by unwashed hands or by flies.	Food infections Typhoid fever
Endamoeba histolytica	Water contaminated at the source— defective plumbing. Food contaminated by unwashed hands or by flies.	Amebic dysentery
Shigella group	Water contaminated at the source. Dishes or silverware contaminated by a carrier. Food contaminated by unwashed hands or by flies.	Bacillary dysentery
Trichinella spiralis	Insufficiently cooked pork.	Trichinosis
Clostridium botulinum	Home-canned foods improperly prepared.	Botulism
Streptococcus group	Raw milk contaminated at the source.	Septic sore throat and scarlet fever
Diphtheria bacillus	Dishes or silverware contaminated by a carrier. Sneezing, coughing, and spitting.	Diphtheria

techniques. Education and inspection are supplemented by law enforcement. It must be stressed, however, that there is no substitute for health education when food handling is involved.

Community Education

Education is fundamental to the application of all other control measures. This involves dissemination of appropriate and feasible information, communication, and intrinsic motivation. Too often local and official health agencies assume that they merely must provide vaccines or medical services; they neglect the adequate planning and preparation necessary to launch a community education program. Parents and children must be continually and emphatically informed of the need for disease protection. In many instances, parents are apprehensive about immunizations because of reports of reactions and failures, indifference, or "fear of the needle." Too often motivation for immunization is extrinsic; for example, a sudden rise in the number of poliomyelitis deaths and cases in a city usually results in a rise in the number of persons requesting polio immunization in that city. However, the authors believe that with the increasing use of vaccines in the form of a pill, candy, a drink, or airborne vaccines, the number of persons immunized will increase markedly. The polio live-virus vaccine, which is taken by mouth, is most promising and will supplement Salk's vaccine.

Education is necessary to help prevent most diseases. For example, the following diseases can be prevented by education:

DISEASE	PREVENTION BY EDUCATION
Typhoid fever	Personal hygiene
Bacillary dysentery	Personal hygiene
Infectious hepatitis	Personal hygiene
Botulism	Proper home canning procedure
Salmonellosis	Keep food hot or cold
Poliomyelitis	Immunization
Encephalitis	Eliminate mosquito breeding areas
Trichinosis	Cook pork
Syphilis	Eliminate promiscuity; blood test
Tuberculosis	Periodic chest x-ray
Rabies	Immunize dogs

Another illustrative example involves the many persons who continually complain about the number of mosquitoes and flies present around their homes each summer; these persons may actually be contributing to the cause of the problem by way of their fish ponds or rain barrels in the former case, or by piling grass clippings or manure in their yards in the latter case.

Legal Aspects of Disease Control

Primary responsibility and authority for public health is vested in the states. The first state health departments were established primarily for the prevention and control of communicable disease. State disease-control functions range from consultation and advisory services to the direct operation of complex statewide programs. During the past half century much of the states' responsibility for public health services has been delegated to local health departments; the state continues to supply technical advice, consultation services, and emergency assistance. The federal government has necessarily assumed responsibility for communicable disease control in three broad functional areas: (1) preventing introduction of disease from abroad; (2) limiting the spread of disease across state lines; and (3) assisting states when health problems exceed state resources. As far as possible, federal activities for disease control are integrated with activities at state and local levels.

Each state has adopted laws relating to the health and safety of its citizens. These laws are basic minimum requirements and standards that must be met by each local health department. However, local officials and citizens may enact additional health legislation to meet the changing and increasing health needs in their area. Usually the enforcement of these laws is no problem, but occasionally the services of the local sheriff or chief of police are necessary to protect the health and safety of the citizens within a community. Examples of these situations may include an active tuberculous recalcitrant patient; a restaurant owner who consistently refuses to comply with the suggestions of the sanitarian and health officer; and the farmer who refuses to pasteurize his milk before distribution to the public. Sanitarians are plagued with nuisance calls, most of which can be tactfully and diplomatically solved. It must be stressed, however, that *education, tactfulness,* and *diplomacy* are key words in promoting public health efficiency, coordination and cooperation. Public health laws are utilized only when these three methods have failed.

Venereal Disease and Tuberculosis

Venereal disease and tuberculosis will be discussed in this chapter because these diseases are two important and challenging community health problems. They emphasize the epidemiological approach and community teamwork, and are characteristic of the transition in the communicable disease program.

The purpose of this chapter is not to discuss the various communicable diseases in detail. One can refer to the communicable disease handbook for a complete analysis of 118 diseases.[1] Instead the chapter is designed to introduce the area and discuss two diseases that are major current public health problems.

QUESTIONS FOR REVIEW

1. Have the number of communicable disease cases and deaths in the United States increased or decreased since 1900? Since 1950? Why?
2. What are the five leading communicable disease killers today?
3. List five major zoonoses, the animals involved, the mode of human infection, and prevention.
4. How can we prevent:

   a) rabies,
   b) encephalitis,
   c) psittacosis,
   d) trichinosis,
   e) infectious hepatitis,
   f) measles,
   g) influenza?

   Which of the above diseases is the greatest problem in your community? State? Why?
5. What are the causes of food poisoning? What is the difference between

staphylococcus food poisoning and salmonella food poisoning? How can we prevent food poisoning?
6. Give five examples of how health education can help prevent specific diseases.
7. Briefly discuss the legal aspects of communicable diseases.
8. Discuss the following statement: "We prefer to educate food handlers first —examine them later."
9. Which diseases are reportable by law in your state?
10. Discuss the communicable disease-control program provided by your local and state health departments.

VENEREAL DISEASE

For many years syphilis has been accepted as a public health responsibility, and its management has been concentrated to a greater extent than that of most diseases in public health clinics supported entirely or partially by public health funds. This can be explained by the fact that a large number of patients are in the lower socioeconomic groups and by the fact that the epidemiology of infectious syphilis is a public health responsibility. Under these circumstances, it is inevitable that control of the disease depends largely on the adequacy of public health programs and is best conducted by public health personnel. However, no program of disease control can be successful without the cooperation of the entire medical profession. The diagnosis and treatment of syphilis have never been confined to clinics; like other diseases, syphilis has always been a responsibility of general medicine.

The importance of venereal disease is reflected in the 3,870 syphilis deaths and 120,000 reported syphilis cases in 1959. The problem is magnified when we consider the physical and mental impairment, sterility, and economic loss resulting from venereal disease. For example, in 1960 there were 33,000 persons in mental institutions in this country because of syphilitic psychoses at a direct cost of maintenance of about $47 million per year. We continue to institutionalize paretics at the rate of about 1,200 new admissions per year. Although there were only 16 deaths from gonorrhea in 1956, there were 233,593 reported cases. Even though the syphilitic case rate has declined markedly during the past 15 years, it now appears that the number of reported cases of primary and secondary syphilis are on the rise again. (See Figure 35.) For example, in 1959 there was a general venereal disease rise in 29 states and 49 major cities. For the country as a whole, the syphilis rate was up 1.2 per cent, and the gonorrhea rate was up 6.3 per cent. Health officials found 22.8 per cent more cases of syphilis in its

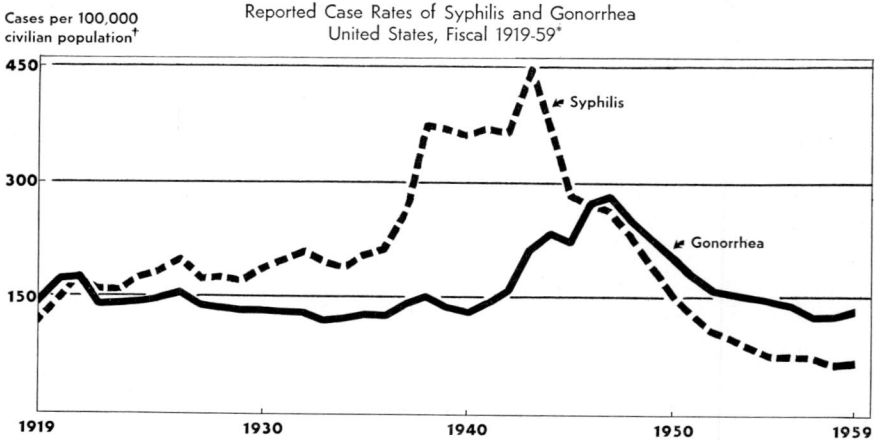

Figure 35. Syphilis and gonorrhea in the United States. (Various reports by the the Venereal Disease Branch, Communicable Disease Center, U.S. Public Health Service. Modified from Research Series Eleven, Health Information Foundation.)

  * Reporting states only, 1919–38. Data relate to fiscal year July 1 to June 30 of year named.

  † Excludes military cases after 1940; for syphilis only, excludes cases reported among Mexican agricultural workers diagnosed in the United States, 1957–59.

early infectious stages, forming a pattern that threatens faster rises in the near future. However, venereal disease case figures may be misleading because of the inconsistencies and fluctuations in reporting. At any rate there are an estimated 2,000,000 persons in the United States today with undiscovered or inadequately treated syphilis. Our successes in case-finding and treatment are being offset by the occurrence of approximately 60,000 new cases a year. If these people are not treated, one in 200 will become blind; one in 50 will become insane; one in 25 will become crippled or incapacitated to some extent; and one in 15 will die with a syphilitic heart ailment.[2] Venereal disease is not peculiar to any particular race, social group, or area of the country, and frequently is found where it is least expected.

Venereal Diseases in Adolescents

Today more than one half of the total infectious cases of venereal disease reported are in the teen-age and young adult groups. In 1957, for example, 49,484 cases, or over 22 per cent of the total number of venereal disease cases reported that year, were in persons under 20 years of age. In 1959 New York City health officials reported that syphilis had increased 78.3 per cent among the 15 to 19 year olds. Several suggested reasons for the venereal disease problem in this youthful group include: lack of parental love, respect, and concern; misinformation by the boys; insecurity in the space age; little sex education; poor church attendance; younger marriages and more divorces; weak civic group membership; increase in cars and spending money per teenager; and the security in knowing that there is a quick, easy, and complete cure in penicillin.

Major Causes

The major source of spread of venereal disease today is the casual relationship or "pick-up," which accounts for 50 to 60 per cent of all infections acquired. Between 1950 and 1957, recorded illegitimate births in the United States increased from 142,000 to 202,000. This was an increase of 42 per cent in illegitimacy, while the total number of women of childbearing age was increasing only 2.6 per cent. Other major sources are the "going steady" or engaged couples who account for 25 to 30 per cent of all infections, and prostitution, which accounts for only 5 to 10 per cent of all infections. The remainder are familial; the husband or wife transmits the disease to the marital partner.[3] Other reasons which may be responsible for the tragic increase in venereal disease include the increase in the number of divorces, a more mobile and rootless population, and the increasing and changing metropolitan centers.

New Problems in Venereal Disease Control

One major and alarming problem in this area revolves around the fact that venereal disease control and case finding programs have been weakened. This has resulted mainly because the number of public health diagnostic and treatment facilities decreased as the venereal disease problem diminished. For example, in 1958, nearly 40 per cent of the total reported cases of early syphilis and about 17 per cent of the total cases of gonorrhea were reported by local physicians. It is estimated that only about 5 per cent of these patients were interviewed by physicians for sex contacts. Thus, very few field investigations were able to find persons exposed to the disease in order to place them under medical supervision. This means that a link in the venereal disease epidemiological chain has been broken and must be repaired in order to control the disease.

Advances in Venereal Disease Control

Nevertheless, great strides have been made in the prevention and control of venereal disease during the past 15 years. The syphilis case rate in the United States was reduced from 234.7 cases per

100,000 population in 1948 to only 68.5 cases per 100,000 population in 1958. Similarily the gonorrhea case rate was reduced from 252 cases per 100,000 population in 1948 to 129.3 cases per 100,000 population in 1958. This progress has resulted from a well-organized and aggressive public health program; the introduction of improved methods of therapy, principally penicillin; and perhaps decreased sex promiscuity. This latter factor may reflect our nation's transition from two wars during the past 15 years to peace time today.

Community Programs

Venereal disease is by no means eradicated, and physicians and public health officials must remain alert to the possibility that syphilis may still produce disability, financial ruin, dementia, and death. In 1956, for example, there were 3,000 patients in New York State mental hospitals because of general paresis. Rapidly declining rates over the past several years have prompted the optimistic demobilization of venereal disease control forces; reassignments of personnel and reduction of case findings; and reduction of diagnostic and treatment facilities, leaving many areas without means to discover cases or to combat sudden outbreaks.

Perhaps health officials must reinforce the weakened venereal disease program and reorient venereal disease control programs to meet the changing needs. Although the American Social Health Association has done an excellent job of disseminating information and aiding groups, sex education requires community teamwork and positive attitudes by all concerned. Special emphasis must continue to be placed on case finding in selected population groups with high-incidence and in areas of high-prevalence.

Control programs must be based on long-term community efforts, and the private physician and local health department must initiate, nurture, and guide those efforts. Perhaps weaknesses in the program are best explained by the fact that physicians and health officials " . . . have the diagnostic tools and the therapeutic agents to control and even eradicate syphilis. But we are failing because of our own complacency about the disease; because of neglected education programs, especially for the teenagers; and because of lack of interest or funds to find and treat the affected persons."[4]

QUESTIONS FOR REVIEW

1. Is venereal disease a major problem in your community? State? Explain.
2. Is venereal disease increasing among adolescents? If so, why?

3. Discuss the differences between syphilis and gonorrhea in terms of etiologic agent, signs and symptoms, prevention, mode of transmission, number of cases, number of deaths, and methods of control.
4. How can we strengthen venereal disease control programs in our communities?
5. How does syphilis relate to mental illness and prenatal health?
6. Discuss briefly the relationship between venereal disease community education programs and the socioeconomic aspects of the community.
7. What do we mean by "breaking the link in the chain of infection"?
8. Discuss the prevention and present treatment of venereal disease.
9. What is the function of the local and state health department in connection with venereal disease?

TUBERCULOSIS

Although the tuberculosis death rate has decreased markedly, the disease still kills more persons in the United States than all other infectious diseases combined, with the exception of influenza and pneumonia. In 1956, tuberculosis claimed 14,061 Americans, and in 1959 the disease claimed 12,000 lives. (See Figure 36 for newly reported tuberculosis cases and tuberculosis deaths in the United States from 1930 through 1957.) Presently, tuberculosis leads the list as a cause of death in 28 countries and territories, which total one-sixth of the world's population, e.g., India, Korea and Pakistan; the disease alone accounts for 75 per cent of all deaths from infectious diseases occurring after age 15.[5] Although the reduction in deaths over the years may be reason for optimism, many new cases are still being reported. For example, 60,000 new active cases were reported in 1959. Furthermore, 150,000 Americans now know they have active tuberculosis, and 250,000 Americans know they have inactive tuberculosis; 100,000 others also have the disease in its active, infectious form, but they may *not know* they have the germ.[6] It is estimated that one-fourth to one-third of the American people are infected with live tuberculous germs.[7] Many of them will eventually develop active tuberculosis. This disease is costly to the family, community, state, nation, and world. The United States spends more than $700,000,000 per year to care for tuberculosis patients. This sum includes only the money spent for tuberculosis and does not include the economic loss to the nation that results from persons being incapacitated or dying from the disease. The major expenditures for tuberculosis are hospitalization, rehabilitation, and compensation.

New drugs and antibiotics have shortened the infectious period and have saved many lives. All the factors that have brought about the striking decline in the death rate from tuberculosis are not known. However, it has been established that public health control

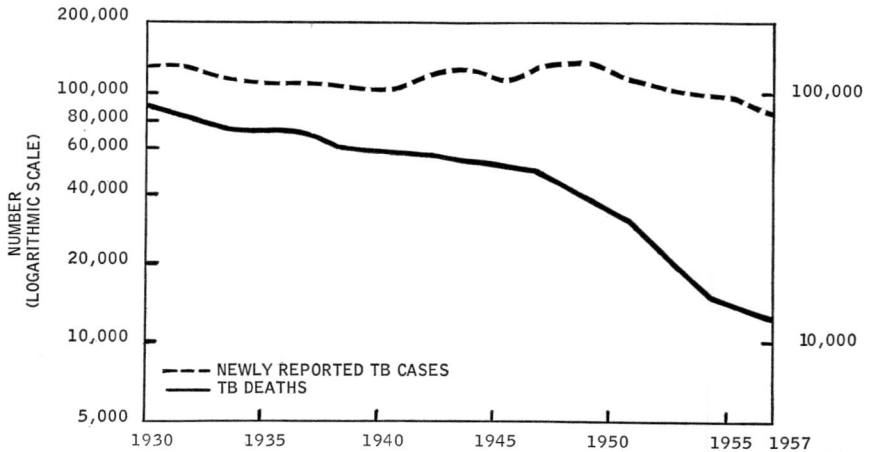

Figure 36. Newly reported tuberculosis cases and tuberculosis deaths in the United States, 1930–1957. The rate of decline in tuberculosis deaths has been greater in the past decade than in earlier years, but newly reported cases have not declined as rapidly as deaths. While the sharp decline in tuberculosis deaths is an indication of gains being made in one aspect of the control of tuberculosis, the continued high level of new cases reported points to the vast amount of work which is yet to be done. Some caution is needed, however, in the interpretation of data on newly reported cases, because such data are affected not only by the incidence of tuberculosis, or the number of new cases developing each year, but also by changes in reporting practices in various states and by the extent of case-finding activities. (From *Tuberculosis Chart Series—* 1958 Revision, Public Health Service Publication No. 639, U.S. Department of Health, Education and Welfare, page 4.)

measures, including mass health education, early diagnosis, mass case finding, public health nursing, efficient case register systems, improvement in living conditions, and advances in therapy have been important factors.

Treatment

It is now agreed that virtually all patients in need of treatment for tuberculosis should receive specific antibacterial drugs. Any two of the three principal drugs, including streptomycin, isoniazid, and p-Aminosalicylic acid (P.A.S.), will effectively suppress the growth of the bacilli. This gives the body's own protective forces a chance to defeat the germs.

Bed-rest programs, so fundamental to tuberculosis treatment in past generations, have now become greatly modified. But bed rest has not been abandoned by most conservative physicians, although the period of rest has been relatively shortened and the degree of restriction considerably relaxed. A balanced, wholesome diet and rehabilitation are important and necessary adjuncts for successful treatment.

Prevention

Prevention of tuberculosis can be accomplished by the following measures:

1. Early case-finding
2. Isolation of persons with known active disease
3. Education of the public
4. Public health supervision of patients
5. Protection of workers against inhalation of silica dust
6. Economic assistance to the families of tuberculous patients
7. Betterment of living conditions among lower income groups
8. Facilities for rehabilitation and aftercare
9. Elimination of tuberculosis in dairy cattle.[8]

Tuberculosis vaccination has shown great popularity with the World Health Organization and in many countries other than the United States. The tuberculosis vaccine BCG derives its name, Bacillus Calumette-Guérin, from two French scientists who pioneered its development over 30 years ago. Although many authorities in this area claim that the vaccine is safe, well-standardized, and effective, other specialists claim that BCG is not safe or effective, and reduces the usefulness of the tuberculin test. Selected readings on this controversial area are listed in the bibliography at the end of the chapter.[9-17]

New Trends and Problems

In the past 20 years the tuberculosis problem has changed radically. There are some areas of the country where active tuberculosis is almost nonexistent; there are many other areas where tuberculosis continues to be a serious public health and medical problem. As the number of cases of communicable tuberculosis becomes fewer through case-finding and effective treatment, the relative importance of the uncooperative patient becomes greater. Each patient who resists isolation and treatment increases the menace of the disease.

The trend in tuberculosis control is now toward more selective case-finding.[18] Mass x-ray surveys are now being planned to concentrate on those areas and among those groups with the highest incidence. Jail inmates, aged persons in boarding homes, patients admitted to hospitals, low-income groups, patients and employees in mental hospitals, migrant laborers, alcoholics, and others are known to have high-scale tuberculosis incidence. (See Figure 37 for yield of active tuberculosis cases in chest x-ray case-finding programs from 1954 through 1956.) However, every community should

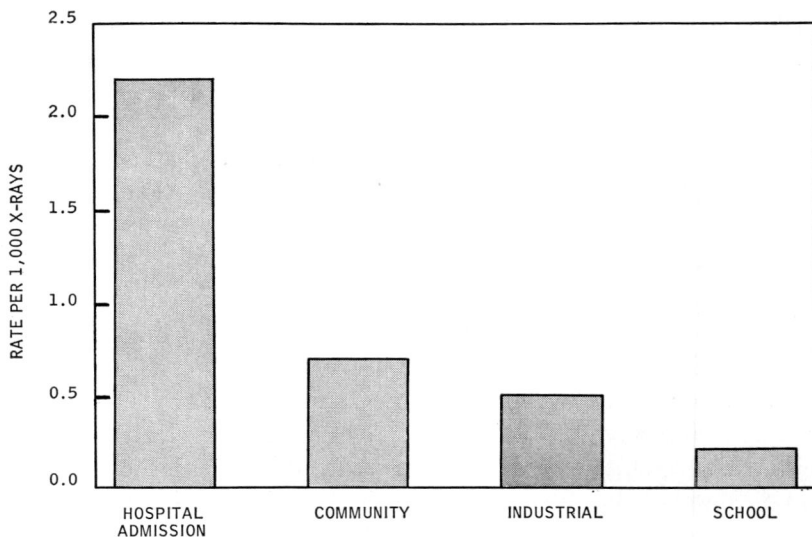

Figure 37. Yield of active tuberculosis cases in chest x-ray case-finding programs, 1954–1956. This chart shows the average yield of new active tuberculosis to be expected from one of the high risk groups—admissions to general hospitals—as contrasted with the yield from three groups not considered at high risk—community, industrial and school—where the prevalence of active disease is not as great. (From *Tuberculosis Chart Series*—1958 Revision, Public Health Service Publication No. 639, U.S. Department of Health, Education and Welfare, page 9.)

evaluate its tuberculosis problem, needs, and resources on a continuing basis so that local x-ray surveys may have efficient use and maximum effect. Further consideration should be given to the tuberculin test as an initial screening device in low-prevalence areas.

Although early diagnosis of tuberculosis has been urged for many years, the response has not been impressive. Year after year statistics reveal that about 80 per cent of newly found cases have already become either moderately advanced or far advanced. Too often, far advanced tuberculosis shows up in a person who had a demonstrated "spot on the lung" some years previously and the condition was neglected. Frequently " . . . that neglect was due to the patient's ignorance and indifference, or to the physician's failure to impress him with the dangerous potentialities of an originally symptomless 'spot'. Inactive tuberculosis is prone to relapse; healing is characteristically incomplete; and immunity is not dependable. No substitute exists for careful, repeated observation of supposedly inactive and apparently healed lesions. Once a lesion is known to be present, it should be followed up at appropriate intervals for the rest of the patient's life."[19]

Another major change in the field is that tuberculosis is no longer primarily a disease of adolescents and young adults. In general, a large proportion of the cases found each year are among the elderly. This is shown in Table 12 in comparing the new cases and deaths from tuberculosis in 1956.

Tuberculosis is becoming more and more a disease of older ages, but it is still very much a foe of youth as well. The rate of newly reported cases for the 15–24 age group is almost as high as the rate for total population of the United States, the younger age groups having below average rates of newly reported cases and those above 25 having above average rates. For the United States the median age for newly reported active cases is approximately 44 years, half of the newly reported cases being under 44 and the other half over 44. The high mortality rate among older adults appears to be due to a combination of a decrease in the effectiveness of treatment and poor case-finding and reporting. This seems to be true even though the older adults have the highest morbidity rates. (See Figure 38 for age-specific rates for newly reported active tuberculosis cases and tuberculosis deaths in the United States in 1956.) Although the gradual decrease in deaths during the most productive years of life represents a great social gain, tuberculosis is more difficult to treat in the older patient. There has also been a shift toward an increasing number of cases in males. Various explanations for this wide-spread phenomenon have been examined; it is thought that the increase in male cases was a temporary one caused by the Second World War. During this period older men returned to work in industry and their resistance to tuberculosis was thereby lowered. In some coun-

Table 12.   New Cases and Deaths from Tuberculosis in 1956*

AGE	RATE PER 100,000 POPULATION	
	NEW CASES	DEATHS
Under 5	13.8	1.7
5–14	7.5	0.2
15–24	34.1	1.2
25–44	50.1	6.0
45–64	64.2	16.6
65 and Over	78.2	34.5
All Ages	41.2	8.4

* *Tuberculosis Chart Series*—1958 Revision, Public Health Service Publication No. 639, U.S. Department of Health, Education and Welfare, page 6.

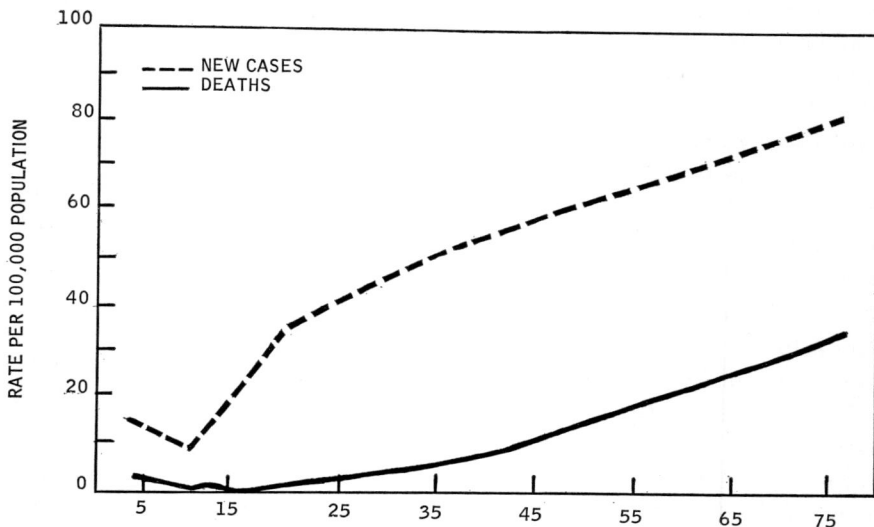

Figure 38. Age-specific rates for newly reported active and probably active tuberculosis cases and tuberculosis deaths in the United States, 1956. (From *Tuberculosis Chart Series*—1958 Revision, Public Health Service Publication No. 639, U.S. Department of Health, Education and Welfare, page 6.)

tries nutritional deficiencies served to lower resistance, and as a result of population movements, exposure to tuberculosis also increased.[20]

Large-scale tuberculin testing is now being used increasingly among preschool and school groups, so that adult cases can be located among the home contacts of the children found to have positive reactions to the tuberculin test.[21] Because so few children are tuberculin positive today, a positive reactor stands out as a warning signal, thus pinpointing the location where an intensive search for tuberculosis should be directed. The advent of isoniazid has made possible the prevention of tuberculosis sickness by early drug therapy of primary tuberculosis. This calls for intensive tuberculin testing programs to seek out infected children in order to afford them the protection of modern drug therapy. Family-contact investigation is still considered one of the most effective methods of finding tuberculosis today.

New advances in tuberculosis, as in other areas of health, have created new problems. For example, new drug therapy has shortened the period of hospitalization, but early discharge has increased the amount of home care supervision by the local health departments. If local health departments are expected to handle this new responsibility adequately, they will need additional personnel and financial support. Furthermore, the use of the newer drugs in tuberculosis therapy has clouded the laboratory diagnosis of the tubercle bacillus. Some of the antibiotics have the effect of changing the characteristics of the bacillus so that it loses its ability to infect laboratory animals.

Recent years have seen a changed attitude regarding the use of hospitals for tuberculous patients. Although the need for tuberculosis hospital beds is decreasing with the new therapy, treatment is becoming increasingly complex, and tuberculosis units need to be integrated more closely with general hospitals. Then an orderly transition can be made to the use of those beds for other illnesses when they are no longer needed for tuberculous patients. It is interesting to note here that some areas of the United States still have an insufficient number of hospital beds for the isolation and treatment of active cases of tuberculosis. Properly equipped tuberculosis diagnostic centers are lacking, and the number of trained professional persons necessary to care for tuberculous patients and provide community tuberculosis control services is inadequate. The trend is away from the small isolated tuberculosis sanatoriums; the aim is toward the coordination of hospital services.[22]

Tuberculosis presents many socioeconomic problems. The patients' diagnosis and treatment are frequently hampered by pressing emotional and psychological problems, family responsibilities, and economic stress. Many individuals fail to take advantage of diagnostic facilities even when these are available to them without charge; many refuse treatment when tuberculosis is discovered; and many tuberculous patients leave hospitals against medical advice before the completion of treatment. In addition, low economic status, which is usually accompanied by malnourishment, overcrowded living conditions, and poor personal hygiene, contributes to susceptibility and to development of the disease.[23] The current migration of American families from state to state further complicates the problem. Residence requirements in many states and local laws prevent persons without legal residence from obtaining necessary hospitalization.

Community Programs

The role of the national, state, and local tuberculosis associations in tuberculosis control is extremely important. The local tuberculosis association is a voluntary health agency composed of public spirited citizens devoted to the fight against tuberculosis. Funds are obtained by the sale of Christmas seals. There are about 2,750 local tuberculosis associations throughout the United States, Guam, Virgin Islands, and Puerto Rico. The local tuberculosis association disseminates information and helps find solutions to problems associated with the disease that confront patients, their families, and the entire community. The organization also takes the lead in encouraging new case-finding and rehabilitation techniques, and agency representatives work closely with many other community groups.

Every effort must be made to continue to reduce the many known cases and to find undiscovered cases early. In spite of favorable advancements and trends, there is no reason for complacency. Strong cooperation and coordination must continue among physicians, the health department, and the tuberculosis association.

QUESTIONS FOR REVIEW

1. How is tuberculosis transmitted or spread? What organs are affected by the germ?
2. Is tuberculosis a problem in your community? State? Explain.
3. Discuss the prevention and present treatment of tuberculosis.
4. Briefly discuss three new trends in relation to tuberculosis control programs.
5. Is tuberculosis increasing among the elderly? Why?
6. What is the value of large-scale tuberculin testing among preschool and school groups?
7. Briefly discuss the relationship between tuberculosis community education programs and the socioeconomic aspects of the community.
8. What is the function of your local tuberculosis and health association?
9. What is the function of the local and state health department in connection with tuberculosis?
10. In what ways does the public health nurse help in the fight against tuberculosis?
11. Discuss the major issues involved in the use of the BCG vaccine.

REFERENCES

1. American Public Health Association: *Control of Communicable Diseases in Man.* New York, The American Public Health Association, 1960.
2. Brown, W. J.: *Let's Stamp Out V.D. Now.* This Week Magazine, Sept. 18, 1960, Page 20.
3. Fiumara, Nicholas F.: *Venereal Diseases—Present and Future.* Am. J. Health, *43:* 1143–1151, 1953.
4. Beerman, Herman: *The Problem of Syphilis Today.* In Archives of Dermatology, Chicago, American Medical Association, 1958.
5. World Health Organization Fact Sheet No. 7. Geneva, Switzerland, World Health Organization, 1958.
6. U.S. Department of Health, Education and Welfare, Public Health Service: *Tuberculosis Chart Series, No. 3, 1958 Revision.* Washington, D. C., U.S. Government Printing Office, 1958, Page 1.

7. National Tuberculosis Association: *Facts About Tuberculosis*. Washington, D.C., National Tuberculosis Association, 1959, Page 3.
8. Commission on Chronic Illness: *Chronic Illness in the United States, Volume I, Prevention of Chronic Illness*. Massachusetts, Harvard University Press, 1957, Page 226.
9. Calez, Rene: *The Birth of the Bacillus Calumette-Guerin*. World Health, 13:27–28, 1960.
10. Medical Advisory Committee of Research Foundation: *Why Have We Not Accepted BCG Vaccinations?* J.A.M.A., 164:951–54, 1957.
11. Medical Research Council: *BCG and Vole Bacillus Vaccine in Prevention of Tuberculosis in Adolescents: First Progress Report to Tuberculosis Vaccine Clinical Trials Committee*. Brit. Med. J., 1:413–27, 1956.
12. Leggot, P. O.: *BCG Vaccine*. Brit. Med. J., 2:74, 1959.
13. Irvine, W.: *The Present Status of BCG*. Practitioner, 183:289–93, 1959.
14. Hartston, W.: *Uncommon Skin Reactions After BCG Vaccination*. Tubercle, 40:265–70, 1959.
15. Finland, Maxwell: *Tuberculosis Mortality and Morbidity and the Problem of BCG Vaccination in the United States*. New England J. Med., 261: 699–702, 1959.
16. U.S. Department of Health, Education and Welfare, Public Health Service: *Tuberculosis Chart Series No. 3, 1958 Revision*. Washington, D. C., U.S. Government Printing Office, 1958.
17. Rosenthal, Sol: *BCG Vaccination Against Tuberculosis*. Boston, Little, Brown and Co., 1957.
18. *X-ray Case-Finding Programs in Tuberculosis Control*. Pub. Health Rep., 73:83–84, 1958.
19. Hinshaw, H. Corwin: *Tuberculosis Problems Facing the General Physician*. Merck Sharp and Dohme, Seminar Report, 2:17, 1957.
20. Monk, Mary A., and Terris, Milton: *Increase of Tuberculosis Mortality in Elderly Men from 1940 to 1950*. Am. J. Pub. Health, 48:1029, 1958.
21. Hsu, K. H. K.: *The Tuberculin Test as a New Approach to the New Era of Tuberculosis Control*. Dis. Chest, 33:23–27, 1958.
22. Hunt, M. Estelle: *Challenge of Communicable Disease Today—Tuberculosis Control*. Am. J. Pub. Health, 49:863, 1959.
23. Commission on Chronic Illness: *Chronic Illness in the United States, Volume I, Prevention of Chronic Illness*. Massachusetts, Harvard University Press, 1957, Page 224.

SUGGESTED READING

American Public Health Association: *Communicable Disease Control in Man*, 8th Ed. New York, American Public Health Association, 1960.

Anderson, Gaylord W., and Arnstein, Margaret G.: *Communicable Disease Control*. New York, The Macmillan Co., 1956.

Badger, T. L.: *Medical Progress—Tuberculosis*. New England J. Med., 261:30–35; 74–81; 131–39, 1959.

Barnouw, Eric, and Clark, E. G.: *Syphilis: The Invader, A Public Affairs Pamphlet*. Washington, D. C., American Public Health Association, 1958.

Clark, E. A.: *Challenge of Communicable Disease Today—Venereal Disease Control*. Am. J. Pub. Health, 49:865–68, 1959.

Dooley, Thomas A.: *The Edge of Tomorrow*. New York, Farrar, Straus and Cudahy, 1958.

Dublin, L. I.: *Cause of Tuberculosis Mortality and Morbidity in the United States*. Am. J. Pub. Health, 48:1439–48, 1958.

Galdston, Iago, M.D., Editor: *The Epidemiology of Health*. New York, Health Education Council, 1953.

Hilleboe, Herman E., and Larimore, Granville W.: *Preventive Medicine, Principles of Prevention in the Occurrence and Progression of Disease*. Philadelphia, W. B. Saunders Co., 1959.

Hunt, M. E.: *Challenge of Communicable Disease Today—Tuberculosis Control*. Am. J. Pub. Health, *49*:857–61, 1959.

Maxcy, Kenneth, Editor: *Preventive Medicine and Public Health*. New York, Appleton-Century-Crofts, Inc., 1956.

Mustard, Harry S.: *Introduction to Public Health, 3rd Ed*. New York, The Macmillan Co., 1953.

Roueché, Berton: *Eleven Blue Men*. New York, Berkley Publishing Corp., 1956.

Smith, Geddes: *Plague on Us*. New York, The Commonwealth Fund, 1941.

Snow, John, M.D.: *Snow on Cholera*. New York, The Commonwealth Fund, 1936.

Stiles, William W., M.D.: *Individual and Community Health*. New York, Blakiston Co., 1953.

The Shattuck Report: *Report of the Sanitary Commission of Massachusetts: 1850*. Reprinted by The American Public Health Association, New York, 1950.

Zinsser, Hans: *Rats, Lice and History*. Boston, Little, Brown and Co., 1935.

Chapter VIII

Safety Education

ACCIDENTS are the fourth leading cause of death in the United States today, and are outranked only by heart, cancer, and cerebral hemorrhage fatalities. Accidents are the leading cause of death in children five to 14 years of age in the United States and 12 other countries in the Western Hemisphere.[1] They also account for about 100,000 deaths each year, and injure, disable, and cripple another ten million persons.

Many parents are more concerned about the child's diet, a rash, or some mild disease than they are by the fact that accidents claim the lives of more than 15,000 children every year. Accidents kill more children each year than polio, cancer, heart disease, pneumonia, tuberculosis and kidney diseases combined. Approximately 40,000 to 50,000 children are permanently crippled by accidents in the United States each year.

During the bloody second world war the United States suffered

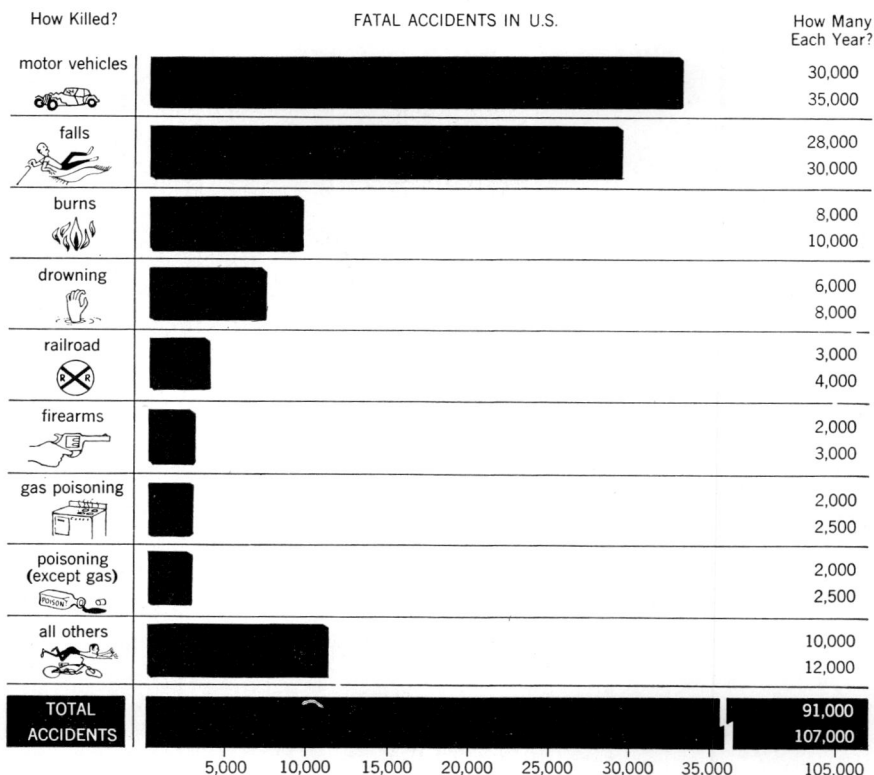

How Killed?	FATAL ACCIDENTS IN U.S.	How Many Each Year?
motor vehicles		30,000 / 35,000
falls		28,000 / 30,000
burns		8,000 / 10,000
drowning		6,000 / 8,000
railroad		3,000 / 4,000
firearms		2,000 / 3,000
gas poisoning		2,000 / 2,500
poisoning (except gas)		2,000 / 2,500
all others		10,000 / 12,000
TOTAL ACCIDENTS		91,000 / 107,000

5,000   10,000   15,000   20,000   25,000   30,000   35,000   105,000

Figure 39. (From Schifferes, J. J., *Essentials of Healthier Living,* John Wiley and Sons, 1960.)

an average of 65,330 combat dead and 149,077 combat wounded each year; during peaceful 1959 the accident toll was 91,000 dead and 9,100,000 injured. What other nation in history has managed to be more deadly at work and play than it has been at war? The number of Americans killed accidentally during 1960 was nearly triple the number of American fighting men killed during the entire Korean War.

If this is a normally "safe" week, 1,800 Americans alive this morning will be dead seven days from today. They will die in accidents, most of them avoidable. Another 173,000 will be hurt in avoidable accidents. During that average week, 11 hunters will either kill themselves by careless handling of their own guns or be shot to death by companions who mistake them for four-footed game; 31 other firearm deaths will include children between five and 14 years of age. Among the do-it-yourself handy men 18 will be electrocuted doing home repair jobs because they forgot to turn off the current. Approximately 385 persons, most of whom are 65 and older, will suffer fatal falls on slippery pavements, in bathtubs, and highly polished floors. Fires will claim another 121 lives, and many victims will be smokers who lit their last cigarette in bed just before falling asleep. About 50 will die from leaking gas or poisons taken by mistake. The leading accident killer, motor vehicles, will claim about 731 persons per week. Drownings, which claim about 6,500 persons each year, will account for 138 fatalities during the average week. Varying only slightly from year to year, the annual accident toll amounts to approximately 90,000 fatalities and 9,050,000 injuries, 120,000 of which result in permanent disability.

Health department officials added accident prevention and safety education to their programs long ago. These programs include health education, epidemiological investigations, pilot studies, and research. Accidents can be prevented and the lives of many can be prolonged.

Causes of Accidents

There is no single cause for accidents, nor is there a single cure. Mechanical and personal failures, environmental hazards, inadequate knowledge, insufficient skill, and improper attitudes and habits are prime causes of accidents. Of all accidents in recent years, 85 per cent could have been prevented if the victims had reacted properly to their environment. Man has not learned to live safely with the powerful forces at his disposal. He drinks while driving; he recklessly speeds to and from work or vacation; he fishes indifferently in a deep lake without knowing how to swim well; he hunts without exercising proper precaution, and carelessly throws away his cigarettes. Furthermore, he does not take preventive measures to protect the elderly person in his home from falling. Year after years, falls are the second leading cause of accidental deaths, and claim about 20,000 persons each year; about 73 per cent of these persons are 65 years of age and older.

Although safety education is stressed today, many persons have not learned common safety facts. Accidents may also be caused by people who attempt to perform feats beyond their ability; who are emotionally disturbed or intoxicated; who have faulty vision or hearing, and who are fatigued. Faulty or negative attitudes, procrastination, and lack of supervision all add to the death toll. Many of these factors are interrelated, and in many cases, faulty attitudes relate to lack of knowledge. Since our daily lives are surrounded by a multitude of hazards, and since most of us find it necessary to "take a chance" or "play the odds" occasionally, motivation and communication must be emphasized in this area.

CHILDHOOD SAFETY

Safety education begins in the home; only parents can immunize their children against accidents. Accidents remain the foremost cause of death among school-age children and account for many more fatalities than are attributed to any single disease. Parents must protect infants from burns, drowning, poisoning, falls, and machinery. When the child begins school, the parent must depend upon the child's knowledge, attitude, skill, habits, and behavior to protect himself. Therefore, parents must be effective teachers and must set good examples for their children.

Children must be motivated to develop and practice protective skills and acquire the habit of conscientiously observing general as well as specific safety principles. Education should engender in every child the desire and the ability to shield himself from potential danger in all circumstances, including those that are new to him and that involve hazards he has not previously encountered. Safety education must be extended to all students in the school and be given proper emphasis in the school curriculum. First aid, swimming instruction, driver training, and bicycle training should be included in the safety education program.

Accidental Poisoning in Children

One of the most important and increasingly common causes of childhood accidents is poisoning. A lengthening list of deodorants, depilatories, detergents, herbicides, insecticides, rodenticides, petroleum products, stimulants, sedatives, and analgesics contribute to the magnitude of the problem.

Poison control centers are established to help meet this problem. These centers maintain 24 hour telephone service and offer frightened parents immediate information concerning the contents, toxicity, and means of combating the accidental poisoning of the child. Further and more complete treatment is given at the center. The public health nurse later visits the family at home, and tries to determine the cause of the accident and suggest ways to remove hazards and prevent future accidents. The first poison control center was organized in Chicago in 1953 by the American Academy of Pediatrics, the Chicago Board of Health, the Illinois State Toxicology Laboratory, the University of Illinois, and six major teaching hospitals. Since then, over 200 centers have been established throughout the country.[2]

These centers will provide a long term study of frequency and causes of poisoning as they occur, so that better methods of prevention can be devised. This program will promote education and cooperative planning, which are two essential ingredients of any successful program.

Recent cumulative studies indicate that the major toxic agents responsible for poisoning cases are aspirin and other internal medications.[3] Flavored baby aspirin is a frequent cause of salicylate poisoning. Other poisons include lead external medications, rodenticides, insecticides, and household preparations, including bleach, petroleum products, lye, disinfectants, detergents, polishes, and solvents. Chemical poisoning in children occurs most frequently in the kitchen. The bedroom and bathroom are also rooms with possible poisoning hazards.

The prevention of poisonings revolves around education, legislation, additional poison-control centers, and continued efforts among physicians, health department personnel, and others. Manufacturers of household preparations and internal and external medications might firmly attach legible labels listing the active poisonous ingredients, warning the users concerning the hazard, and describing appropriate antidotes. Many manufacturers are experimenting with hard-to-open safety closures for containers in an effort to protect small children against potentially harmful substances.

An example of needed legislation is a law to prohibit the sale of kerosene in other than a distinctive container equipped with a label warning about flammability. The danger of putting kerosene into vessels intended for food and beverages is the possibility of fatal pulmonary damage following ingestion.[2] Federal controls are lacking that require proper labeling of household, commercial, and industrial products, such as cosmetics, soaps, detergents, solvents, waxes, deodorizers, paint, ink, dyes, paint thinner, and other substances with a high toxicity rating.[4]

The poisoning problem and the steps necessary to prevent it must continually be brought before the public and especially parents. Parents can help prevent poisonings by keeping poisonous and "questionable" substances locked up or out of reach of children. Parent-teacher associations and service club meetings offer excellent opportunities to discuss the problem.

A few precautions necessary to prevent poisoning are:

1. Keep all drugs, poisonous substances, and household chemicals out of the reach of children.
2. Do not store nonedible products on shelves used for storing food.
3. Do not transfer poisonous substances to unlabeled containers.
4. Never reuse containers of chemical substances.
5. Do not leave discarded medicines where children or pets might get at them.
6. Never tell children you are giving them candy when you are actually giving them medicine.
7. Read labels before using chemical products.
8. Never give or take medicines in the dark.

Safety Education

Most traffic and safety experts recommend a four-pronged attack to reduce teen-age murder and suicide on the highway: (1) increasing the number and quality of high school driver education courses; (2) encouraging parents to set better examples behind the wheel; (3) making dangerous driving socially unacceptable among youngsters; and (4) whenever possible, enforcing traffic rules through student government.

The death rate for children between the ages of five and 14 has shown a remarkable reduction since safety education was introduced into school programs. The decreasing number of pedestrian accidents and the continuing low rate of bicycle accidents almost certainly reflect the school's efforts to promote safety in these areas, particularly the increasing use of student traffic patrols.

Although the death rate for young people between the ages of 15 and 24 has shown little change during the last 20 years, more than 50 per cent of all fatalities in this group are due to automobile accidents, with drowning and firearm accidents responsible for most of the rest. If driver education courses, a relatively recent addition to the school curriculum, become more widespread, however, the death rate for adolescents and young adults should also be reduced. At present over two million students are enrolled in these courses, which are offered by 15,000 high schools. Statistics show that both the accident rate and the incidence of traffic violations are lower among these students than other drivers of the same age.[5] On a proportionate basis, five times more infractions are committed by the untrained group than by the trained group.

In stressing the relationship of safety education to the community, Drs. Florio and Stafford, safety educators, noted:

"If safety education is to meet its challenge, it must be extended not only to more and more students, but to their parents as well—in fact to all members of the community. The school's program functions best when it is supported by outside agencies; the effectiveness of classroom instruction is weakened when parents do not support the program, e.g., permitting a child to ride a bicycle in the street before he has acquired sufficient skill and knowledge. When a student brings home a check list of home hazards, it is important that his parents pay attention, for any indifference or opposition on their part may negate the value of what he has learned. The training students receive at school must be strengthened by their outside experiences; otherwise they may take the proper precautions only when they are closely supervised. It is far easier to induce children to behave safely at all times if adults set a good example."[*]

Research Studies

A research study was conducted in the state of Oregon on student injuries in the secondary schools.[6] The purpose of the study was to analyze and evaluate the reported injuries occurring to pupils who were protected by the Student Mutual Benefit Plan Insurance. The enrollment included 28,878 children in the insurance plan and of this number, 1,815 injuries were reported. There were slightly more than six injuries for every 100 students that were insured.

The findings of the study were as follows:

1. Of the 28,878 insured students in the study, 1,815 injuries were reported with a ratio of 6.2 per 100 students.

2. The time of the day accounting for the greatest number of injuries was from 3:00 P.M. to 4:00 P.M., with 14.5 per cent of the total injuries.

3. The month of February was found to have the greatest amount of injuries, with 13.3 per cent of the total.

4. Physical education classes, with 52.9 per cent of the total injuries, more than doubled all other organized and unorganized school activities combined. Others in order of frequency were: school building, 13.8 per cent; school grounds, 7.7 per cent; shop, 6.3 per cent; to and from school, 5.2 per cent; classroom, 3.6 per cent; noon-hour activities, 3.3 per cent; extracurricular activities, 2.3 per cent; intramurals, 2.0 per cent; and dressing room and showers, 1.7 per cent.

5. Sprains accounted for 31.3 per cent of the total injuries, contusions were

[*] Florio, A. E., and Stafford, C. T.: *Safety Education.* New York, McGraw-Hill Book Co., Inc., 1956, Page 15.

second, with 24.5 per cent; fractures and lacerations with 13.3 per
cent and 12.6 per cent respectively.

6. Ankles accounted for the greatest number of sprains with 33.1 per cent of
total injuries. The fingers accounted for 17.7 per cent and the back
13.2 per cent of the sprains.

Physical educators might help to prevent accidents by keeping
participants in superior physical condition; by giving prompt and
expert treatment of injured players; by requiring complete physical
examinations before participation; and by maintaining safe and
proper equipment.

A survey of 92 public schools in New York State in 1955 on the
nature and frequency of accidents among elementary school children, revealed the following findings:[7] (1) the greatest number of
accidents occurred during May and October; (2) the fifth grade
had the greatest amount of accidents; (3) the head was the part of
the body most frequently injured; (4) most accidents (about 64.0
per cent) occurred on the playground and in the gymnasium;
(5) the most serious accidents occurred at the bicycle rack, stair-
way, athletic field, doorways, and on school sidewalks.

From these findings it is recommended that teachers show
elementary pupils how to use equipment and supplies safely. The
playground apparatus should be located on some type of resilient
material such as sand; all activities should be properly supervised;
there should be better supervision of the stairways; and all class-
rooms of the future should be constructed on the ground level.

School accident policies should be cooperatively formulated,
printed, posted, and distributed to all employees. It is the teacher's
responsibility to know exactly what to do in case of an accident.
Accident reports must be filed and evaluated in an effort to determine the pattern and thus help reduce and prevent accidents. First
aid courses should be completed by as many persons on the staff as
possible. Parent-teacher association meetings might include a very
interesting and educational safety education program revolving
around the particular safety needs and interests of the school. The
considerations may include school safety evaluations, pupil transportation, liability insurance, and thorough prephysical examinations for athletes.

HOME SAFETY

Home accidents account for approximately 27,000 deaths each
year. Falls and fire burns account for more than 60 per cent of these

accidents in the home. Most falls in the home occur in the bedroom and involve aged persons. Home-fire deaths occur most frequently in helpless infants and aged persons; they are mainly caused by smoking, faulty cooking stoves, faulty house and water heaters, and faulty electrical equipment.

There is convincing evidence that certain types of home accidents can be prevented through state and local health department programs. The W. K. Kellogg Foundation promoted research on this subject by providing funds to certain select local health departments for developing methods of preventing home accidents. The San José City Health Department of California was one of the few local health departments selected, and the project began by defining these objectives:

1. To find methods for obtaining statistical data for home accidents. Sources included the emergency first aid stations, death certificates, coroner's reports, and initiation of hospital reporting programs.

2. To find ways in which home safety can be integrated into the regular activities of the health department. For example, public health nurses and sanitarians promoted home safety education by disseminating information, and participating in home safety check-list evaluations during routine nursing home visits or sanitation inspections.

3. To determine the responsibilities a local health department can accept in stimulating a community home safety program. These responsibilities included:

    a. Provide the necessary stimulus in the development of a community organization for the home safety program.

    b. Assist in the coordination of home safety activities undertaken by other community agencies.

    c. Provide statistical data and information to community groups.

    d. Offer consultation and guidance to community groups in program planning for home safety.

    e. Provide facilities, services, and personnel to work with community groups.

4. To develop awareness of the people in the community to home safety problems and to encourage community acceptance of safe home practices. This is best accomplished by stimulating community participation in the home safety program, by assisting in the development of in-service training program for community groups, and by jointly planning with community groups.

Today, over half of the state health departments and many local health departments have created special departments or divisions with qualified personnel to work in this special area of increasing importance. Cooperation with local agencies and organizations will continue to reduce accidents and prolong lives.

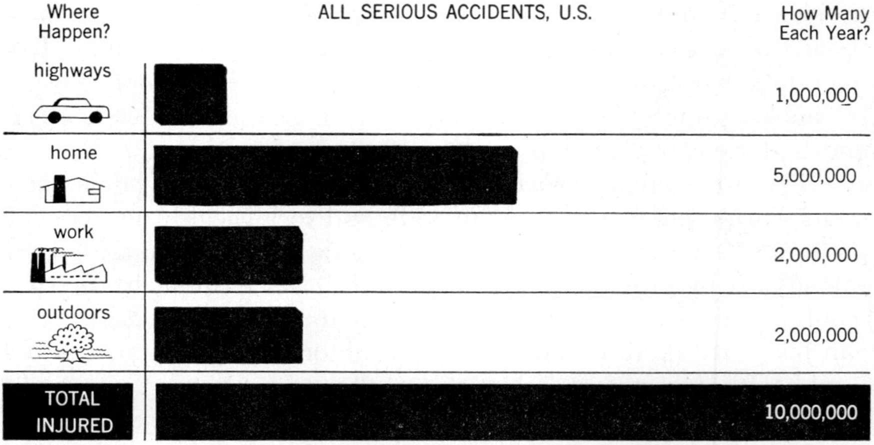

Figure 40. (From Schifferes, J. J., *Essentials of Healthier Living,* John Wiley and Sons, 1960.)

MOTOR VEHICLE SAFETY

It is the concensus of most experts in the field of safety education that the number of accidents on our public highways has killed more Americans since the advent of the automobile than were killed in all the wars of our country. Year after year, approximately 40,000 Americans are killed in motor-vehicle accidents. In those states where the motor-vehicle accident rate is decreasing, officials point to the rigid enforcement of the following safety measures:

1. Increasing the number of police patrons on highways (This has top priority in most states.)

2. New laws—or harsher enforcement of existing laws—calling for suspension of licenses and/or fines and imprisonment for motorists convicted of drunk driving, "chronic" negligence and speeding

3. Tighter examinations for vehicle licenses and mandatory auto inspection programs

4. Use of National Guard troops or sheriff's deputies to reinforce regular highway police during peak travel periods, such as holiday weekends

5. Periodic roadblocks—with massed troops stopping all cars and checking on licenses, intoxication and vehicle condition

6. Expansion of the use of radar devices in apprehending speeders

7. Establishing state speed limits where they are not already in force.

Governor C. Mennen Williams, noting Michigan's decrease from 2004 traffic deaths in 1955 to 1725 in 1956, declared: "The main weapons we have used are increased state police patrols; better control of driver licensing and suspension of licenses from dangerous drivers; use of National Guard troops to reinforce state patrol and sheriffs' road patrols, and widespread publicity."

Connecticut is another example of a state that found the key to its safety program with the rigid enforcement of the State's speed laws. The most potent weapon in that program is suspending the licenses of convicted speeders for a period of 30 days. The experiment has proved that people will slow down to save their drivers' licenses, *not* their lives. Governor Abe Ribicoff of Connecticut insists that a good traffic safety program should include the following:

1. Continuing accurate analysis of the traffic problem

2. Strict control of drivers through good examination and licensing as well as fearless use of suspension and revocation

3. Stringent law enforcement by police and courts

4. Proper education and training of all drivers to develop knowledge, attitudes, and skills

5. Improved vehicles and roads.

The State of Iowa has initiated an experiment that is being tested throughout the state, and it may prove to be one answer to the reckless driver problem that plagues the nation. Motorists charged with driving violations are given the choice of license suspension for a month or attendance at a "safe driving" school conducted by the State Safety Department. Tuition at the school is five dollars, and absenteeism is not allowed. Following the course, which stresses driving problems and motives of reckless drivers, the "students" are placed on one-year probation. The school is not a substitute for fines which are levied in addition. At present, the school obviously is not an adequate answer to the State's needs along this line, but it is a beginning. Other states might well consider a similar project to reeducate chronic traffic violators in the art of safe driving, and, at the same time, probe some of the psychological "drives" and attitudes that lead to reckless driving.

Causes

No one can say exactly how many motor-vehicle accidents are due to a particular circumstance. Most accidents are due to a combination of several circumstances, and few accidents are investigated carefully enough to determine exactly what the underlying causes were. However, about one of every 13 drivers involved in fatal accidents have a physical condition that could have been a contributing factor; fatigue or lack of sleep was the condition in two-thirds of the cases; defective eyesight, illness, and defective hearing ranked next in order. Some drugs, especially the antihistaminics often used by hay fever victims impair coordination and judgement, or cause drowsiness. Alcohol is also responsible for a large percentage of motor-vehicle accidents in the United States.

Certain physical disabilities should motivate the conscientious person to stop driving. Many, but not all, persons with heart disease, diabetes, epilepsy, and other disabling illnesses should put themselves in the nondriver category. Drivers with poor vision and hearing will add to public safety if they refrain from driving automobiles. Excessive nearsightedness, night blindness, and "tunnel vision", ability to see only what is directly in front of him, are particularly dangerous. Persons with sight in one eye only often have difficulty judging distance and getting a clear perspective. They tend to be unsafe drivers. Glaucoma steals eyesight slowly; at least 800,000 Americans are losing their sight because of glaucoma without realizing it. Many automobile operators, especially those past 40 years of age, may have glaucoma and not be aware that the disease is present. If the disease has progressed, the victim may not see a car approaching from the extreme left or right. As we grow older our eyes often change and become more vulnerable to defects and disease; the highest proportion of poor vision occurs among people past middle age. Yet, only a few states (Michigan, Iowa, and Colorado) require eye tests for drivers' license renewal. Most states believe that if the driver has good vision at 17 years of age, his vision will be good at age 65. States should enact a law whereby each driver *must* have his eyes rechecked each year. Defective hearing cases should also be investigated. Age itself is not necessarily a ban to driving; a fortunate few retain alert senses and good muscular coordination even up to the age of 70. However, almost everyone should give up the wheel at that age, as indicated by Dr. W. W. Bauer of the American Medical Association: "The automobile plays such an important part in our lives that to ask an individual to refrain from driving because of physical or emotional infirmity is demanding a serious sacrifice. Yet we would not permit such people to operate busses, streetcars, cranes or heavy machinery. Why then should they be allowed to cause death and destruction on our highways?" Perhaps the largest group of persons who should give serious consideration to whether or not they are fit to drive is that group with recognized emotional instability. The excitable, the quick-tempered, the absent-minded, the "touchy", and the easily upset persons become a serious threat behind the wheel of a fast moving vehicle.

The Automotive Crash Injury Research Project conducted at Cornell University has amassed a large volume of data since 1952. An analysis is made of injuries and fatalities incurred by occupants in accidents involving passenger cars in relation to agent factors such as speed of the vehicle, nature of impact, ejection, and internal structure of the automobile. Several important facts derived from these studies include:[8, 9, 10]

1. If ejection of passengers from automobiles involved in motor vehicle accidents could be prevented, a 25 per cent reduction in fatalities would result; an estimated 5,500 lives would be saved in the United States each year.

2. In "paired comparisons" of similar accidents, the frequency of injury of all degrees was two and one half times greater in occupants without seat belts than in those with seat belts, or a reduction in risk of injury among seat belt users of 60 per cent.

3. In comparing injuries sustained by ejected persons with those sustained by nonejected persons wearing seat belts in similar types of accidents, the mortality was eight times greater in those ejected, or a reduction in mortality of 87 per cent in the seat belt group.

Although these facts are encouraging, a recent survey has revealed that public interest in this safety device, never really widespread, has deteriorated to virtual indifference. It is estimated that seat belts are used by fewer than one percent of American drivers.[11] Furthermore, only nine of 41 brands tested met federal specifications.

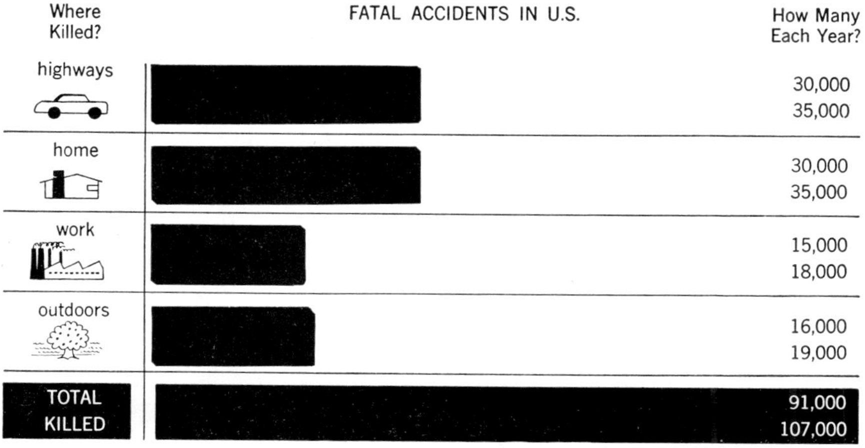

Where Killed?	FATAL ACCIDENTS IN U.S.	How Many Each Year?
highways		30,000 35,000
home		30,000 35,000
work		15,000 18,000
outdoors		16,000 19,000
TOTAL KILLED		91,000 107,000

Figure 41. (From Schifferes, J. J., *Essentials of Healthier Living*, John Wiley and Sons, 1960.)

Prevention

Safety educators and safety engineers will continue to have a difficult time preventing accidents, saving lives, and extending the scope of safe living until the public is fully aroused. The organization of the Committee on Highway Safety of the National Governors' Conference shows great promise in striving for uniformity and promoting safety education. At the forty-eighth Conference of Governors, held in 1956, a committee of governors was appointed to undertake an immediate study to make recommendations for the adoption of:

1. A uniform set of motor-vehicle laws for the fifty states (including signs, speed limits, traffic lights, signals, etc.)

2. Uniform enforcement of motor vehicle laws

3. Nationwide reciprocity in upholding convictions and penalties from the enforcement of motor vehicle laws

4. The development of state and community-wide programs for safety education.

Various methods for studying this problem of motor-vehicle accidents have been proposed; a few have been carried out. Many experts suggest that the epidemiological approach, so familar to health departments in other programs, may be applied advantageously to studying causation and possible prevention of motor-vehicle accidents. The epidemiological approach includes study of the host factors such as behavior and attitudes; motor and sensory defects; effects of fatigue, alcohol, and drugs on driver responses; and environmental factors, e.g., seasonal, geographic, climatic, and urban versus rural incidence.

Prevention of accidents can be grouped under the three E's— Education, Enforcement, and Engineering. The process of learning to live safely involves understanding the many hazards that one must encounter in his various daily activities; developing attitudes and behavior patterns that predispose one to adjust properly to his environment; and mastering skills that enable one to cope with particularly dangerous situations.

It is essential to motivate and educate people to assume the role of responsible citizens; to cooperate with authorities and others in upholding the law; and to make the home, school, community, factory, and highway safe places for all.

Safety Council

A school-community safety council can help prevent accidents and help develop social and civic responsibility. Perhaps no other phase of the school program offers students a greater opportunity to prepare for citizenship and "to learn by doing" than do these organizations. A school may organize a safety council to coordinate all safety matters brought to its attention; to coordinate the various school activities concerned with accident prevention; and to establish safety regulations regarding such matters as the use of bicycles, motor vehicles, and safe conduct in and around the school. A school-community safety program should be concerned not only with teaching children and adults how to avoid accidents, but with eliminating the physical hazards that endanger them. All members and agencies in the community should cooperate and actively participate in promoting safety. The local safety and health council must maintain a continuous education program, and find and eliminate safety hazards in an effort to prevent accidents.

QUESTIONS FOR REVIEW

1. Compare the number and kinds of accident fatalities in the various age groups in the United States.
2. List and briefly discuss the major causes of accidents.
3. Discuss accidental poisoning in children.
4. (a) What part does the local health department play in accident prevention?
   (b) State health department
   (c) United States Public Health Service
   (d) World Health Organization
   (e) Local Safety Council
   (f) National Safety Council
5. How can we prevent:
   (a) auto accidents,
   (b) home accidents,
   (c) school accidents?
6. What is the nature and function of a community safety council?
7. Discuss the following statement: "How can I prevent accidents? It's the other fellow you have to watch."

REFERENCES

1. Goddard, J. L.: *Accident Prevention in Childhood.* Pub. Health Rep., *74:* 523, 1959.
2. Arena, J. M.: *The Problem of Accidental Poisoning in Children As It Exists Today.* J.A.M.A., 159:1537–39, 1955.
3. Jacobziner, H.: *The Accidental Chemical Poisoning Problem.* Postgrad. Med., 22:283–298, 1957.
4. Gosselin, R. E.: *How Toxic Is It?* J.A.M.A., 163:1333–37, 1957.
5. Brody, L., and Stack, Herbert J.: *Highway Safety and Driver Education.* New York, Prentice-Hall, Inc., 1954, Pages 360–361.
6. Haar, Frank, and Martin, Don B.: *Student Injuries in Secondary Schools in Oregon.* Res. Quart., 24:276, 1953.
7. Hase, Gerald J.: *Nature and Frequency of Accidents Among School Children in New York State.* Albany, University of the State of New York, 1957.

8. Tourin, B.: *Ejection and Automobile Fatalities*. Pub. Health Rep., 73:381–391, 1958.
9. Moore, John O.: *Testimony Before Special Subcommittee on Traffic Safety of the House Committee on Interstate and Foreign Commerce*. Washington, D.C., U.S. Government Printing Office, 1957.
10. Cornell University: *Progress Report on Automotive Crash Injury Research*. New York, Cornell University Medical College, 1957.
11. Consumer Report: *Auto Seat Belts*. Washington, D.C., U.S. Government Printing Office, 1960, Pages 82–87.

SUGGESTED READING

American Automobile Association: *Sportsmanlike Driving*, 2nd Ed., Washington, D.C., American Automobile Association, 1948.
American National Red Cross: *Accident Prevention*. Washington, D.C., American National Red Cross, 1958.
American National Red Cross: *First Aid Textbook*. Washington, D.C., American National Red Cross, 1960.
American National Red Cross: *Life-Saving and Water Safety Manual*. Washington, D.C., American National Red Cross, 1958.
American Public Health Association: *Public Health Problems of Accidental Poisoning*. Am. J. Pub. Health, 46:951–58, 1956.
American Public Health Association: *Uniform Definitions of Home Accidents Developed by the Conference on Uniform Definitions of Home Accidents*. Washington, D.C., U.S. Public Health Service Publication No. 577, 1958.
Dearborne, Ned H.: *Safety and Health*. Am. J. Pub. Health, 46:1415–18, 1956.
Flanagan, J. E.: *Labeling Legislation—A Summary Review of Recent Developments*. Am. J. Pub. Health, 50:637–41, 1960.
Florio, A. E., and Stafford, C. T.: *Safety Education*. New York, McGraw-Hill Book Company, 1956.
Harnett, Arthur L., and Shaw, John H.: *Effective School Health Education*. New York, Appleton-Century-Crofts, Inc., 1959.
Hilleboe, Herman E., and Larimore, Granville W.: *Preventive Medicine, Principles of Prevention in the Occurrence and Progression of Disease*. Philadelphia, W. B. Saunders Co., 1959.
Metropolitan Life Insurance Co.: *Incidence of Disability During 1957, Statistical Bulletin*. New York, Metropolitan Life Insurance Co., 1958.
Metropolitan Life Insurance Co.: *Where and How Fatal Accidents Occur, Statistical Bulletin*. New York, Metropolitan Life Insurance Co., 1951.
National Education Association: *Safety Education-Teaching Aids and Materials*. Washington, D.C., National Commission on Safety Education, 1960.
National Safety Council: *Accident Facts*. Chicago, National Safety Council, 1960.
Nemir, Alma: *The School Health Program*. Philadelphia, W. B. Saunders Co., 1959.
Roueché, Berton: *Eleven Blue Men*. New York, Berkley Publishing Corp., 1956.
Seaton, Don Cash: *Safety in Sports*. New Jersey, Prentice-Hall, Inc., 1948.
State Motor Vehicle Department: *State Traffic Code and Driver's Handbook*. Published By All State Motor Vehicle Departments, 1960.
Waterman, T. L., and Lang, V. F.: *Chronic Illness*. St. Louis, The C. V. Mosby Co., 1955.
Whitney, Albert W., Editor: *Man and the Motor Car*. New York, Accident Prevention Division of the Association of Casualty and Surety Association Executives, 1950.

Chapter IX

Mental Health

Mental Illness—What Is It?

Mental illness is a disturbance of the mind and emotions. The illness may be so mild that it is unrecognized, or so severe that it is tragically disabling. Doctors have found that more than one-half of all persons who consult their family or school physicians for treatment of a physical ailment suffer from emotional difficulties.

There are two main categories of mental disease—the neuroses and the psychoses. The chief characteristic of neuroses is anxiety, and it is directly felt or unconsciously controlled by the use of various psychological defense mechanisms. The neurotic person does not lose contact with reality and does not display gross disorganization of personality. He may carry on his business and social affairs as a seemingly normal person; yet inwardly he may be suffering from some anxiety, resentment, fear, or hostility that destroys his capacity for normal, happy living. Actually, there is a fine line between the neurotic individual and the so-called normal person, and experts disagree about where that line is to be drawn.

The psychotic person loses contact with reality. The chief characteristic of this illness is personality disintegration with disorientation for time, place, or person; and hospitalization is usually required. The psychotic person may live in a dream world, perhaps unaware of his own identity or surroundings, or he may be unable to control his behavior. He may have fantastic ideas (delusions), or he may misinterpret what he sees and hears (illusions). He may see, hear, feel, taste, or smell things that are not there (hallucinations). Two common psychoses are schizophrenia and the manic-depressive psychoses. Schizophrenia (reality disturbance) accounts for about one-half of the hospitalized cases of mental illness; most victims are young adults. The schizophrenic withdraws and has daydreams, delusions, and hallucinations. The manic-depressive has prolonged periods of high excitement and deep depression, and he may alternate from one to the other.

Possible contributing factors to mental illness include emotional experiences in infancy and childhood, increasing pressures in a fast age of insecurity, and certain chemical changes in the body. Most authorities agree that there is insufficient evidence to single out one factor.

Advances and Problems

Mental illness is one of the most challenging unsolved public health problems today. The growing size of the mental-illness problem, the suffering it causes, and the staggering cost of care and treatment make the search for more effective preventive measures an urgent necessity. An estimated 20,000,000 Americans are now suffering from some form of mental illness; 3,000,000 men, women, and children are treated in mental hospitals, at psychiatric clinics, or by private psychiatrists each year. While new treatments are shortening the period of hospitalization, more than 50 per cent of the nation's hospital beds are occupied by psychotic patients, particularly schizophrenics. (See Figure 42.) At least 800,000 more mental patients need hospital treatment, but have not been admitted to the already overcrowded institutions. It is estimated that one out of every ten babies born today will be hospitalized with mental illness at some time during his lifetime. Because many emotionally disturbed persons do not see a doctor, there are no reliable statistics on the number of Americans with psychoneurotic problems like depression, anxiety, acute lack of self-confidence, hypochondria, and hysteria. The number of people so afflicted is large and may be growing because of the stress and unpredictability of modern life. Another reason may revolve around the fact that mental illness is being detected earlier, and patients are seeking help earlier.

The proportion of elderly people in our mental hospitals is increasing at an alarming rate. Of all patients admitted to mental hospitals, 40 per cent are over 60 years old; 30 per cent are over 65 years of age. About 94 per cent of all mental patients over 65 will remain in the hospital until death. Although many of these older persons have had a mild stroke or may be senile due to cerebral arteriosclerosis, many of these patients are simply custodial cases with no place else to go and no family to care for their simple needs; they are not treatable and are not really mentally ill. In order to cope with this problem, Kentucky, Ohio, and several other states, spurred by a combination of humanitarian motives and a desire to save tax money, are screening patients and are placing elderly persons who are not mentally ill in boarding and nursing homes. This program saves the state money because the patients promptly become entitled to federal old-age benefits, and the federal government also shares the cost of operating the nursing homes. Although the increase in the number of older age persons may be a factor in this problem, perhaps the nature of our present competitive, tract-home, restless, mobile, status-seeking society may be involved. It is interesting to note that at present it is estimated that a new patient has about a fifty-fifty chance of leaving a mental hospital within twelve months. After two years the odds against leaving rise 16 to one, and after 5 years the odds increase 99 to one.

The increase in the number of youngsters afflicted with mental illness parallels the aged problem. The rise in mental illness among children is probably due to more accurate diagnosis. In the past, many of these mentally ill youngsters roamed the streets or were sent to reform school. It is estimated that more than 10 per cent of the nation's public school children are emotionally disturbed and need guidance. Children as young as five years of age may develop schizophrenia.

Great strides have been made through the years in the prevention of mental illness. For example, patients suffering from pellagra once filled mental hospitals in the South. Today, pellagra patients

MENTAL PATIENTS OCCUPY SLIGHTLY MORE THAN ONE OUT OF EVERY TWO HOSPITAL BEDS

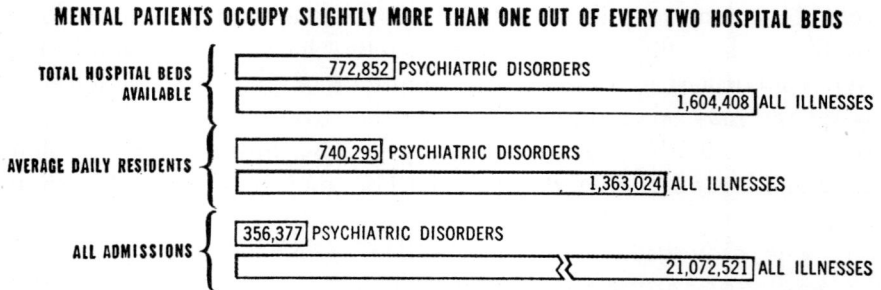

TOTAL HOSPITAL BEDS AVAILABLE	772,852 PSYCHIATRIC DISORDERS
	1,604,408 ALL ILLNESSES
AVERAGE DAILY RESIDENTS	740,295 PSYCHIATRIC DISORDERS
	1,363,024 ALL ILLNESSES
ALL ADMISSIONS	356,377 PSYCHIATRIC DISORDERS
	21,072,521 ALL ILLNESSES

Figure 42. (From Therapeutic Notes. Parke, Davis and Co., December, 1957.)

have practically disappeared because it was discovered that the disease is caused by a dietary deficiency. Another important example is the tremendous reduction in admissions to mental hospitals from advanced cases of syphilis since penicillin treatment was instituted in 1943.* Furthermore, much has been done to prevent brain damage (encephalitis) caused by unnecessary exposure to lead and other heavy metals by certain workers. Mental cases following accidental injuries are far fewer than formerly. Even with these advances, however, there has been a steady increase in the mental hospital population. (See Figures 43 and 44.) Factors contributing to the increase in mental illness are the country's increased urbanization and industrialization; the higher proportion of older persons in the population; and the greater longevity of mental patients.

During the past 25 years, the growth of mental health clinics has been of great importance. They serve as mental first-aid stations where the public may obtain help for emotional problems before these problems become too serious. The clinics play a particularly vital role in preventing mental illness at the source or formative years of childhood. Early recognition and prompt treatment are as important in mental illness as they are in physical illness.

Although there are over 1,200 mental health clinics in the entire country, approximately one-half of these give only parttime service. There should be at least one full-time mental health clinic for every 50,000 persons or a total of about 3,600 clinics. One state has no clinic; some states have only one or two clinics. More than 50 per cent of the clinics are located in the Northeast, which has only about 25 per cent of the total population. It would seem advisable to increase the number of mental health clinics as part

* Nevertheless, in 1960 the cost was 47 million dollars a year for maintaining the syphilitic insane confined in publicly supported mental hospitals.

of the out-patient services of general hospitals. Patients who need help are often reluctant to seek out the clinic of a mental hospital and may often be deterred by both distance and the stigma attached to the name "mental hospital."

There is a particular need for well-supported and carefully planned research on all aspects of mental health. Prevention of mental disease may revolve around the same epidemiological principles utilized in preventing other diseases. For example, we must determine how many persons have the disease, what kind of people they are, and under what conditions they get the disease. This information can then furnish clues for intensive investigation of the causes.

Mental health programs and activities in the states received a great stimulus as a result of the passage of the National Mental

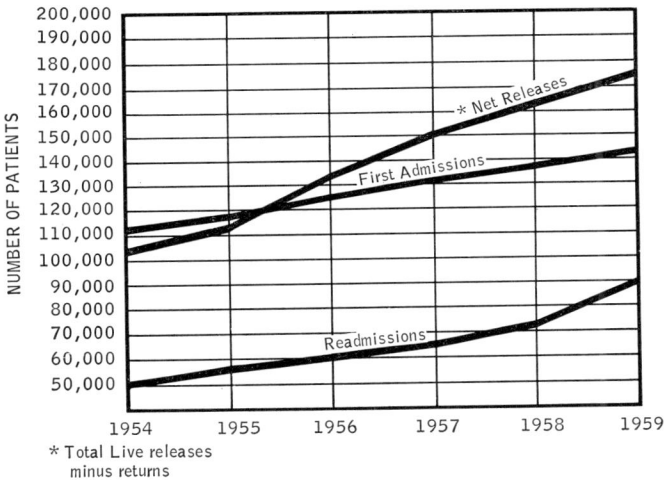

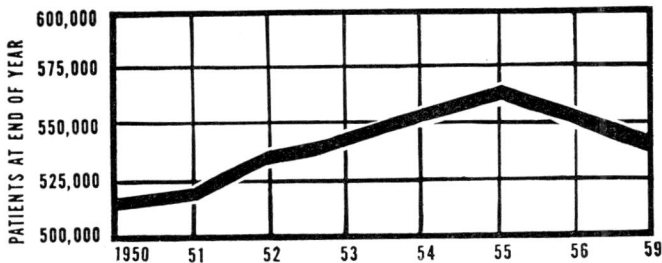

Figures 43 and 44. Downward trends in public mental hospital population began in 1956 with 7,095 fewer patients than in 1955. This change reflects an increasingly greater percentage of patients discharged, despite gains in first admissions and readmissions. (From U.S. Public Health Service.)

Health Act in 1946. This act provided for federal grants-in-aid to states for research, for training, and for assisting with the establishment and development of community mental health programs. Although federal funds are helpful and stimulating, the major responsibility for mental health programs rest with the states. When the National Governors' Conference on Mental Health was held in 1954, it was revealed that less than 1 per cent of the states' total mental health budgets was allotted to research; the remainder was allotted for care and treatment. The annual expenditures from all sources for research in the mental health field amounted to only approximately $27,000,000 in 1957. The assembled governors urged that state legislatures take steps to remedy this situation. Steps were taken by the federal government, and in 1956 Congress adopted new legislation which provided grants to state mental institutions to develop improved methods of care, treatment, and rehabilitation. At this time, however, state allocations for mental health are still small, and measures for handling the problem are still far from commensurate with its magnitude.

New admissions to mental hospitals are soaring, and readmissions of relapsed patients have also shown an alarming increase. (See Figure 43.) Patients are returning to mental hospitals in growing numbers because they are unable to make the transition from organized hospital life to the pressures and complexities of society, they fail to continue taking the drugs that helped them recover, or they may have been released too soon. In America there are more than 50,000 narcotics addicts, more than 5,000,000 problem drinkers, and at least 16,000 suicides each year. These are signs of a mentally and emotionally disturbed nation. Other problems in this area include a lack of mental hospitals and treatment facilities, and a shortage of psychiatrists and other aides. It is encouraging to note, however, that the number of patients in the nation's mental hospitals has consistently decreased from 1956 through 1959. For example, there were 542,721 patients in 277 mental hospitals at the end of 1959. This is a decrease of 2,142 patients since 1958. The current decline is the result of the fact that discharges from the hospitals are being made faster than admissions. This indicates that improved methods of treatment, the use of tranquilizers and other drugs, and earlier treatment of patients, are leading to faster rehabilitation. Partly as a result, average daily expenditure on each patient rose 18 per cent from 1956 to 1958, or from $3.74 to $4.42.

In 1956, the annual outlay from all sources for research in mental health amounted to about $30,000,000; this amount comprised only 3 per cent of all medical research funds. On the other hand, the annual cost of mental illness during the same year was estimated at about $5,000,000,000. (See Figure 45.) The country's major psychiatric research program is that of the United States Public Health Service's National Institute of Mental Health at Bethesda, Maryland. The Institute conducts intensive research and provides research grants to universities and other groups.

The Veterans Administration has become the largest single psychiatric hospital program in the nation. In the past 15 years it has grown tremendously and now offers about 70,000 psychiatric beds and 40 mental hospitals. Veterans Administration mental hospitals are staffed by about 600 psychiatrists and have been erected in 32 states.

One of the major problems in mental health is that the public reaction and attitude toward discharged mental cases is poor. No amount of medical support can alter the suspicion felt by some communities against the man or woman who has been in a mental hospital. Accordingly, the man or woman often returns to the hospital after being tragically rejected by society.

ANNUAL COST OF MENTAL ILLNESS IS ESTIMATED AT $4,172,124,955 (1956)
An Average of $1,190 for Each Patient

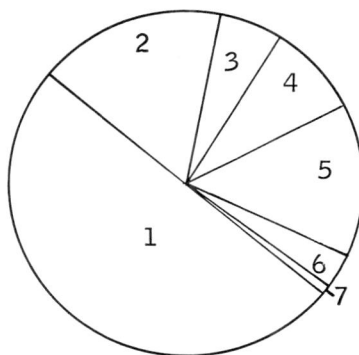

$2,061,526,350	loss in patients' earnings and federal income tax revenue—1
662,146,372	public mental hospital maintenance—2
238,000,000	care and maintenance of mentally ill in veterans' hospitals —3
284,240,844	compensation and pension payments to mentally ill veterans —4
750,000,000	construction and renovation of state mental hospital facilities —5
157,908,029	hospital care for mentally defective and epileptic patients —6
18,303,360	public assistance for mentally ill and defective persons—7

Figure 45. Only $27,265,577 is spent on mental disease research. (1956) Average yearly cost per patient $37. $15,353,000 of this money comes from federal funds for National Institute of Mental Health and Veterans Administration. $11,912,577 comes from state allocations and funds from foundations and associations. (From *Mental Health, A Paramount Problem,* Therapeutic Notes, 64:288-89, December, 1957).

Treatment

Recognized types of psychiatric treatment are:

SUPPORTIVE THERAPY. An effort to work with the patient's "conscious" mental facilities by direct influence from the psychiatrist. This technique requires reeducation and little probing of the patient's emotions.

FREUDIAN PSYCHOANALYSIS. This treatment involves the study of the emotions through free association and dream investigation in an effort to dredge the hidden and often hindering depths of the mind or "unconscious."

SHOCK THERAPY. There are three principal methods of shock therapy: insulin coma, the Metrazol drug convulsion method, and electric shock, which is the least complicated technique. Cure rates in some studies are as high as 80 per cent, particularly in manic-depressive psychoses.

PREFRONTAL LOBOTOMY. Early in 1936, Dr. Egas Moniz, of Lisbon, Portugal, began using this psychosurgery on psychotics. Two small holes are bored in the forehead, and a slender rod, ending in a small sharp knife, is inserted into the frontal lobe area, called "the seat of apprehension." The surgeon cuts the connecting brain fibers and disconnects the frontal lobe area from the rest of the brain centers. Patients undergo a complete personality change marked by lack of apprehension and indifference to fears. Since 1940, thousands of these operations have been performed, but always as a last resort in hopeless cases.

GROUP THERAPY. This is a type of psychological treatment used to enable patients to work out problems they have with other people, mainly with their so-called "peer relationships," such as schoolmates, associates on a job, friends, or relatives. The group encourages an individual to learn about himself, and to learn more satisfying and appropriate ways to react to other people. Understanding of one's self also leads to respect for self and others. Thus, individuality is strengthened within a group setting.

As a type of treatment, group therapy has two main attributes. First, it allows an individual to express his ideas and feelings, to "let out" his specific inhibitions and conflicts; it relieves emotional pressure and leads to self-understanding as emotionally he gains awareness of his problems. And second, the group therapy session becomes an actual practice period for an individual; it teaches him specific skills and techniques in dealing more effectively with other people. He "learns by doing."

DEEP ENCEPHALOGRAPHY. This therapy involves boring small holes in the patient's skull and implanting tiny electrodes in specific subcortical regions of the forebrain. Later, the therapists stimulate these areas electrically, in the hope of altering any abnormal circuit in the brain's switchboard.

PSYCHOSOMATIC TREATMENT. This treatment involves cases in which an emotional conflict in the unconscious is revealed in the form of a physical disturbance. Psychiatrists use a combination of sympathetic persuasion and psychological rehabilitation. Over one-half of the patients suffer from physical ailments caused or complicated by mental or emotional factors. Gastric ulcers, migraine headaches, backaches, arthritis, and high blood pressure, for instance, can have both emotional and physical origin.

GERIATRIC PSYCHIATRY. The remarkable rise in longevity has created a tremendous demand for old-age psychiatry. The highest rate of first admissions to mental hospitals is for elderly men and women; major causes include senile psychosis and psychosis from cerebral arteriosclerosis. The psychiatrist who treats the aged can help many patients adjust to growing old by stimulating their interest in new activities.

DRUGS. New tranquilizing drugs have revolutionized psychotherapy. Two drugs ushered in the new era: the first was chlorpromazine, which is a synthetic compound; the second was reserpine, a pure alkaloid from the juices of the snakeroot plant (Rauwolfia serpentina), crude extracts of which had been used for centuries by medicine men in India. Both drugs became available in the United States in 1953. These drugs have appeared under such brand names as Thorazine, Serpasil, Miltown, Frenquel, and Raudixin. Designed primarily to calm disturbed patients and make them amenable to regular psychotherapy, tranquilizers neither cure nor act as a substitute for therapy. Mental institutions throughout the nation have reported a remarkable shortening of the acute phases of illness when these drugs were administered. Utilization of these drugs has also changed the types of treatment given patients. Use of physical restraints, seclusion rooms, and other outmoded treatments has greatly diminished. Perhaps the most dramatic result is the great number of patients granted increased hospital freedom.

Mental Health Organizations and Societies

Various professional organizations are endeavoring to meet the problem of nervous and mental disease. The American Psychi-

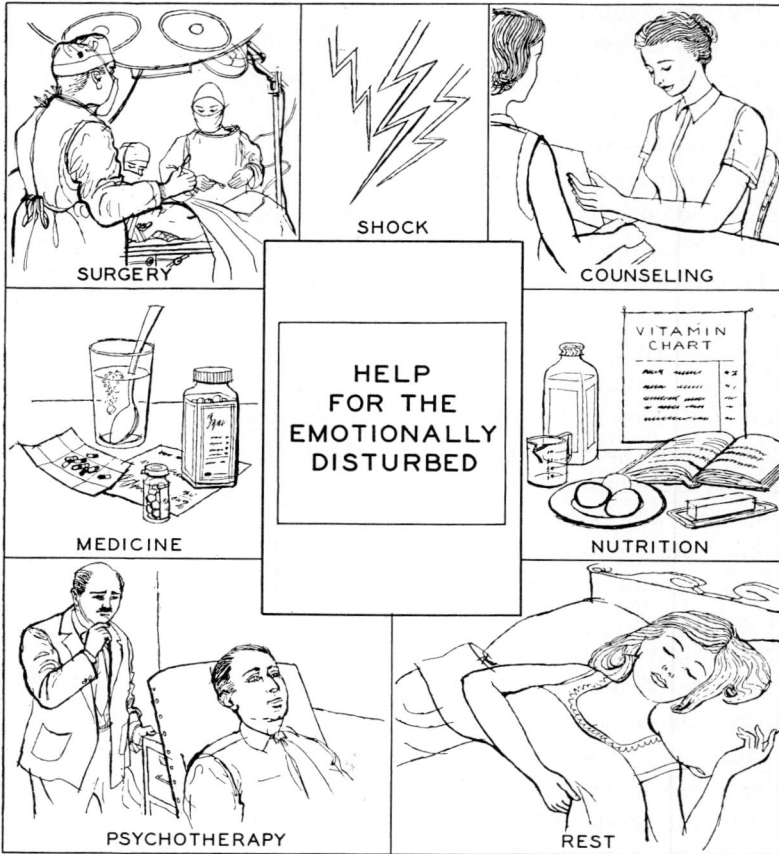

Figure 46. Help for the emotionally disturbed. (From Byrd, *Textbook of College Hygiene,* 2nd ed., 1957.)

atric Association sets up standards for care in psychiatric hospitals and encourages the training of psychiatrists, psychiatric nurses, and psychiatric aides. It furthers psychiatric education and research and devotes much time and effort to the development of out-patient clinics and all other agencies concerned with the social and legal aspects of mental disorders. The Committee on Hospital Care, a branch of the American Hospital Association, is encouraging the development of psychiatric wards in general hospitals. Training centers are being established to train psychiatrists and nurses. One such center is the Menninger Foundation School of Psychiatrists at Winter General Hospital and the Topeka State Hospital, both located near Topeka, Kansas. The Menningers trained 500 psychiatrists from 1946 to 1956.

State and local societies for mental health and other citizen groups are active in expanding facilities in their local communities for the treatment and care of the mentally ill. Many of these local mental health organizations are sponsored by the Community Chest and may include the adult and child guidance clinic, family service agency, day center for the aging, and community service organization. There is usually a long waiting list applying for these services. Some state societies are organized by professional persons; in others laymen carry on the work. In many communities various organizations, clubs, lodges, parent-teacher associations, and churches have programs that are concerned either directly or indirectly with mental health. These programs include presentation of facts, exchange of ideas, problems and their partial solutions; and surveys to discover local mental health problems. Each group actively cooperates in an effort to solve its problems. Such groups also work for the improvement of mental institutions, strive for enlightened legislation, help to establish centers for prevention and research, and educate others regarding the steps leading to good mental health.

National organizations have developed programs of public education for the improvement of services to the mentally ill. The National Committee for Mental Health works for the conservation of mental health, the reduction and prevention of mental disorders and defects, improved care and treatment of persons suffering from mental diseases, special training and supervision for the feebleminded, and the issuing of reliable information concerning these subjects. The National Mental Health Foundation sponsors a nation-wide program of public education to create a better understanding of mental disorders, and methods of prevention and cure. Its purpose is to correct false beliefs about mental ailments, to cooperate with other agencies in stimulating research and training, to provide better care and treatment for the mentally afflicted, and to replace outmoded laws with enlightened legislation.

Mental health is a problem of the entire world; this fact precipitated the adoption of international measures for mental health. The Expert Committee on Mental Health of the World Health Organization had its first meeting in 1949 to formulate and agree upon principles and priorities in mental health work. In view of the tremendous needs and the present shortage of psychiatric personnel and facilities throughout the world, the Committee decided that it would be impossible to provide therapeutic facilities for all the needy people in the world. The Committee therefore suggested preventive measures for the ultimate solution of the mental-illness problem. The group emphasized the importance of public health and community programs to promote mental health.

Other international organizations involved in promoting mental health include the UNESCO (United Nations Education, Scientific, and Cultural Organization) Project on International Tensions, which is probably the most elaborate international project involving psychiatric factors, and the World Federation for Mental Health, which is a group of nongovernmental organizations concerned with promoting mental health.

Prevention

Mental illness can be prevented. Prevention depends partly upon providing a healthful environment during childhood and partly upon helping the emotionally disturbed child early in his life. Other primary preventive measures include protection of the central nervous system from damage, facilitating the development of strong and mature personalities, providing help at critical periods in one's lifetime, e.g., puberty, military service, marriage, and retirement, and alleviating stress in the home, school or on the job.

The National Association for Mental Health lists the following ten signs of good mental health:

1. A tolerant, easygoing attitude toward yourself as well as others
2. A realistic estimate of your own abilities—neither underestimating nor overestimating
3. Self-respect
4. Ability to take life's disappointments in stride
5. Liking and trusting other people and expecting others to feel the same way about you
6. Ability to give love and consider the interests of others
7. Feeling part of a group and having a sense of responsibility to your neighbors and fellow men
8. Acceptance of your responsibilities and doing something about your problems as they arise
9. Ability to plan ahead and formulating realistic goals for yourself
10. Putting your best efforts into what you do and getting satisfaction out of doing it.

Certain guide lines are essential for maintaining good relations and mental health in community work. They are:

1. Basic honesty—Relate personal matters openly and relieve yourself of such pent-up emotions as love, hatred, and insecurity.
2. Attention and interest—Be sympathetic and a good listener; maintain a sincere and genuine interest in people; try to understand a person's actions, reactions, and interests.
3. Attempt to understand yourself and others in interaction with you.

Currently, researchers are investigating new methods of electroshock and psychosurgery. Scientists have learned how to analyze blood flowing through the living brain; this may lead to important discoveries. It is thought by some that the adrenal glands of the schizophrenics do not function as do those of normal people; certain chemicals produce false psychotic symptoms. The immediate future may belong to the biochemists and pharmacologists.

Other factors involved in preventing and solving our mental illness problem include our fast pace of life and the fact that many persons do not take the time to formulate a philosophy and to determine objectives in life. Once having formulated the objectives, we fail again if we do not strive to attain those goals we set for ourselves. In this respect, one famous psychiatrist commented that the truth of the matter is that most Americans today exist without purpose and without significance. They have no articulate philosophy; they do not live within any frame of reference. Some people are able to achieve their goals by themselves, but for most people religious faith plays an increasingly important role. Religious leaders, physicians, teachers, counselors, social workers, parents, and others are beginning to emphasize the importance of integrating all the factors of personality, environment, and emotional status when dealing with children and adults. The above groups are also beginning to understand and inform others about the meaning of the preamble to the constitution of the World Health Organization —"Health is a complete state of physical, mental, and social well-being and not merely the absence of disease or infirmity."

As with every health problem, when the citizens become fully aware of the need, the battle is half won. The outlook for a concentrated attack on the problem of mental illness looks promising in most states; interest is gaining, and more people are openly facing the problem.

Community Programs

Broad expansion of community mental health services took place during 1957 as a result of the large volume of state legislation aimed at stimulating mental health programs in the communities and at improving conditions for the mentally ill. During that year, many states passed laws providing grant-in-aid for community mental health services. Most bills provided for the following phases of a mental health program:

1. In-patient care—psychiatric hospital or county hospital
2. Out-patient care—community clinics
3. Rehabilitation
4. Consultation
5. Education.

Out-patient clinics included county health departments, family service agencies, and adult and child guidance clinics. Each program utilizes the mental health team approach, which usually consists of a psychiatrist, a psychologist, and a social worker. Most mental health programs emphasize the need for group interest and group education in an effort to gain further financial support from state and local government officials, as well as support from the public.

A new and different type of rehabilitation program has been operating successfully in San José, California. The "Quarters" is a temporary home for 25 men who have been released from mental hospitals. Here they are given a chance to draw that second breath, become adjusted, and find jobs before they tread the accustomed streets once again. Savings to taxpayers plus the expatients' earnings far exceed the small rehabilitation cost. Operating funds are obtained from voluntary contributions.

Although *early diagnosis* and *prompt treatment* are key phrases in the prevention of mental illness, new techniques and approaches are proving to be successful. A few include:

1. Immediate attention is being given to patients when they need it the most. In Amsterdam, Holland, for instance, a person in need of mental first-aid dials a certain telephone number. Shortly thereafter a consultant appears on the scene and becomes involved with the patient's problem at a very important and critical time.
2. Involving the entire family during treatment often solves certain problems of unknown origin. Actions and reactions within a family group are very difficult to isolate.

3. We may reach more persons in need of help by utilizing voluntary indoctrinated consultants, such as nurses, teachers, clergy, health educators, therapists, recreation leaders, physical educators, and others.

4. Attractive "problem clinics" placed strategically in a city where people may drop in to discuss their problems with sympathetic and understanding persons is proving successful. For example, Los Angeles opened a Suicide Prevention Center in 1958. This center is devoted to detecting possible suicide victims, including persons who are either threatening suicide or who have tried to commit suicide before and have failed. The center provides patients with psychiatric and psychological aid.

5. Certain advanced areas maintain placement centers for older and retired people. As our life expectancy increases the problem of keeping the aged active and productive becomes magnified.

Schools have begun to take a long, new look at mental health problems. The mental health team, including the psychiatrist, the psychologist, and the psychiatric social worker, have offered the following solutions to various school mental health problems:

1. A typical problem case is presented, discussed, and solved or concluded by the mental health team. Sometimes the problem is presented in the form of a sociodrama.

2. Individual consultation is designed to help the child and teacher understand each other.

3. Regular scheduled meetings with counselors enforces the school counseling and guidance program in many ways.

4. Case seminars are conducted where teachers present, discuss, make recommendations, and follow up certain cases.

5. On the job group therapy provides help for teachers, since all teachers have problems. Often informal discussions help clarify such problems, e.g., the reasons one particular student makes a teacher angry.

QUESTIONS FOR REVIEW

1. Define:
    (a) health
    (b) mental health
    (c) psychoses
    (d) neuroses
    (e) schizophrenia.

2. Discuss the merits of the following statement: "Mental health programs must place more emphasis upon treating and caring for the great number of mentally ill persons rather than providing mass prevention programs."
3. In what ways can we promote mental health and prevent mental illness?
4. Name and briefly discuss five recognized types of psychiatric treatment.
5. What agencies and organizations in your community are helping to promote mental health and prevent mental illness?
6. What are some of the various causes of mental illness?
7. Briefly discuss three new techniques and approaches in the prevention of mental illness that have proved successful in the community or school.
8. What are the purposes and function of a community mental health association?
9. How can the teacher help prevent mental illness?
10. "There was more mental illness in 1900 than there is today." Discuss this statement.

SUGGESTED READING

Blanton, Smiley: *Love Or Perish.* New York, Simon and Schuster, 1956.
Clausen, J. A., and Kohn, M. L.: *The Ecological Approach in Social Psychiatry.* Am. J. Sociol., 60:140–149, 1954.
Coleman, J. V.: *Relations Between Mental Health and Public Health.* Am. J. Pub. Health, 46:805–11, 1956.
Cummings, E., and Cummings, J.: *Closed Ranks.* Massachusetts, Harvard University Press, 1957.
Farnsworth, Dana, M.D.: *Mental Health in College and University.* Massachusetts, Harvard University Press, 1957.
Gorman, Mike: *Every Other Bed.* New York, World Publishing Co., 1956.
Hilleboe, Herman E., and Larimore, Granville W.: *Preventive Medicine, Principles of Prevention in the Occurrence and Progression of Disease.* Philadelphia, W. B. Saunders Co., 1959.
Hollingshead, A. B., and Redlich, F. C.: *Social Class and Mental Illness: A Community Study.* New York, John Wiley and Sons, 1958.
Jenkins, Richard L., M.D.: *Breaking Patterns of Defeat.* Philadelphia, J. B. Lippincott Co., 1954.
Kotinsky, R., and Witmer, H., Editors: *Community Programs for Mental Health.* Massachusetts, Harvard University Press, 1955.
Lemkau, Paul V.: *Mental Hygiene in Public Health.* New York, McGraw-Hill Co., 1955.
Lystad, M. H.: *Social Mobility Among Schizophrenic Patients.* Am. Sociol. Rev., 22:288–292, 1957.
Menninger, Karl, M.D.: *The Human Mind,* 2nd Ed. New York, Alfred A. Knopf, Inc., 1942.
Noyes, Arthur P., M.D., and Kolb, Lawrence C., M.D.: *Modern Clinical Psychiatry,* 5th Ed. Philadelphia, W. B. Saunders Co., 1958.
Rennie, T. A. C., Srole, L., and Opler, M. K.: *Urban Life and Mental Health.* Am. J. Psychiat., 113:831–836, 1957.
Reusch, Jurgen, M.D., and Bateson, Gregory: *Communication: The Social Matrix of Society.* New York, Norton Publishing Co., 1951.
Rose, A. M., Editor: *Mental Health and Mental Disorder.* New York, Norton Publishing Co., 1955.
Steiner, Lee R.: *A Practical Guide for Troubled People.* New York, Greenberg Publishing Co., 1952.

Strecker, Edward A., and Appel, Kenneth E.: *Discovering Ourselves, 3rd Ed.* New York, The Macmillan Co., 1957.

Tashman, Harry F.: *Today's Neurotic Family.* New York, New York University Press, 1957.

Williams, W. S.: *Class Differences in the Attitudes of Psychiatric Patients.* Social Problems, 4:240–244, 1957.

Chapter X

Environmental Sanitation

History

Many important sanitation principles had their beginnings in England. Slow sand filtration of community water supplies was initiated in England in 1829 by the Chelsea Water Company; Edwin Chadwick initiated the establishment of a board of health in 1848 to combat environmental hazards; and in 1849 John Simon and John Snow demonstrated conclusively that a community water supply polluted with human wastes could be dangerous.

The foundation for public health and sanitation in America was laid in 1850 with the publication of the Report of the Sanitary Commission of Massachusetts, 1849, by the Commissioners appointed under a resolution of the Legislature of Massachusetts and commonly called the Shattuck Report.[1] In the report, Lemuel Shattuck had strongly urged the formation of a state board of health in Massachusetts; however, it was not until 1869 that this state organ-

182

ized the second state health department in the country. In 1872 Stephen Smith founded the American Public Health Association, and in 1874, state laws concerning food sanitation were initiated by the state of Illinois. The Rockefeller Sanitary Commission, established in 1909 to combat hookworm, aided states in the establishment and organization of full-time county health departments and advanced sanitation programs. Although many sound sanitation principles were advanced early by a few pioneers, there has always been a social lag between discovery and adoption of these principles.

Through the years, the inventions of man have created new causes of pollution in his environment. The new, more subtle, insidious contaminants are the man-made undesirable by-products of technological progress. New, ubiquitous, and rapidly increasing chemicals, drugs, air pollutants, and water pollutants are finding their way into the air people breathe, the water they drink, and the food they eat. Although the problem is enormously complex and difficult, the gap between technology and biology must be closed quickly. In the last analysis, however, progress in this area will depend upon the attitudes and values of the people; these may be reflected by some citizens demanding "reasonably clean air and water at reasonable costs," and other citizens demanding "clean air and water at all costs." In either case, it is necessary for all to realize that water, air, and food respect no city or state boundary, and cooperation, coordination, and support of local bond issues are necessary to further the growth, development, and health of the nation.

The sanitarian of today understands and practices modern sanitation principles, and his services range from restaurant inspection to the all-inclusive nuisance abatement. Other areas of interest to the sanitarian are milk and food sanitation, air and water purity, garbage and rubbish disposal, and many other conditions of civilized living. In order to keep pace with the increasingly complex environment, the sanitary *engineer* has become a very important person in community health. Inspection, education, and enforcement must be supplemented by principles of sanitary engineering. A masters degree in public health sanitary engineering can be obtained at most of the approved schools of public health.

COMMUNITY WATER SUPPLIES
Sources of Water

The average American uses over 147 gallons of water each day. With the increase in population and the increase of per capita use

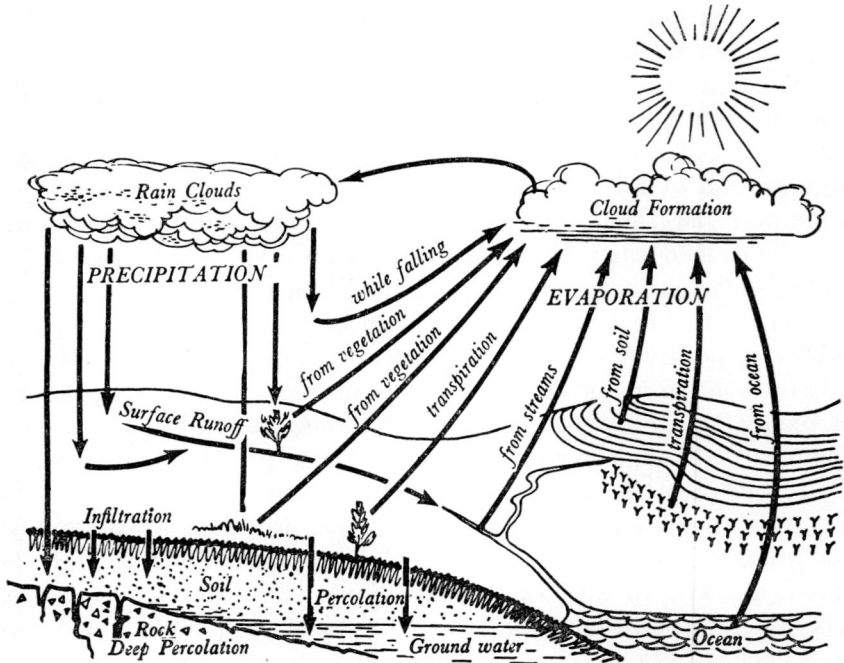

Figure 47. *The hydrologic cycle.* (Reprinted from the *Yearbook of Agriculture,* 1955, United States Department of Agriculture.)

of water, it is estimated that this figure will rise to over 225 gallons per day by the year 2000. Many large cities use the water from the rivers or lakes on whose shores they were founded. (See Figure 47.) Many communities depend on underground sources such as wells and springs for their water supplies. Some cities like New York and Los Angeles transport water from distant upland sources: e.g., water from the Colorado River is carried 400 miles through aqueducts as large as 16 feet in diameter to supply Southern California. Various sources of water are discussed on the following pages.

LAKES AND RESERVOIRS. Since lake water is clearer and less polluted than water from most streams it is the most satisfactory source of surface water. The term lake, often called a reservoir, means a large body of open fresh water fed by small tributary streams or springs. Lakes may be either natural or man-made. The clarity of lake water arises from the fact that lakes used for drinking water generally have forested watersheds and are fed by short tributary streams flowing in rocky channels. Storing water in lakes permits clarification by natural sedimentation, and the substantial removal of objectionable bacteria by time and sedimentation. Most lake water requires no treatment other than chlorination; a prominent example is the New York City supply. An auxiliary value of the lake may be its location at a higher elevation than the city served. The cost of pumping water is thus saved, and occasionally, electric power may be generated as well.

Certain limiting factors prevent the extensive use of lakes and reservoirs as sources of supply. Frequently, suitable sites and catchment areas within an accessible distance are lacking. Lake supplies are often costly, because of the large investments in land having watersheds for sanitary protection, long aqueducts, and sometimes cost of pumping. Slightly turbid lake waters may be more difficult to filter than more turbid stream waters. Seasonal taste and odor from plant growth are other problems.

STREAMS. Streams are the most common source of surface supply because more cities are accessible to an adequate stream source than to lakes and reservoirs. They are also the most common source of supply for cities above 25,000 population in this country, because adequate ground water resources are less frequently available. Stream supplies include brooks, creeks and rivers. Many mountain side spring-fed brooks, serving small communities, compare favorably in water quality with lake and reservoir supplies, and they do not require filtration. Most creek supplies and practically all river supplies must or should be filtered and chlorinated because of turbidity, color and pollution.

GROUND WATER. Ground water is obtained from below the surface of the ground. Such supplies include wells, springs, and infiltration galleries, the latter being rare. Wells and springs are the most common sources of supply for communities up to about 600 population. (See Figure 48.)

Water-Borne Diseases

Contaminated water may carry infection from human or animal waste or may have been rendered unwholesome by poisonous chemical compounds; this contamination can be easily checked by field or laboratory analysis. The greatest danger of pollution is from the discharges from the human body; there is very little danger of infection from lower animals or from the organic matter of plant life. Organisms discharged from humans are grouped as "colon bacilli" and are called the "coliforms." These are always present in human

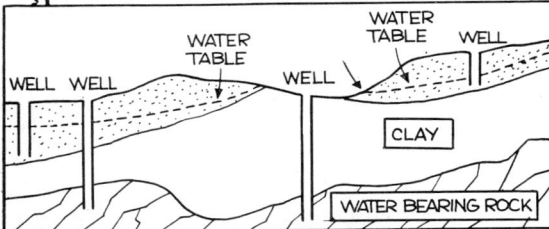

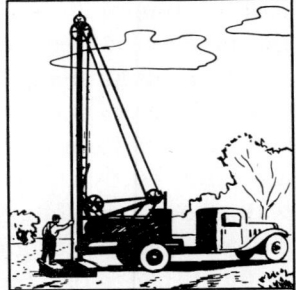

IF YOUR WATER SUPPLY COMES FROM UNDERGROUND SOURCES IT WILL USUALLY REQUIRE LESS TREATMENT, AS THE GROUND ITSELF WILL PERFORM MUCH OF THE FILTRATION AND PURIFICATION

WELLS DRAW WATER FROM POROUS UNDERGROUND FORMATIONS RESTING ON TOP OF NONPOROUS FORMATIONS DEPENDING ON THE GEOLOGY OF THE AREA. THE GROUND WATER MAY BE AT ANY DEPTH — IN SOME PLACES CROPPING OUT ABOVE THE SURFACE IN SPRINGS AND POOLS AND AT OTHERS SINKING TO MANY HUNDREDS OF FEET BELOW THE SURFACE

FROM THEIR KNOWLEDGE OF THE UNDERGROUND STRUCTURE OF AN AREA, BY THE SINKING OF TEST WELLS, AND BY USE OF GEOPHYSICAL EQUIPMENT, GEOLOGISTS CAN DETERMINE THE BEST LOCATIONS FOR DRILLING WELLS.

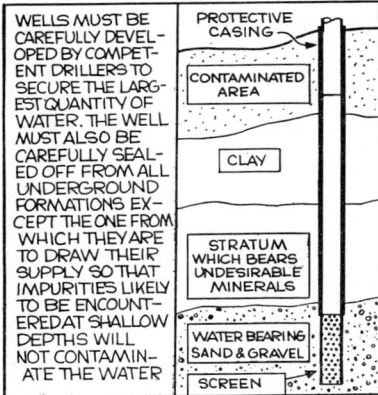

WELLS MUST BE CAREFULLY DEVELOPED BY COMPETENT DRILLERS TO SECURE THE LARGEST QUANTITY OF WATER. THE WELL MUST ALSO BE CAREFULLY SEALED OFF FROM ALL UNDERGROUND FORMATIONS EXCEPT THE ONE FROM WHICH THEY ARE TO DRAW THEIR SUPPLY SO THAT IMPURITIES LIKELY TO BE ENCOUNTERED AT SHALLOW DEPTHS WILL NOT CONTAMINATE THE WATER

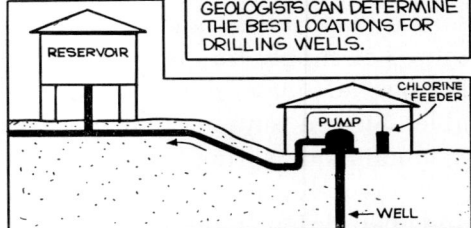

BETWEEN THE TIME THE WATER EMERGES FROM THE WELL AND THE TIME IT IS PUSHED OUT INTO THE REGULAR DISTRIBUTION SYSTEM BY THE WELL PUMP, IT RECEIVES SUCH TREATMENT AS THE LOCAL CONDITIONS REQUIRE. WHEN ONLY CHLORINATION TO DESTROY HARMFUL BACTERIA IS REQUIRED, A SIMPLE FEEDER IS USUALLY HOOKED UP TO OPERATE WITH THE PUMP.

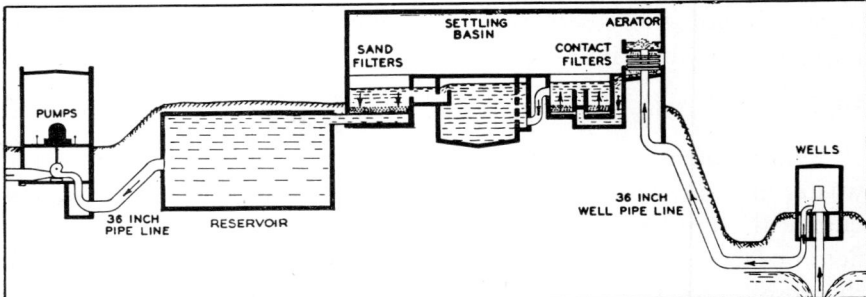

ELSEWHERE THE TREATMENT MAY BE MORE ELABORATE, REQUIRING SOFTENING, REMOVAL OF STAINING MINERALS AND IMPROVEMENT OF TASTES AND ODORS.

Figure 48. (From *The Story of Water Supply*. New York, American Water Works Association, 1957.)

intestines and feces and their presence indicates water contamination. A laboratory technician can test for this pollution by placing a water sample in a tube of lactose broth, and then incubating it at a temperature of 37 degrees Centigrade for 48 hours. The coliforms will ferment lactose and their presence is indicated by gas in the tube.

The most common of the water-borne diseases from pollution are typhoid fever, paratyphoid fever, the dysenteries (amebic and bacillary), gastroenteritis, infectious hepatitis, schistosomiasis, and Asiatic cholera. Typhoid, paratyphoid, dysenteries, gastroenteritis and Asiatic cholera are transmitted by urinary and intestinal discharges of ill persons and human carriers. Gastroenteritis is a diarrheal disorder involving the alimentary tract; infectious hepatitis is caused by a virus and could be transmitted by direct personal contact or from food, water, or milk. Poliomyelitis is also a virus disease which has been found in the feces of infected persons and in sewage; schistosomiasis organisms are parasites which have their life cycle in certain species of water snails. These organisms can leave the snail and are able to enter the skin of bathers or swimmers using the water for recreational purposes.

Water Treatment Methods

Since most lakes, reservoirs, streams, and ground water are subject to pollution, many community water supplies are purified and periodically analyzed for chemical or bacteriological contamination. The most common type of water treatment is the rapid sand gravity filtration method that consists of chemical addition and mixing, flocculation and sedimentation, filtration, and chlorination. The first three steps are designed to remove turbidity and color, although flocculation and sedimentation assist in the removal of bacteria and other organisms such as algae and protozoa. Filtration removes most impurities from the water, and effective filters include sand, diatomaceous silica, and anthracite coal. (See Figure 49.)

Disinfection of water depends upon the number and nature of organisms present, temperature, time of contact, pH (potential of hydrogen), oxidation potential, and the type of disinfectant used. Chemicals that have good disinfecting qualities include potassium permanganate, copper, silver, ozone, chlorine dioxide, and the halogens.

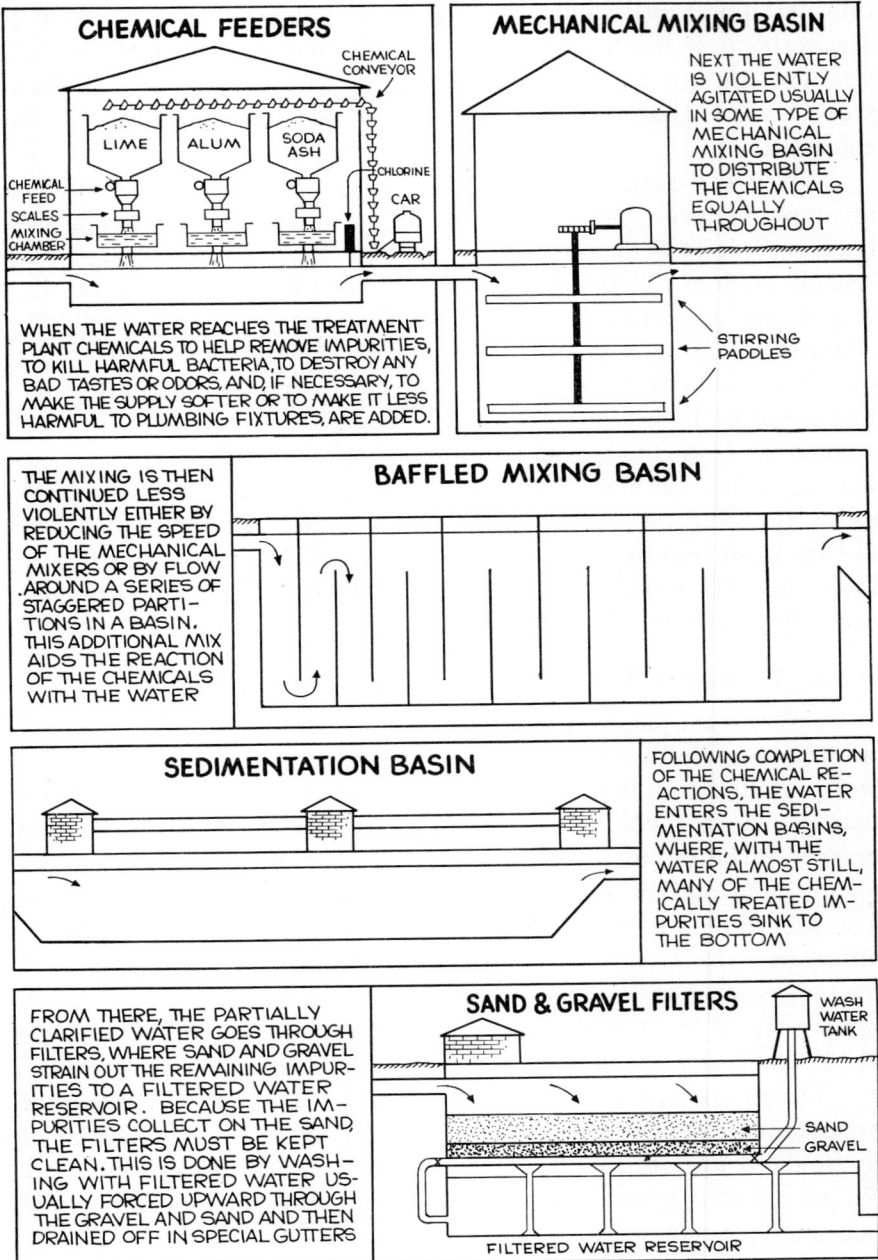

CHEMICAL FEEDERS

CHEMICAL CONVEYOR

LIME   ALUM   SODA ASH

CHEMICAL FEED SCALES

MIXING CHAMBER

CHLORINE

CAR

WHEN THE WATER REACHES THE TREATMENT PLANT CHEMICALS TO HELP REMOVE IMPURITIES, TO KILL HARMFUL BACTERIA, TO DESTROY ANY BAD TASTES OR ODORS, AND, IF NECESSARY, TO MAKE THE SUPPLY SOFTER OR TO MAKE IT LESS HARMFUL TO PLUMBING FIXTURES, ARE ADDED.

MECHANICAL MIXING BASIN

NEXT THE WATER IS VIOLENTLY AGITATED USUALLY IN SOME TYPE OF MECHANICAL MIXING BASIN TO DISTRIBUTE THE CHEMICALS EQUALLY THROUGHOUT

STIRRING PADDLES

THE MIXING IS THEN CONTINUED LESS VIOLENTLY EITHER BY REDUCING THE SPEED OF THE MECHANICAL MIXERS OR BY FLOW AROUND A SERIES OF STAGGERED PARTITIONS IN A BASIN. THIS ADDITIONAL MIX AIDS THE REACTION OF THE CHEMICALS WITH THE WATER

BAFFLED MIXING BASIN

SEDIMENTATION BASIN

FOLLOWING COMPLETION OF THE CHEMICAL REACTIONS, THE WATER ENTERS THE SEDIMENTATION BASINS, WHERE, WITH THE WATER ALMOST STILL, MANY OF THE CHEMICALLY TREATED IMPURITIES SINK TO THE BOTTOM

FROM THERE, THE PARTIALLY CLARIFIED WATER GOES THROUGH FILTERS, WHERE SAND AND GRAVEL STRAIN OUT THE REMAINING IMPURITIES TO A FILTERED WATER RESERVOIR. BECAUSE THE IMPURITIES COLLECT ON THE SAND, THE FILTERS MUST BE KEPT CLEAN. THIS IS DONE BY WASHING WITH FILTERED WATER USUALLY FORCED UPWARD THROUGH THE GRAVEL AND SAND AND THEN DRAINED OFF IN SPECIAL GUTTERS

SAND & GRAVEL FILTERS

WASH WATER TANK

SAND
GRAVEL

FILTERED WATER RESERVOIR

Figure 49. (From *The Story of Water Supply.* New York, American Water Works Association, 1957.)

Tracing the Origin of Polluted Water

The classical method of detecting and tracing typhoid carriers is by investigation of probable typhoid cases, followed by an analysis of individual fecal or rectal swab specimens. These procedures are complicated, time consuming, and require extensive contact with large numbers of people. The newer sewer swab technique provides a simplified and impersonal screening procedure for reducing the suspected area in which the carrier will probably be found with a minimum of community disruption. Typhoid organisms are traced to a specific sewer, then a specific area, and finally toilet swab tests are conducted in the homes in that area. A positive swab test is confirmed by analysis of stool specimens provided by individuals living in that particular home.

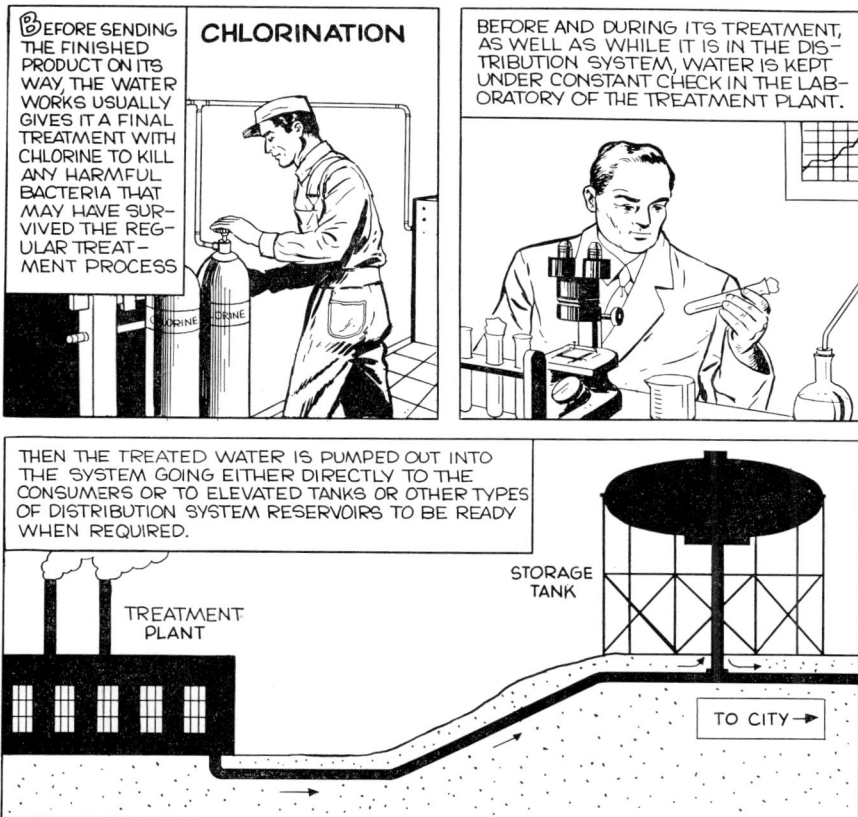

BEFORE SENDING THE FINISHED PRODUCT ON ITS WAY, THE WATER WORKS USUALLY GIVES IT A FINAL TREATMENT WITH CHLORINE TO KILL ANY HARMFUL BACTERIA THAT MAY HAVE SURVIVED THE REGULAR TREATMENT PROCESS

CHLORINATION

BEFORE AND DURING ITS TREATMENT, AS WELL AS WHILE IT IS IN THE DISTRIBUTION SYSTEM, WATER IS KEPT UNDER CONSTANT CHECK IN THE LABORATORY OF THE TREATMENT PLANT.

THEN THE TREATED WATER IS PUMPED OUT INTO THE SYSTEM GOING EITHER DIRECTLY TO THE CONSUMERS OR TO ELEVATED TANKS OR OTHER TYPES OF DISTRIBUTION SYSTEM RESERVOIRS TO BE READY WHEN REQUIRED.

STORAGE TANK

TREATMENT PLANT

TO CITY →

Figure 50. (From *The Story of Water Supply*. New York, American Water Works Association, 1957.)

Polluted water may be detected by the use of dyes to help trace the movement of water underground. *Fluorescein,* also called uranin, is considered a harmless organic dye, which can be removed by the use of filtration. The solution is mixed by adding one pound of fluorescein to one pound of caustic soda in ten gallons of water. If surface pollution of a well is suspected, some of the solution is sprinkled on the surface and the water is observed for color.

Fluorescein dye is also commonly used as a tracing agent in sanitary field practice, for:

1. Tracing the flow patterns and estimating rates of flow in sewers and streams
2. Estimating the detention times in sewage settling tanks
3. Detecting cross-connections between potable and nonpotable water supplies
4. Detecting the entry of surface of contaminated ground water into supply wells
5. Determining the zone of influence of waste discharges in receiving waters
6. Detecting emergent flows of waste effluents from subsurface disposal fields.

Care should be taken in the use of fluorescein and it should be avoided when the community may have contact with it in heavy concentrations. Care should also be taken to see that the dye does not enter potable water supplies of the community.

Under normal sanitary uses, the dye will be low in toxicity. The public should be protected from contact with heavy concentrations of the dye and water supplies should be diluted so that the dye is not detected by the naked eye. Precautions and expert handling of the dye should be followed carefully.

Rural Water Supplies

Rural water supplies are usually obtained from simple, shallow, and unprotected wells. The great increase in infectious hepatitis in the United States can be traced to shallow wells that have become polluted by inadequate disposal systems or ineffective septic tanks. Inadequate sanitary laws, and the lack of public health education, very often lead to poor sanitation conditions in the rural or suburban areas of a state.

The tops of driven wells should be carefully protected since polluted water may run down the sides of the pipe in the well. The well should have a heavy top bolted tightly to prevent loosening of the joints. The ground should slope away from the well and the area around the well should be kept clean.

Most county or state health departments have adopted specifications for property owners to follow in constructing wells. They will gladly send a consultant to help plan the well in order to prevent pollution. Basic well construction measures include:

1. The well should be of considerable depth to avoid excess seepage from the ground.
2. The well should be cased, in order to prevent shallow levels of water from seeping in.
3. A concrete collar should be constructed around the upper part to prevent surface washing from seeping in.
4. There should be a covering on the top to prevent tampering, and to keep dirt from entering.
5. The water should be lifted by means of a pump instead of a rope and bucket.

Chemicals in the Water

Chlorine is added to the water to kill the harmful or pathogenic bacteria that it may contain. (See Figure 50.) Chlorine is universally used in water purification because it is reliable, inexpensive, and easy to administer. Chlorine plus water yields hypochlorous acid plus hydrochloric acid, $Cl_2 + H_2O \longrightarrow HCl + HClO$. Hypochlorous acid is a very efficient disinfectant, especially at low pH values.

Copper sulfate is added to water to control the algae growth. It is applied in a proportion of 0.1 to 1.0 part per million parts of water. Some of the copper precipitates, settles to the bottom of the tank and is then removed from the water. Copper is not an accumulative poison; it is found even in the milk that we drink.

Physicians have experienced a problem with patients for whom they must prescribe strict sodium-free diets. Because public water supplies contain this mineral in varying degrees, many states and communities are now busy determining the sodium content of most of the public water supplies. With this knowledge, a physician will be able to determine whether or not a patient on a sodium restricted diet can drink from his usual source of water, or if distilled water must be prescribed.

Safe Community Water Supplies

When planning a safe community water supply, the following criteria should be considered:

1. The community should be able to obtain water at nominal water rates; have adequate methods of distribution; and provide minimum requirements adopted by the local health department.

2. A concentration of from 0.7 part per million to 1.5 parts per million of fluoride should be added to the water supply in order to give protection against tooth decay. Fluoridation has been approved by the American Dental Association, The American Medical Association, and The American Public Health Association in the United States. Research studies have proved that fluoridation of public water supplies in various communities has resulted in as high as a 65 per cent reduction in dental caries in children.

3. All water supplies should be chlorinated with a concentration of 2 parts per million to 5 parts per million. This procedure reduces the water-borne diseases to a minimum.

4. If surface water is used, it should be inspected and controlled at the watersheds.

5. The water supply intake should be located to reduce the possibility of pollution.

6. Plumbing codes should be designed to regulate plumbing cross-connections and prevent back siphonage.

The public health department, the city or county housing and planning commission, builders' organizations, and professional health organizations should all cooperate to provide safe water for the community.

WATER POLLUTION

Pollution of American rivers, lakes, and harbors is spreading an evil and potentially dangerous blight over the nation. Countless cities and towns flush their raw, untreated sewage into once beautiful streams. Over 15,000 industrial plants dispel millions of tons of poisonous, corrosive chemicals into the drinking water; over 100 million Americans depend on surface streams for drinking water. Polluted water is not only a health menace, but also decreases property value, destroys fish, and eliminates many recreational activities. It is estimated that the economic loss caused by water pollution amounts to over 1 billion dollars per year.

The burden on America's rivers and lakes grows with increasing industrialization, exploding population, and modern conveniences such as dishwashers and garbage disposals. The amount of sewage in the United States, which is estimated at over 50,000,000 pounds of solids per day, has increased 70 per cent in the past 20 years. The United States Public Health Service reveals that at least 10,000 new municipal and industrial treatment plants must be built, and 1,700 more plants must be modernized to handle the overload. The problem increases in complexity and importance with the increasing number of new synthetic chemicals, radioactive wastes, and detergents pouring into the water.

Inadequate Sewage Treatment Plants

Sewage treatment plants and chlorinated water have prevented disease for many years. However, many cities have inadequate sewage treatment plants; over 30 million Americans live in cities with no water treatment facilities. Most cities have only primary sewage treatment plants, whereby there is only a 30 to 40 per cent reduction in polluted material. The remainder of the pollution is discharged and stabilized by the stream itself. With increased population and industry, sewage treatment must be increased. Many sewage treatment plants, effective as they are against most germs, cannot cope with germs such as the virus of hepatitis and microscopic worms called nematodes. Sewage treatment plants were primarily designed to control bacteria pollution and break down and eliminate organic wastes. Present sewage treatment methods cannot cope adequately with detergents used widely by housewives, toilet paper, or chemical wastes from industries. These substances are soluble in water and go through the best treatment plants. (See Figure 51.) It is not uncommon in some areas to see a sudsy "head" appear when a glass of water is drawn from the tap. The harmful effects and toxicity of these detergents and chemicals is questionable and presently under investigation. Officials are, however, concerned with the potential long range chronic dangers.

A United States Public Health Service study in 1960 revealed that drinking water taken from 13 United States rivers contained nematodes that can carry disease-causing bacteria or viruses.[2] Many of these nematodes are able to withstand filtration and chlorination and serve as carriers of disease by ingesting and protecting pathogens. Investigators believe that the nematode population in any water supply can be reduced by using superchlorination on the raw water before treatment, and by having a more efficient flocculation process.

Prevention

The majority of states have laws which give authority to the state boards of health to make and enforce regulations governing

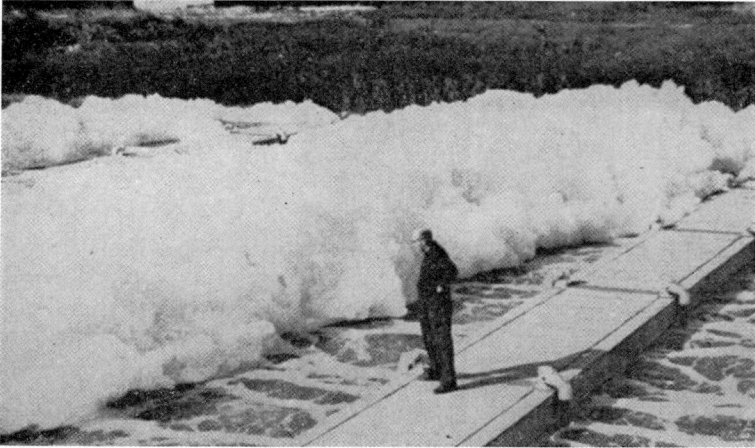

Figure 51. Billowing suds in one city's sewage plant reveal a growing problem. Present methods of treatment can't cope with detergents now used widely in American homes. (From *How Pure Is Your City Water?* U.S. News and World Report, Feb. 29, 1960.)

the quality of public water supplies. Standards that are recommended by the United States Public Health Service are usually followed. Some states have an additional agency; Oregon, for example, maintains a State Sanitary Authority. This committee works closely with the Oregon State Board of Health in controlling water pollution in the State.

In 1948, the Congress of the United States passed a Federal Water Pollution Control Act. This act gives the Surgeon General of the United States Public Health Service the authority to supervise stream pollution in the United States; the enforcement of this act, however, is delegated to each individual state. The act also provides for Federal research and consulting services to states, interstate agencies, municipalities, and industries throughout the United States. An amendment to the Federal Water Pollution Control Act in 1956 empowers the Public Health Service to call a conference of state agencies involved in a pollution problem, make recommendations, and establish a schedule for construction of treatment facilities by the offending cities and industries. Although this procedure usually brings results, the Secretary of Health, Education and Welfare may go further; he may call a public hearing and issue a formal notice to stop interstate pollution. If the notice is defied, the federal government, with the consent of the state pollution agency, may take the case to court in order to compel obedience.

To lighten the financial burden on cities, and to motivate state and local governments to take action, the federal government instituted a program of sewage-plant construction grants in 1956. It provides 30 per cent of the cost of any single project up to $250,000. By 1961 the federal government had invested $194,000,000 against local funds totaling nearly $1,000,000,000.

Although more than 40 states have enacted antipollution legislation, many communities have refused to finance the construction of sewage treatment plants. At the present time, primary sewage treatment can be provided at a cost of about 35 dollars per capita. Advanced or secondary treatment will cost from 80 to 150 dollars per capita. Citizens must unite and promote the construction of these plants in order to protect their health, and to restore the purity and beauty of their lakes, rivers, and streams. The Ohio River Valley offers an excellent example of what can be done in this area. In 1950 the basin's 17 million residents had few sewage treatment plants, and five million persons eliminated raw sewage directly into the river system. A small group of interested citizens organized the Ohio River Valley Water Sanitation Commission and initiated an educational attack followed by a fund raising campaign. The Junior Chamber of Commerce, Boy Scouts, newspapers, and other civic minded organizations supported local bond issue campaigns. River testing stations gained active cooperation from industry. The Commission gained the support of 1,000 basin towns and cities to build modern sewage treatment plants that cost up to $150 per capita. Today, treatment plants serve ten million residents, and new plants are being added rapidly. The results are already measurable in terms of clean, new beaches, fishing, boating, and water skiing.

In addition to the need for improved water treatment methods to deal with the problem like the nematodes, research experts at the Sanitary Engineering Center in Cincinnati, Ohio, are trying to find new methods of sewage treatment. Further research is also needed in capturing materials present in water, identifying the recovered material, and determining the effect of these materials in the body. Water monitors made to detect radioactivity and other pollutants must be installed in all water supplies.

As suburbs continue to grow, contagious disease hazards increase because of poor and inadequate sanitary facilities. Since no public sewer system exists in many suburban areas, many people are using septic tanks for sewage disposal. Where improper soil conditions occur, proper absorption of septic tanks effluent is impossible, and the effluent may find its way into wells or main drainage ways. The logical solution to this problem in suburbs is annexation to the nearest city and installation of public sewer systems. People must realize that any increase in taxes can be small compared to hospital bills.

Sewage Treatment

Although Lemuel Shattuck recommended that cities install sewer systems as a sanitary measure in 1850, there were only ten municipal sewer systems in the United States by 1860. By 1880 this number had grown to over 200. These sewers were all discharged into lakes or streams without any previous purification. In the cities, individual households gradually installed water closets that were drained into cesspools. This device was a large, closed, bricklined tank which was buried in the back yard, and was emptied at night at appropriate intervals with attempts at secrecy.

This system of sewage disposal met with general community disapproval because of the bad odor that was created. In 1851, when President Millard Fillmore first installed a permanent bath and water closet in the White House, these innovations met with great popular disapproval. The major objection to the installation of sewers was the fact that it was believed that sewer gas was poisonous and a source of infection.[3]

Today, disposal of sewage into the waterways is considered a privilege rather than a right. Nevertheless, raw sewage is drained into many rivers and bays throughout the country, and many sewage treatment plants are inadequate and ineffective in coping with the increased sewage, chemicals, and detergents. Sewage treatment plants should at least provide primary and secondary treatment in larger communities. (See Figure 52.)

Primary sewage treatment consists of screening and sedimentation. Screens may be coarse or fine and help remove large objects that may damage the pumps. Sedimentation, which takes place in settling tanks, allows the solids to settle when the velocity or flow of the turbid liquid is reduced or stopped. The solid portion of the settling tank, called sludge, is then transported to the digestion tank, where sludge particles support a colony of anaerobic bacteria, initiate biochemical oxidation of the sludge, and release the gases carbon dioxide and methane; these gases supply the energy to generate the pumps. The sewage is transported to open-air drying beds, and is then buried, burned, dumped, or sold for fertilizer.

Meanwhile, the liquid portion of the settling tank is transported to a secondary treatment tank, such as the open-air trickling filter type. In this tank, the sewage is sprayed on top of a large, deep, open bed of coarse stones, and the droplets trickle from stone to stone to the bottom of the bed, where they collect and flow into an underground drainage system, and the cycle is then repeated. This system utilizes aerobic bacteria, air, water, and sunlight that help oxidize and purify the liquid portion of the sewage. It is then chlorinated to reduce bacterial content and odor, and transported to the river or bay. This same sewage flows downstream, and may be the source of another community's water supply.

AIR POLLUTION

Smog and other forms of contaminated air, previously considered a local annoyance, are now recognized as a national problem and a menace to the future health of this country. Evidence from disastrous occurrences elsewhere, and from available data, though limited, are indicative that air pollution poses a significant public health problem. Further investigation reveals that air pollu-

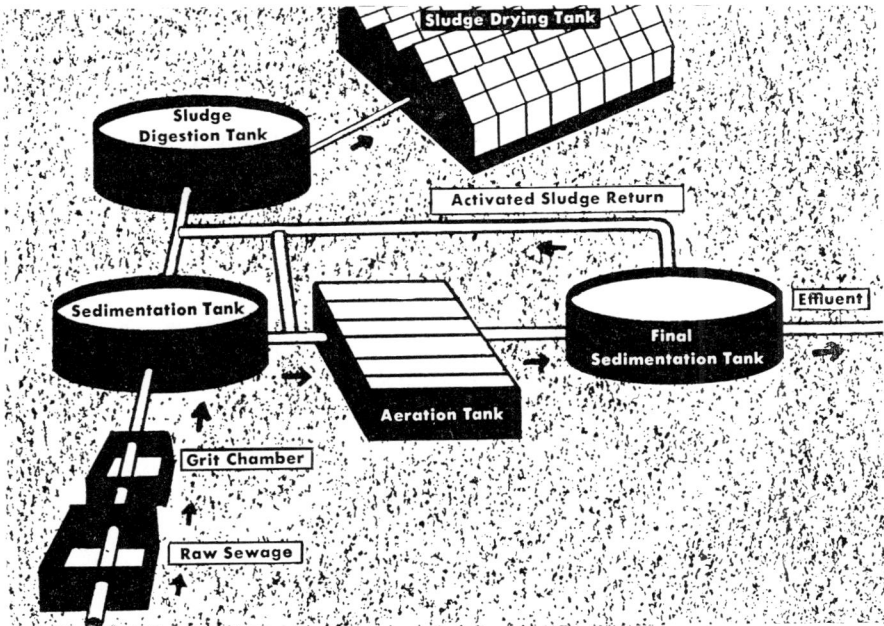

Figure 52. This activated sludge type of sewage treatment is used by many large cities. Solid matter is broken down by action of bacteria and air after it settles. (From Rosenblum, Marcus, *Public Health,* Merit Badge Series, Boy Scouts of America, 1956.)

tion is injurious to agricultural crops and livestock, and is hazardous to air and ground transportation.

At present, over ten thousand communities in the United States have some kind of an air pollution problem. Each year additional communities find it more difficult to keep the air supply fresh and healthful for people to breathe. This should be a major consideration, since each of us breathes in about 15,000 quarts of air per day. But the tendency to associate the smoking industrial stack with prosperity has consistently allayed community rebellion. This popular concept is now waning; people all over the industrialized world are awakening to the air pollution hazard.

Air and Health

There is no conclusive evidence that concentrations of community air pollution are producing severe harmful effects on the average person. However, studies reveal that air pollution may cause reduced visibility, eye irritation, respiratory irritation, damage to certain rubber and plastic products, crop damage, and discomfort. Other medical studies link air pollution with lung cancer, emphysema, and certain other diseases. In London, for example, chronic bronchitis-emphysema, an irreversible pulmonary disorder that can cause eventual heart failure, is the third leading cause of death (behind heart diseases and cancer) of men over 45 years of age. Many British doctors attribute its rapid rise to polluted air.

Three episodes of acute air pollution have been characterized by sudden death. These tragedies occurred in Belgium's Meuse Valley in 1930, in Donora, Pennsylvania in 1940, and in London in 1952. In each case a heavy fog had settled over the area and did not lift; in each case the phenomenon was produced by a temperature inversion or a layer of warm air over a layer of cold air; and in each case there was a heavy concentration of smoke and pollutants. During these periods, 63 deaths in Meuse Valley, 20 deaths in Donora, and three thousand deaths in London were attributed to air pollution. Most of those who died, however, were elderly people already suffering from diseases of the respiratory or circulatory systems.

Sources of Air Pollution

Three general types of substances are known to pollute the atmospheres of all industrial environments. These are chemical, radioactive, and biologic substances. Chemical pollutants are becoming the major concern because of expanding industrial, automotive, and domestic wastes. But we must also keep in mind the radioactive pollutants which add to the total exposure in both urban and rural air. Biologic dusts and pollens likewise may cause harmful effects, especially in persons who react to them with hay fever, asthma, and other allergies. The accidental industrial fumigation of the Mexican town, Poza Rica, during a temperature inversion in 1950 poisoned 329 persons and killed 22 in the immediate vicinity of an oil refinery. This catastrophe showed that hydrogen sulfide can diffuse through the air in concentrations sufficient to kill individuals in normal health. Other immediate lethal concentrations can occur to a degree far above tolerance levels.

Two major causes of air pollution are the steady and rapid industrialization and urbanization, and the weather. More than 40 foreign substances have been identified in the atmosphere of California coastal cities. The principal sources of some of these substances are identifiable: e.g., hydrocarbons in the atmosphere arise from motor vehicle exhausts, petroleum refinery processes, the storage and marketing of petroleum products, and from other sources; nitrogen oxides occur in exhausts from autos, household and industrial fuel, and oil and gas burners; smoke may be traced to domestic incinerators and fuel oil burners; dusts and fumes result from certain mineral and earth processes, metal industries, grain and feed processes and a wide variety of chemical industries; sulfur oxides are emitted from fuel oil burners, petroleum processes and chemical processes.

Tests made with air filters give an idea of the extent to which the atmosphere is being filled with dust, oxides, lint, chemicals, and substances that cannot be identified. For example, a study made in Louisville, Kentucky, revealed that a daily average of 440 tons of man-made substances are thrown into the air over the city's main industrial section; in Seattle, Washington, autos and trucks alone were found to be putting 100 tons of hydrocarbons, 20 to 80 tons of nitrogen dioxide, and four tons of sulfur dioxide into the city's air each day; in Chicago, the Illinois Institute of Technology found that each month, dust fall, a measure of air contamination, was averaging 52.9 tons per square mile compared with 71 tons in the same period of the year when industrial activity was significantly higher.[4]

Several organizations have made estimates of the kinds and amounts of air pollution originating from urban areas in California, particularly Los Angeles. More than 12,500 tons of pollutants are discharged (80 per cent by autos) into the air each day in the Los Angeles basin. This figure would be 3,300 tons higher without the city's severe industrial controls. Toxic substances include lead, acids, sulfur dioxide, oxides of nitrogen, organic substances, hydrocarbons, ozone, aldehydes, and carbon monoxide. Average carbon monoxide content in Los Angeles has risen from 5.5 parts per million in 1956 to 9 parts per million in 1960. Under Los Angeles air pollution control system, an alert would be called if carbon monoxide ever reached a level of 100 parts per million parts of air. It is estimated that a concentration of 200 parts per million for two hours is necessary to produce minimal effects in humans. Major contributors to air pollution include motor vehicles, oil refineries, fuel oil and fuel gas, gasoline marketing and distribution, refuse incineration and disposal, manufacturing, processing, chemical industries, exotic sources, combustion of fuels other than petroleum products and gas, locomotive and aircraft fuel combustion, and material from abrasion of rubber tires.

Many rural areas are now engulfed by air pollution. Unlike the air pollution problems in cities, however, the rural problems differ greatly in character from place to place. They reflect the nature of localized agricultural and industrial activities. Principal rural air pollution problems include: dust storms, smoke and charred sawdust from sawdust burners, dust clouds in delta lands, dust from cement plants, smoke, irritating vapors from hot road mix plants, odors from faulty disposal of organic industrial wastes, toxic aerosols from the use of insecticides, and smoke from orchard heating.

The Cost of Air Pollution

City officials and businessmen have learned how expensive air pollution can be. They count the billions of dollars damage from smog in cleaning bills, corrosion, crop losses, and lowered property values. Economic damage alone is estimated at five billion dollars per year. This can be expected to increase if toxic substances in the air are allowed to rise. Devices designed to "launder" the air used in manufacturing and utility plants have doubled in the last several years at a cost of about 300 million dollars per year. California alone appropriated a total of five million dollars during 1956 to fight air pollution; more money is being appropriated each year for this cause. Private industry is now spending about five hundred million dollars per year on air-pollution control work, and much more will be spent in the future.

Prevention and Control

Present control programs are aimed at reducing the quantity of waste materials disposed into the air because no other method of improving air quality has yet been developed. Before a community can intelligently plan an air pollution control program, it must have an understanding of the quantity of air available, a knowledge of the kind and amount of pollutants, and an understanding of the reactions that take place in the atmosphere.

To narrow the gap between the known and unknown factors in the air pollution problem, investigations are being carried on by many groups. Effective control of smog is not now possible because of a lack of fundamental information. No simple, inexpensive solution is at hand, but all groups involved in air pollution are working toward a solution and realize that they must:

1. Identify the compounds that cause typical smog conditions
2. Extend scientific studies to determine the nature of reactions taking place in the atmosphere, the substances entering into these reactions, and the compounds formed
3. Learn more about the adverse effects of air pollution on humans and identify the specific substances responsible
4. Develop additional knowledge so that standards for air quality can be established and hazards to health and damage to vegetation can be prevented
5. Devise reliable and practical means for continuously measuring air quality
6. Develop practical and effective means of controlling certain emission (particularly hydrocarbons from motor vehicles).[5]

Research

Many organizations are involved in air pollution research in an effort to find answers to certain problems. The Taft Sanitary Engineering Center in Cincinnati, Ohio, is involved in many studies, and also coordinates the National Air Sampling Network, which has over 170 stations throughout the country. The National Cancer Institute is also investigating the relationship between certain pollutants and cancer. The result of work carried on by the Franklin Institute of Philadelphia under the sponsorship of the American Petroleum Institute during 1956 is significant. Here, a unique long path infrared spectrophotometer study of smog-producing gas mixtures resulted in the identification of a compound which is believed to play an important role in the generation of large amounts of ozone. Almost all the investigations of several agencies into the reactions that produce smog have emphasized the importance of nitrogen dioxide as a key compound in its formation; the major sources of nitrogen dioxide are known. They are generated in the combustion processes in which nitrogen and oxygen from the air combine at elevated temperatures. For example, the automobile engine is a combustion engine, and power plants and heaters use the combustion processes. However, the exact manner in which nitrogen dioxides are formed, how they can be controlled, and what effect their control will have on smog formation is only partly understood.

The significance of all combustion processes in air pollution has been highlighted by research at the University of California in Berkeley. Here it was shown that whenever the combustion of fuel, including the very simple hydrocarbons, is incomplete, many complex substances are generated.

Many agencies and organizations are involved in air sampling programs, consisting of measuring and recording air contaminants; establishing background levels for measuring pollutants; and studying air quality, nature of emissions, meteorological conditions, and effects of air pollution. Meteorologists assigned by the United States Weather Bureau conduct studies of wind projections to determine the origin of the air that passes over the remote air sampling stations. Studies to determine the health effects of air pollution include: analyses of mortality data of exposed populations to determine whether or not such pollution contributes to death; study of the sickness experience through special surveys of the exposed general population, of school and industrial groups, and of patients admitted to hospitals; investigation of the effects of air pollution on the frequency and intensity of attack of hay fever, asthma and other respiratory illnesses; and studies of the effects of air pollution on normal activities of individuals.

Engineering

The solution of a community's air pollution problems will depend in part on the successful application of these engineering principles:

1. Control of air pollution emissions at the source. For example, internal combustion engines, electrostatic precipitators on smoke stacks, auto exhaust filters.
2. Substitution of materials and methods. For example, sanitary land fill in place of backyard incineration.

3. Zoning in locating new industrial plants.

4. Improving ventilation of communities by thermal, catalytic, or mechanical methods.

5. Neutralizing the pollutants in the atmosphere.

6. Governing emissions according to meteorologic conditions, relayed in advance perhaps, by a weather detector photographic satellite.[6]

Legislation

Local or regional government has the prime responsibility for regulating and controlling air pollution. Yet, only about three hundred communities have active, operating control programs, and only 15 states have comprehensive air pollution legislation. It is apparent that additional legislation is needed to achieve state-wide air pollution control programs. In most states the director of public health has the power to summarily abate public nuisances creating a public health hazard. The Attorney General may also bring a civil action to abate a public nuisance such as smog for the protection of public rights and interests. However, the power of each official is restricted because it is extremely difficult to determine who is polluting the air, whether the pollution constitutes a public nuisance, and whether there is imminent danger of irreparable damage to vital plant and animal life.[6]

A new and interesting example of state legislation in the fight against smog is reflected by the law enacted by the California legislature in April, 1960, which requires every new car registered in the state to be equipped with an antismog device or "afterburner" within a year after the Motor Vehicle Pollution Control Board approves at least two such devices. Within three years after approval, practically all cars and trucks in the state will be required to have the devices. The afterburner is a device or attachment that will oxidize or burn the fuel in the automobile exhaust more completely. Without the afterburner about 5 to 10 per cent of the automotive fuel is not burned, and is discharged into the air.

The first federal law relating to air pollution was passed in 1955. The Federal Air Pollution Act authorized the United States Public Health Service to make studies of air contamination in states and cities, and appropriated a sum of five million dollars per year for a five-year period. The United States Public Health Service conducts a vast research program, trains people in the technical phases, and extends technical assistance and consultation to states and localities. Nevertheless, the major responsibility for regulatory control of air pollution remains, as it should, at state and local levels. One major problem, however, is whether unified multicounty districts are more effective and practical than local enforcement of anti-smog regulations. Proponents of the district plan contend that the district has the responsibility for curbing smog, and that smog does not respect government boundaries. They further claim that the use of local smog policemen would counterbalance the strength and position of the district by placing smog control at the mercy of local politicians and thus make enforcement a matter of local political manipulation.

Most municipalities and counties under state constitutions have extensive police power to abate air pollution by the enactment of air pollution control ordinances. Unfortunately air pollution does not respect political boundaries. Local smoke-control ordinances and adequate provisions for waste disposal to stop backyard burning and excessive air pollution by industry, however, are clearly necessary and proper.

OCCUPATIONAL HEALTH

History

Medical history reveals that the health of the individual was often influenced by his occupation. Many match sellers and glass blowers were afflicted with eye trouble, miners developed lung disease, hat cleaners contracted psychic disturbances, musicians developed hernia, and flute players had lung edema. Hippocrates described diseases in the metal workers in the year 460 B.C. and Pliny, the Elder, is said to have invented the first gas mask, but it remained for farsighted Bernardo Ramazzini to give a comprehensive description of the many diseases associated with occupation. His book, *A Treatise on the Disease of Workers,* is still an authoritative classic, although it was first published in the year 1700.

Modern occupational health is an outcome of the industrial revolution in England in the nineteenth century. At that time numerous laws were passed for the protection of workers as a result of the increasing deplorable work conditions, and the exploitation of women and children in industry. Dr. Alice Hamilton, author of *Industrial Poisons in the United States*, published in 1925, is considered the founder of industrial toxicology in the United States and is recognized as having opened the era for the modern practice of industrial medicine. Medical care for employed groups had its beginnings in 1887, when the Homestake Mining Company of

South Dakota established a medical department with a full-time staff providing complete medical services to employees and their families.

The theory of workmen's compensation as a social answer to legal problems and failure of existing laws originated in England and gradually spread throughout the world. The first workmen's compensation law in the United States was enacted in 1908 and covered certain injuries and disease of federal employees. New York, Maryland, California, and Wisconsin were the first states to enact workmen's compensation laws. The slow progress, in this area, however, is illustrated by the fact that today, 19 states have only partial coverage, two states have no provisions, and about half the states limit medical benefits in occupational disease cases.

Present Concepts

Occupational health is primarily a preventive program aimed at the protection and promotion of health of the employed workers. The objectives of the occupational health program as advanced by the American Medical Association Council on Industrial Health are:

1. Detection, evaluation, and correction of hazards to health imposed by environment and materials of work

2. Medical examination of employees to effect suitable job placement and to discover health impairments caused by work surroundings. Ideally, health education, and counseling are included.[7]

Such programs have been found to help improve employees health morale and good will, and they have also resulted in savings from decreased workmen's compensation costs, lower insurance premiums, increased efficiency, fewer infections and disease, better placement and less turnover, improved working conditions, better health education and diminished absenteeism. For example, the National Association of Manufacturers reported that health costs in the average company with ordinary risks of accident and disease are:[8]

"A 500 man plant has an expectancy of 335 days of disability due to industrial accident and disease, and 4,500 days due to nonoccupational injury and illness. Translated into money, this represents an average wage loss of $48,350 to employees, based on a daily wage of $10. Proportionately, in a 200 man plant the wage loss is $20,000 per year; in a 100 man plant, $10,000 per year."

Industrial health programs are increasing in large industries that can afford facilities and personnel for such a program. Industrial medicine is a growing specialty, and there are over 2,000 physicians working in this field. A good industrial health program may include preemployment and periodic physical examination for employees, counseling and guidance, prevention of industrial health hazards and disease, health education, and immunization and rehabilitation programs. This program usually involves the services of a physician, nurse, and industrial hygiene or safety engineer.

Official Agency Programs

Official agency programs were initiated because occupational diseases and deaths were increasing throughout the nation and most of these were preventable. Funds for occupational health programs were allocated to state and local health departments as a result of the Social Security Act in 1935. Renewed interest in this field developed after certain industrial tragedies occurred that could have been prevented by such a program. The continued existence of these programs is related to rapid industrial expansion and the daily introduction of complex health hazards in the form of chemicals or processes.

The first state occupational health programs were initiated by New York and Ohio in 1913. The following year The Office of Industrial Hygiene and Sanitation was created as a branch of the United States Public Health Service. An occupational health division may include a physician, nurse, industrial hygiene engineer, industrial hygiene chemist, and public health educator who work as a team in an effort to protect and promote the health of the workers in the community. Today, most state health departments and a few local health departments have occupational health divisions. In some states occupational health matters are the joint concern of the Department of Public Health and The Division of Industrial Relations. However, the state occupational health divisions generally are hampered by lack of funds and personnel, and are able to reach only about 10 per cent of the nation's workers each year.

The scope of the local health department's occupational health program is broad since it includes all occupations, but most programs direct their major efforts toward the manufacturing segment of industry; more people are employed in this category and the number of hazards is greater. Services of the occupational health division may include periodic physical examinations of government employees, prevention of industrial health hazards and disease, consultation, and education. The Federal Environmental Health Center located at Cincinnati, Ohio, now employs hundreds of scientists and technicians, and is leading the way in environmental health research and field investigations. In general, the local health department may be divided into engineering, medical and nursing, and laboratory services.[9]

1. Engineering services include: review of plans for new procedures or processes or for proposed changes in established operations; engineering survey of an entire plant or selected operations for job hazards; consultation on industrial waste disposal and air pollution problems; consultation and assistance in the design of engineering control measures including industrial exhaust systems.

2. Laboratory services refer to: analytical chemistry determinations in connection with any of the engineering studies; consultation concerning chemical methods of control or concerning the development of laboratory testing procedures related to occupational health, and the analysis of materials of known or suspected toxic composition.

3. Medical and nursing services include: consultations concerning the need for, or the organization and conduct of, employee health plans; assistance in planning medical facilities and in the selection of equipment; consultation and assistance in defining causal relation of diseases noted in the working environment and in the prevention, diagnosis and management of occupational diseases. In addition, the division actively promotes on-the-job rehabilitation beginning with the injured employee and progressing through the plant nurse and all of the agencies involved.

4. Special studies relating to possible occupational disease or hazards in certain groups is of particular concern. An example of such a study is one which has to do with radiation exposure of dentists and dental assistants.

The public health problems in this area are increasing rapidly. A major problem is the increasing production of new compounds and chemicals, many of which may be harmful or injurious to workmen, farmers, and others. Increasing uses of radioactive materials present new and different ocupational health problems. With increased numbers of working women, opportunities for health promotion and protection are being expanded. State and local health departments must continue to expand their occupational health programs in order to cope with these increasing problems, protect and promote the health of the worker, and save the taxpayers' money.

Environmental Agents

One of the major objectives of an occupational health program is the prevention of adverse effects by environmental agents. Environmental agents may be divided into three categories: chemical

Silicosis—still the No. 1 occupational disease.

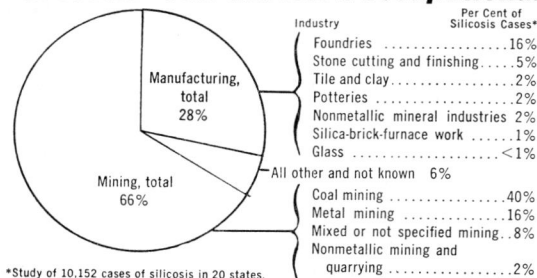

Industry	Per Cent of Silicosis Cases*
Foundries	16%
Stone cutting and finishing	5%
Tile and clay	2%
Potteries	2%
Nonmetallic mineral industries	2%
Silica-brick-furnace work	1%
Glass	<1%
All other and not known	6%
Coal mining	40%
Metal mining	16%
Mixed or not specified mining	8%
Nonmetallic mining and quarrying	2%

Manufacturing, total 28%

Mining, total 66%

*Study of 10,152 cases of silicosis in 20 states.

Despite the accomplishments of dust control measures, silicosis is still the major occupational disease in the U.S. in terms of disability and compensation costs. Silicosis cases, which represent only 3% of claims, account for more than one quarter of all compensation awarded in occupational disease cases by the New York State Workmen's Compensation Board. The latest count of persons with silicosis in 26 states in the U.S. was 12,763; however, this number does not include many persons with nondisabling silicosis. At least half and probably closer to three quarters of workers disabled by silicosis are over 50 years of age.

Dermatitis is a widespread industrial problem.

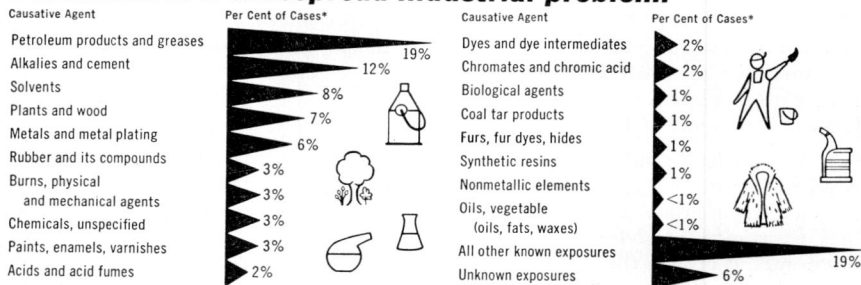

Causative Agent	Per Cent of Cases*
Petroleum products and greases	19%
Alkalies and cement	12%
Solvents	8%
Plants and wood	7%
Metals and metal plating	6%
Rubber and its compounds	3%
Burns, physical and mechanical agents	3%
Chemicals, unspecified	3%
Paints, enamels, varnishes	3%
Acids and acid fumes	2%

Causative Agent	Per Cent of Cases*
Dyes and dye intermediates	2%
Chromates and chromic acid	2%
Biological agents	1%
Coal tar products	1%
Furs, fur dyes, hides	1%
Synthetic resins	1%
Nonmetallic elements	<1%
Oils, vegetable (oils, fats, waxes)	<1%
All other known exposures	19%
Unknown exposures	6%

Figure 53. The most common industrial health problem is occupational dermatitis. Dermatitis of occupational origin tends to be temporary in nature and less costly than most other occupational diseases. Average cost per case in New York is $698. About 90% of dermatoses are caused by contact with chemicals, four fifths of which are primary irritants, the remainder are sensitizers. It is estimated that slightly less than half of occupational dermatitis cases in the manufacturing industries are caused by petroleum products. In the case of dermatitis, 41,628 workers were studied. (From Patterns of Disease. Parke, Davis and Co., January, 1960.)

agents, physical agents, and biological agents. Chemical agents may be the gaseous contaminants, such as carbon monoxide, or particulate matter contaminants such as dust, fumes, mist, and fog. Physical agents include high or low air pressure, temperature and humidity, illumination, radiant energy, mechanical vibration, and noise. Biological agents include many communicable diseases which often have an occupational origin such as anthrax and brucellosis.

Injurious substances reach the body and cause damage by inhalation, skin contact, and ingestion. The nature and degree of injury are determined by the nature of the substances involved, the intensity and length of exposure, and the susceptibility of the person exposed. Despite the accomplishments of dust control measures, silicosis is still the major occupational disease in terms of disability and compensation costs. Dermatitis continues to be the most common industrial health problem. (See Figures 53 and 54.) It is interesting to note that the most dangerous occupations include coal mining, logging, steel erection, and electric light and power work in terms of accidental death and disabling injuries. Nevertheless, occupational diseases and hazards are decreasing due to expanding industrial medical services, legislation, development and use of protective engineering and safety measures and devices, and continuous health education programs.

Industrial Safety Programs

The industrial safety programs have helped reduce the national industrial accident frequency 75 per cent during the period from 1926 to 1954. This reduction was due largely to the application of preventive medicine in industry. During this period absenteeism was cut in half, compensation costs were reduced by two-thirds, and accident sickness costs were decreased 40 to 50 per cent. Many small plants joined medical service plans which served many companies.

Health hazards—from fiber glass to actinic rays.

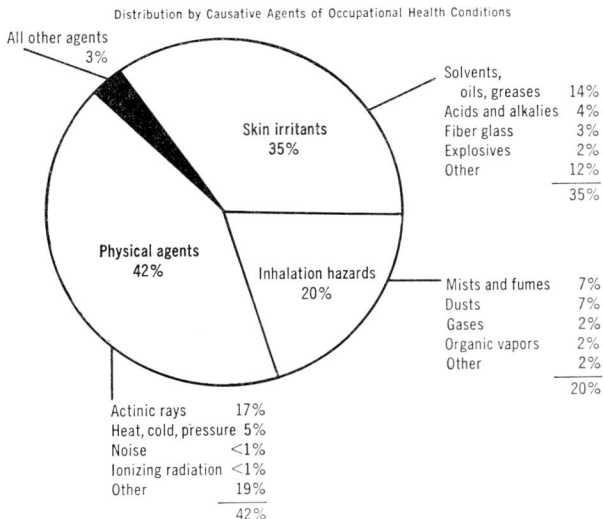

Distribution by Causative Agents of Occupational Health Conditions

All other agents 3%

Skin irritants 35%

Solvents, oils, greases 14%
Acids and alkalies 4%
Fiber glass 3%
Explosives 2%
Other 12%
————
35%

Physical agents 42%

Inhalation hazards 20%

Mists and fumes 7%
Dusts 7%
Gases 2%
Organic vapors 2%
Other 2%
————
20%

Actinic rays 17%
Heat, cold, pressure 5%
Noise <1%
Ionizing radiation <1%
Other 19%
————
42%

Figure 54. Study of 1,733 occupational medical conditions occurring among 314,000 civil service employees during 1957. (From Patterns of Disease, Parke, Davis and Co., January, 1960.)

Industrial accidents are caused by personal or mechanical difficulties. It has been said that 80 to 85 per cent of industrial accidents are due to faulty human actions and less than 20 per cent are due to mechanical design factors. Perhaps safety may be improved if mechanical design is more closely related to the anatomical, physiological, and psychological characteristics of workers. Personal causes include unnecessary exposure, accident proneness, improper starting or stopping of machinery, operating machinery at unsafe speed, lack of skill or knowledge, improper machine guards, hazardous arrangements, and unsafe wearing apparel. A good accident-prevention program in industrial safety includes personnel selection combined with adequate medical examination, human engineering, and job supervision.

FOOD SANITATION

The local health department has the responsibility for protecting the public's health against food contamination. This includes epidemiological investigations, regulation and enforcement of minimum sanitary food standards, supervision of food establishments, and health education. Sanitarians must keep pace with the rapidly changing technology of quick freezing, radiation, and the use of antibiotics in perishable foods. (See Appendix 5 for food and sanitary engineering inspection forms.)

Salmonella and staphylococci germs are very prevalent and multiply rapidly in food, and thus gastroenteritis and "food poisoning" are the predominant infections transmitted by food. Other diseases transmitted by food include the common cold, typhoid fever, amebic dysentery, and bacillary dysentery. Tapeworms and other parasites occasionally contaminate the food supply. However, many other germs may be carried by utensils; the drinking glass is the most important vehicle of transmission, and the poorly operated and managed bar, soda fountain, and luncheonette are the worst offenders among food handling establishments. (See Figure 55.)

Food poisoning symptoms include cramps, diarrhea, and vomiting within three hours to two days after eating contaminated food. Foods that are intimately handled, stored, and mixed after cooking have the highest frequency of food-borne infection. These include salads, sauces, creamed foods, and cream-filled pastries and pies. If food is kept longer than one hour at room temperature before it is eaten, food poisoning may contaminate it. Nine easy rules for safe food are:

1. Keep cold foods cold—hot foods hot. Don't let foods stand at room temperature. (Above 140° Fahrenheit hot; Below 40° Fahrenheit cold.)
2. Keep hands clean and touch food with hands as little as possible.
3. Don't let anyone with a skin infection or a cold handle food.
4. Keep kitchens, dining rooms, or food sale booths free of flies and cockroaches.
5. Protect foods from sneezes, handling, and dust.
6. Be sure poisons are well labelled and kept far away from the place where food is prepared.
7. Wash dishes, glasses, and silver by methods recommended by your health department. Use paper service when possible.
8. Wash fruits and vegetables carefully.
9. Do not keep fruit juices in galvanized containers.

Food poisoning by chemicals frequently encountered include:

1. Cyanide, which is contained in some silver polishing compounds
2. Cadmium and zinc from cooking, storage, and refrigeration utensils and equipment

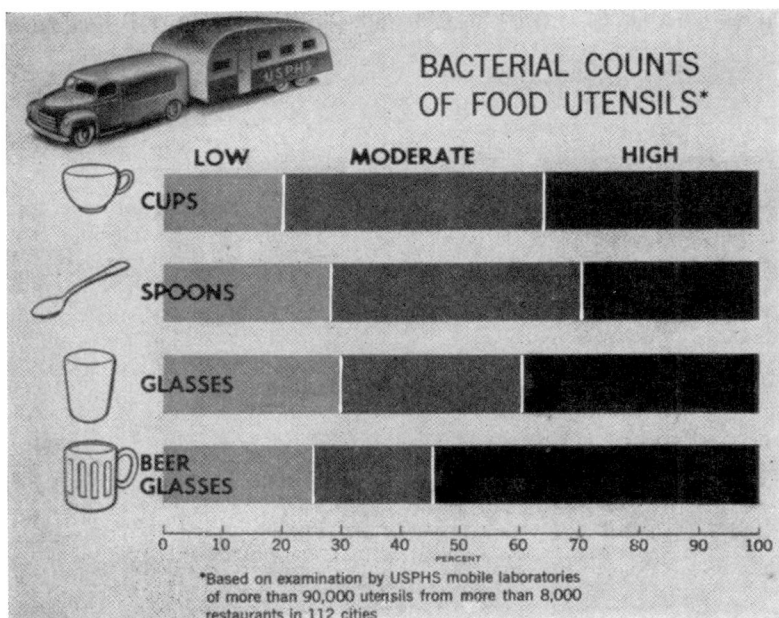

Figure 55. (From *Environment and Health.* U.S. Public Health Service, Washington, U.S. Government Printing Office, 1951.)

3. Arsenic as a spray residue on fruits

4. Sodium nitrite mistaken for the preservative sodium nitrate. With the increased use of new insecticides, fruits and vegetables must be carefully washed.

Botulism, a highly fatal form of food poisoning, usually results from improperly home canned foods. Boiling before serving will destroy the poison but the only specific treatment is the limited botulinus antitoxin. Mussel and clam poisoning is another highly fatal form of food poisoning, which has been kept under control in many shore areas by quarantining mussels during warm months.

The objectives of food control include protecting the consumer from:

1. Food-borne infections
2. Food poisoning by bacterial toxins
3. Poisoning by toxic chemicals and metals
4. Effects of undesirable aesthetic conditions such as dirt in food, utensils, and surroundings
5. Prevention of adulteration.

In order to meet these objectives, sanitarians observe and supervise the following criteria:

1. The food and drink served should be safe.
2. The personal hygiene and food handling practices of the food handlers should be satisfactory.
3. The water supply should be safe.
4. Sewage, other liquid wastes, garbage, and other solid wastes should be disposed of in a sanitary manner.
5. Food should be protected from contamination during production, processing, display and storage.
6. Utensils and equipment should be washed, sanitized and stored in a sanitary manner.
7. The general sanitary maintenance of an establishment should be satisfactory, this includes exclusion of rodents, vermin and flies; refrigeration, handwashing and toilet facilities should be clean; good housekeeping, adequate light, ventilation and satisfactory arrangement of facilities should be provided.

Education and guidance have replaced threats and legal suits in restaurant sanitation; education activities are directed toward the public, management and food handlers. The most significant development in this area has been the establishment of short training courses for food handlers by many health departments. Education of food handlers may be supplemented by periodic physical examinations in order to detect tuberculosis, typhoid fever, and other diseases that may be transmitted by "carriers." Large food companies are now employing trained, experienced public health engineers and sanitarians to supervise food production and promote education. Trained specialists in food sanitation are also employed by restaurant associations and chains in an effort to educate and self-police members and units.

MILK SANITATION

Milk is an excellent food but it is also a favorable culture medium for many diseases. Milk-borne diseases include streptococcal infections, diphtheria, dysentery, tuberculosis, brucellosis, typhoid, and paratyphoid fever.

Opportunities for milk infection are numerous; the first source of infection is the cow. Diseases indigenous to the cow include brucellosis and bovine tuberculosis. Brucellosis and tuberculin testing of cows is standard procedure today. In addition, infected udders are a source of human streptococcal infection, but this perhaps should be considered an exotic disease of the cow since it is generally contracted by the cow as a localized infection from a human milk handler. The usual form of bovine mastitis is caused by other streptococci which are non-pathogenic to man. Opportunity for infection arises with the milk handler who may contaminate the milk through carelessness, lack of personal hygiene, or disease. Other opportunities for milk infection involve unsanitary utensils, equipment, barn, and impure water used in cleaning the utensils and equipment. Nevertheless, milk sanitation programs emphasize education rather than compulsion to achieve results.

Pasteurization

Pasteurization is a bactericidal process which applies heat to milk for a sufficient time-temperature period to kill all milk-borne pathogens without impairing the flavor or nutritive quality of milk. Cooling of milk before and after pasteurization is an important supplemental safeguard. The tubercle bacillus and the Q fever organism seem to be the most resistant germs under most time-temperature combinations. Pasteurization may best be performed in a neutral time-temperature zone.

The most common method of pasteurization is called the Holding Method and involves holding milk at a temperature of between 142° F. and 145° F. for thirty minutes. The newer high-temperature, short time method is a flow-through process whereby milk is heated to 160° F. for 15 seconds.

Pasteurization should not be considered a substitute for proper sanitation, but rather an essential supplementary safeguard for all fluid fresh milk. To the milk sanitarian and other public health workers, properly pasteurized milk is safer than certified raw milk. The necessity for pasteurizing raw milk, even when produced under spotlessly sanitary conditions is highlighted by the fact that no practical system of inspection has been developed that can ensure the noninfectiousness of the cow and the milk handler at all times. Cows may contract brucellosis and human streptococcal organisms between frequently performed veterinary inspections; milk handlers may become harborers of streptococcal and salmonella organisms without evidence of illness, and typhoid carriers are not always detected by single or random stool examination. When milk is produced and handled under other than virtually aseptic conditions, as is generally the case, the argument for effective pasteurization is strengthened.

Sanitary milk tests include:

1. Direct microscopic counts for total bacteria
2. Direct microscopic examination for specific organisms, especially strepto-cocci
3. Plate counts for total bacteria
4. Phosphatase test that determines the effectiveness of the pasteurization process (This enzyme is present in raw milk, but is thermosensitive at pas-turization temperature.)
5. Coliform test (Pasturization kills all coliform organisms.)
6. Reductase test determines the bacterial condition of milk
7. Sediment test indicates the cleanliness of the milk.

Effective control programs are administered by trained city and county sanitarians with the support of state health and agriculture departments and private dairies. Most of their work is guided by basic state laws and supplemented by local ordinances. Individual states have vested authority over milk sanitation in either the health department or the agriculture department. In an effort to standardize milk sanitation and pasteurization regulations, the Public Health Service published a code interpreting the standard milk ordinance. This code has been accepted by many states as the basic regulation for an interstate certification program and an industry-wide education program. In addition, the Public Health Service initiated the interstate Milk Certification Program, which provides for milk shipments to be inspected and rated by state health officials and certified by the Public Health Service. Milk from a certified shipper may then be accepted in other states and municipalities without further inspection.

REFUSE DISPOSAL

Methods of collecting refuse vary according to the size and type of city or county organization; there are several methods that are usually employed. Dumping is one method in which some remote area in the community is selected for disposal leaving the accumulated refuse for decomposition by nature. This, however, makes ideal conditions for rodent and fly breeding. The trenching technique consists of shallow trenches where refuse is deposited and immediately covered with dirt; the same land can be used again about every two or three years. The sanitary fill is a method in which suitable swampy or unused land is selected by a community. The fill is built up to a height of about ten feet. The refuse is then compacted by a bulldozer and covered. This method is employed by the armed forces in their camps and bases throughout the world. Sanitary landfills have been increasing in number throughout many

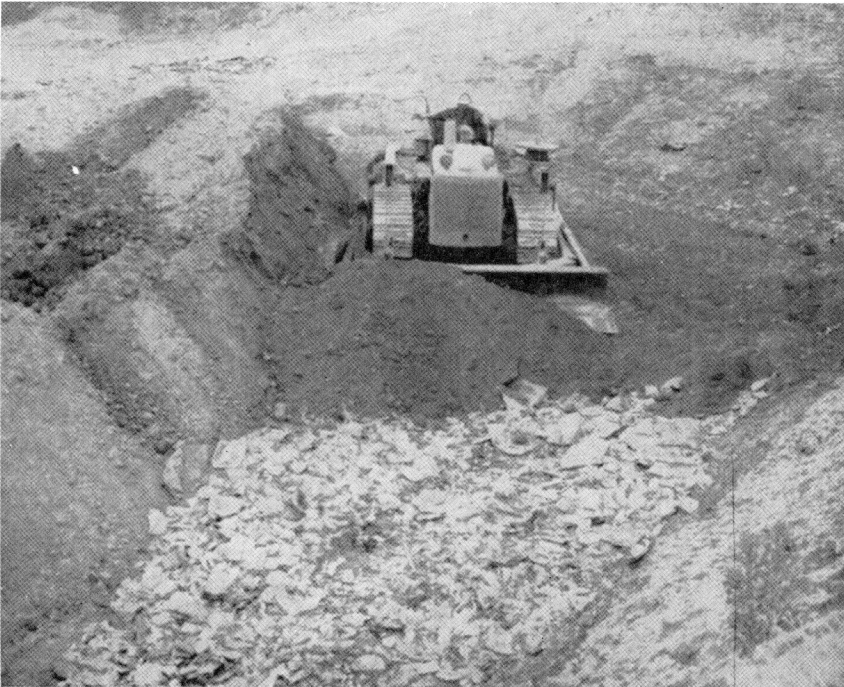

Figure 56. A properly designed and managed sanitary landfill is best at a large camp. This is a landfill that was used at the 1953 national jamboree in California. (From Rosenblum, Marcus, *Public Health*, Merit Badge Series, Boy Scouts of America, 1956.)

states in recent years and this method continues to grow in acceptance by communities. (See Figure 56.) Reduction is a method in which refuse is cooked under steam pressure with recovery of the melted fats and dry solid residue. The fats are used for soap-making, and the residue is used as a fertilizer. Biological digestion consists of placing the refuse into tightly sealed vaults and allowing it to decompose. After about 25 days, the residue can be used as a fertilizer. This method is not a popular procedure in the United States, although some European countries still use it. The incineration procedure burns the refuse at a high temperature.

The collection and disposal of refuse is a proper and important community function and should be controlled by officials of the public health department. In some communities the refuse is collected by a private concern under contract. In either case, refuse collection and disposal should be controlled and regulated by the health department to meet the necessary standards in order to protect the health of the community.

QUESTIONS FOR REVIEW

1. What are the major sources of water in your community? State?
2. What diseases may be transmitted by water?
3. List four chemicals or elements that are added to the water, and explain why each is added.
4. List six criteria to consider when planning a safe community water supply.
5. (a) Discuss the water pollution problem in your community, state and nation.
   (b) How can water pollution be prevented?
6. Explain, step-by-step, the operation of a sewage treatment plant.
7. (a) What part does the local health department play in keeping water safe and pure,
   (b) State Health Department,
   (c) United States Public Health Service?
8. (a) Discuss the air pollution problem in your community, state, and nation.
   (b) How can air pollution be prevented and controlled?
9. Discuss the relationship between air and health.
10. What are the sources of air pollution?
11. (a) What part does the local health department play in preventing air pollution,
    (b) State Health Department,
    (c) United States Public Health Service?
12. What are the present concepts of occupational health?
13. (a) What part does the local health department play in occupational health programs,
    (b) State Health Department,
    (c) United States Public Health Service?
14. Briefly classify and discuss the environmental agents that may be harmful to health.
15. List nine easy rules for keeping food safe.

16. What germs and diseases may be transmitted by food?
17. (a) What part does the local health department play in food sanitation,
    (b) State Health Department,
    (c) United States Public Health Service?
18. Discuss: Botulism, mussel poisoning, chemical poisoning.
19. Is it best to examine or educate food handlers? Explain.
20. Plan, organize, and outline a five hour program to educate food handlers.
21. (a) What part does the local health department play in milk sanitation,
    (b) State Health Department,
    (c) United States Public Health Service,
    (d) Department of Agriculture?
22. What diseases may be transmitted by milk?
23. "Pasteurization destroys certain vitamins and flavor, and is not necessary if milk is produced and handled under sanitary conditions." Discuss this statement.
24. List and briefly discuss five sanitary milk tests.
25. (a) What part does the local health department play in refuse disposal,
    (b) State Health Department?
26. (a) List 5 refuse disposal methods.
    (b) Which is considered best? Why?

REFERENCES

1. The Shattuck Report: *Report of Sanitary Commission of Massachusetts: 1850.* Reprinted by the American Health Association, New York, 1950.
2. United States News and World Report: *How Pure Is Your Water?* Washington, D.C., U.S. News and World Report, 1960, Pages 52–54.
3. Smillie, W. G.: *Public Health—Its Promise for the Future.* New York, The Macmillan Co., 1955, Page 347.
4. U.S. News and World Report: *How To Fight Air Pollution.* Washington, D.C., U.S. News and World Report, October 1958, Page 81.
5. Second Report of the California State Department of Public Health: *Clean Air for California.* California, California State Department of Public Heath, March 1956, Pages 5–6.
6. Initial Report of the Air Pollution Study Project: *Clean Air For California.* California, California State Department of Public Health, March 1955, Pages 42–43, 47.
7. Holland, B. D.: *Scope and Interprofessional Relations of Occupational Medicine.* J.A.M.A., 170:1515, 1959.
8. Occupational Health Series I: *Dollars and Sense.* Santa Clara, California, County Health Department, Division of Occupational Health, 1958, Page 3.
9. *Santa Clara County Health Department Occupational Health Seminars.* California, Santa Clara County Health Department, 1959, Pages 5 and 6.

SUGGESTED READING

Brown, J. A. C.: *The Social Psychology of Industry.* England, Pelican Book A296, 1958.
Century of Progress Through Sanitation, Part 2. Am. J. Pub. Health, 43:6, 1953.
Cleary, E. J.: *Creating Public Awareness and Motivation for Clean Streams.* Am. J. Pub. Health, 49:757–61, 1959.

Ehlers, Victor H., and Steel, Ernest W.: *Municipal and Rural Sanitation*, 4th Ed. New York, McGraw-Hill and Co., 1951.

Environment v. Man, Subtle New Pollutants Endanger Health. Time, Sept. 26, 1960, Pages 66–68.

Harvey, J. C.: *Experience with the Food Additives Amendment.* Am. J. Pub. Health, 50:627–31.

Hilleboe, Herman E., and Larimore, Granville W.: *Preventive Medicine, Principles of Prevention in the Occurrence and Progression of Disease.* Philadelphia, W. B. Saunders Co., 1959.

Hunter, Don: *Health in Industry.* England, Pelican Book A441, 1949.

Phelps, Earle B., et al.: *Public Health Engineering: A Textbook of the Principles of Environmental Sanitation*, Vol. I. New York, John Wiley and Sons, Inc., 1948.

Rogers, S. M.: *Air Pollution Legislation—A Review of Current Developments.* Am. J. Pub. Health, 50:642–48, 1960.

Simpson, D. F., Dunsmore, H. J., Purdom, P. W., Vester, K. G., Senn, C. L., et al.: *Are You Getting the Most Environmental Health Service Out of the Tax Dollar?* Am. J. Pub. Health, 49:729–56, 1959.

Spivak, Jonathan: *Filthy Water—Uncle Sam Steps Up Drive to Halt Pollution by Cities, Industries.* The Wall Street Journal, Nov. 14, 1960, Pages 1, 14.

Toy, Stewart: *Fighting Fumes—Firms Rush to Perfect Auto Anti-Smog Device for California Market.* The Wall Street Journal, July 22, 1960, Pages 1, 13.

U.S. Public Health Service, Federal Security Agency: *Environmental and Health, Publication No. 84.* Washington, D.C., U.S. Government Printing Office, 1951.

What Does Water Pollution Mean? American City, 68:87, 1953.

Chapter XI

Radiological Health

EXAMPLES of radiation or energy are all around us. The colors we see and the noises we hear depend upon the nature of these energy waves. A match, stove, and light bulb release heat and light while radio waves, infra-red lights, and ultra-violet lights release wave light energy and heat. The sun, a magnificent example of heat and light, has available energy to start fires, burn our skins, and cause chemical explosions. These are all examples of electromagnetic or wave light radiations, and the lower-energy, long wave length radio waves cannot penetrate as far, and are therefore not as dangerous as the high-energy, short wave length gamma rays. The other type of radiation or energy is released by streams of atomic particles called protons, electrons, or alpha particles during chemical reactions. These are referred to as corpuscular radiations.

TYPES OF IONIZING RADIATION

All sources of radiation are effective because of ionization. Ionization is the property that enables radioactive particles or rays

219

WHAT RADIATION IS

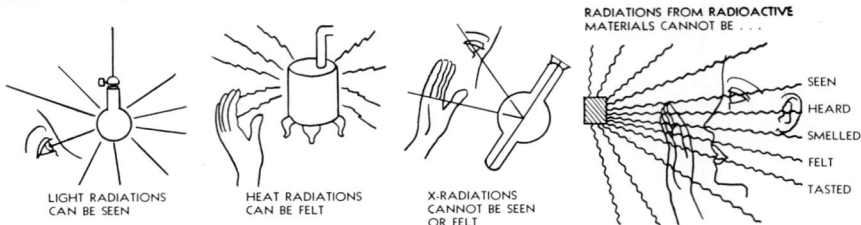

RADIATIONS FROM RADIOACTIVE
MATERIALS CANNOT BE . . .

SEEN
HEARD
SMELLED
FELT
TASTED

LIGHT RADIATIONS
CAN BE SEEN

HEAT RADIATIONS
CAN BE FELT

X-RADIATIONS
CANNOT BE SEEN
OR FELT

RADIOACTIVE RADIATIONS ARE STREAMS OF FAST-FLYING
PARTICLES OR WAVES WHICH COME FROM UNSTABLE ATOMS

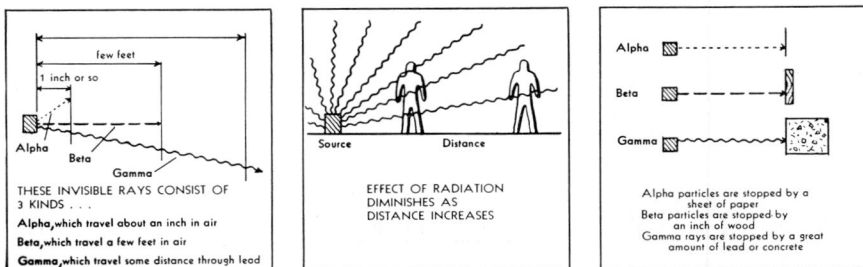

few feet

1 inch or so

Alpha
Beta
Gamma

THESE INVISIBLE RAYS CONSIST OF
3 KINDS . . .

Alpha, which travel about an inch in air

Beta, which travel a few feet in air

Gamma, which travel some distance through lead

Source   Distance

EFFECT OF RADIATION
DIMINISHES AS
DISTANCE INCREASES

Alpha
Beta
Gamma

Alpha particles are stopped by a
sheet of paper
Beta particles are stopped by
an inch of wood
Gamma rays are stopped by a great
amount of lead or concrete

Figure 57. (From *You Can Understand The Atom*. U.S. Atomic Energy Commission.)

to interact with matter and split atoms and molecules into pairs of electrically charged fragments called ions. For example, in the electrolysis of water, H_2O or HOH, it ionizes into the H^+ ion, and the OH^- ion. Ionization of living matter results in tissue changes that may affect health. The extent of tissue ionization depends upon the composition of the tissue and the quantity, type, and energy of the radiation. Tissue damage caused by ionization is partially irreversible.

Alpha Particles

Alpha particles have tremendous ionizing power, 10,000 times that of gamma rays. However, the relatively large alpha particles have both a low penetrating power and range and are easily stopped by a thick sheet of paper or the external layer of skin on the body. As a result, damage due to external exposure generally is not significant. If, on the other hand, an alpha-emitting substance is swallowed, absorbed, or inhaled severe internal damage may result. Radium is a powerful alpha emitter, and, once inside the human body, its retention is practically permanent. Only traces leave the body, mostly in the form of radon gas in expired air, sweat, feces, and urine.

Beta Particles

As negatively charged electrons, beta particles have 100 times the ionizing power of gamma rays, but can travel only a few yards through the air. Ordinarily, they can be stopped by clothing and will penetrate only a fraction of an inch into the skin, affecting it very much like a burn. A thin sheet of plastic, such as lucite, or light metal, such as aluminum, will stop the beta particle. Beta particles are emitted along with gamma rays, generally. However, certain radioisotopes are pure beta emitters. Energetic beta particles are most dangerous following ingestion or inhalation.

Gamma and X-rays

These have quite low specific ionization values, but characteristically are capable of penetrating matter. Lead, steel, and concrete are among those materials that are frequently used to reduce gamma or x-rays to harmless levels. As a group, gamma and x-ray radiations constitute the chief health hazard of external radiation. Only well designed underground shelters could provide good protection from gamma radiation.

Neutrons

Neutrons are uncharged particles weighing about one-fourth as much as an alpha particle. They are incapable of causing ionization by themselves, but are able to impart sufficient energy to hydrogen atoms for them to cause ionization. Neutrons of high energy have a much greater biological effect than do low-energy neutrons. When an atom absorbs a neutron it becomes radioactive, or emits gamma rays to get rid of the excess energy introduced by the captured neutron. High-energy neutrons are normally shielded with concrete, steel, water, or paraffin. Low-energy neutrons are readily absorbed by cadmium or boron. The major sources of neutrons are nuclear reactors.

SOURCES OF RADIOACTIVITY

The application and frequency of use of radiation have increased tremendously in the past several years. This increase is not only the result of new developments in atomic pile-produced radioisotopes, but also the result of an accelerated use of x-radiation and, in a more limited way, natural sources of gamma radiation, principally radium. It is not uncommon to find industrial plants, research laboratories, and hospitals where total exposure to radia-

Table 13. Types of Radiation

TYPE OF RADIATION	PHYSICAL NATURE	DISTANCE OF TRAVEL IN AIR	EFFECTIVE SHIELDING*	USUAL MEANS OF DETECTION	PRINCIPAL HAZARDS
ALPHA (α)	Heavy Particle, Helium nucleus, double positive charge–great ionizing power	Few inches maximum	Skin or thin layer of any solid material	Special laboratory instruments	Extreme hazard when taken into the body by inhalation, injestion, or through open wounds. Little external hazard.
BETA (β)	Light particle, electron, single negative charge	Few yards maximum	One-half inch of any solid material, clothing, Al	Geiger counter, film badge, dosimeter	Moderate internal and external hazards. Can cause skin burns.
GAMMA (γ)	Ray, similar to X-ray–low ionizing power–B particles usually emitted with γ rays	Very long	Lead, other heavy metals, concrete, tightly packed soil	Geiger counter, Ion chamber, Film badge, dosimeter	From sources external to the body–chief health hazard of external radiation.
NEUTRON (η)	Moderately heavy particle, neutral charge–high energy and low energy types	Very long	Water, steel, paraffin, concrete	Special laboratory instruments.	From sources external to the body.

* The best protection from *any* type of radiation is distance from the source of radiation (time and shielding are other factors). Gamma Rays and neutrons are given off at the instant of detonation of an atomic bomb. This is termed *initial radiation*. Alpha, Beta, and Gamma radiating materials remain after the explosion. Radiation from this source is called *residual radiation*.

tion is the summation of the use of x-ray and fluoroscopic machines, radium, and radioisotopes.

The world is radioactive and will always remain so. The atoms of some elements, called the radioactive elements, undergo a spontaneous disintegration and release energy. Some of the common radioactive elements are uranium, thorium, actinium, polonium, and radium. The nuclei of these atoms are unstable and therefore explode. For example, after a series of disintegrations accompanied by radioactive energy, the radium atom finally becomes an isotope of lead, which is a stable element. There are approximately 50 radioactive elements in nature.

Nature

In the earth's crust are found large amounts of uranium, thorium, actinium, and their related elements. There is no portion of the earth's surface free from the radiation produced spontaneously by these materials. A square mile of surface soil one foot thick is conservatively estimated to contain an average of one gram of radium, three tons of uranium, and six tons of thorium, all of which are radioactive.[1] However, some natural places have subsoil rather free from radioactive elements and the earth's contribution to radioactivity is small there. Natural potassium has a radioactive isotope, potassium-40, the activity of which is appreciable. All natural potassium, whether in the earth's crust or as a component of living individuals, is thus radioactive and produces an appreciable increment in the total dose to which people are exposed. Likewise, the carbon which forms a large part of our bodies has a constant fraction, composed of the radioactive isotope of carbon of mass-14. This carbon is originally produced by the action of cosmic rays on the nitrogen of the atmosphere. Food, milk, and water, particularly water from wells and mineral springs, contain traces of radioactive substances detectable by modern, sensitive instruments. The air we breathe contains minute amounts of radon and thoron that are gaseous decay products of radium, uranium, and thorium from the earth.

It is interesting to note variations in background radiation. Total background radiation is least over the open ocean and greatest over granite. The weather, too, affects local conditions of atmospheric radioactivity. For example, radon, thoron and their derivatives attach themselves to dust particles in the air; rainfall brings them down to the ground level; a snowfall prevents their escape from the ground into the air. Similarly, on a cloudy day there is less background radiation than on a clear day. Even man made structures of wood, brick, or concrete emanate measurable quantities of radioactivity, and interior walls of plaster are sufficiently radioactive to affect the function of detecting instruments.

In Kerala, located at the southern tip of India, about 100,000 people live in fishing villages strung along a hundred miles of a geological curiosity—an ocean beach whose black sands are radioactive. The people who live there have always lived in a radiation field about ten times larger than the average radiation field in the United States.

Cosmic Radiation

Cosmic radiation is that radiation coming from outside the earth, much of it from outside the solar system. Gamma rays of the very highest energy content are part of the complex nature of cosmic rays probably formed in the upper atmosphere by collisions of protons from outer space. They seemingly originate within our galaxy of stars—the Milky Way. Exceedingly energetic radiations are thus received from outer space, and all living things on earth are constantly bombarded by this celestial radiation. At high altitudes the amount of cosmic radiation is appreciably increased; at an altitude of 5,000 feet the cosmic radiation is approximately double that experienced at sea level. Persons living at high altitudes are subjected to twice the natural radiation received by persons in nonmountainous areas. Pike's Peak has almost five times as much background radiation as does a point on the Pennsylvania Turnpike, which is designated as the place with the lowest amount of background radiation in the United States. Fortunately, however, the earth's atmosphere filters out most of the cosmic rays before they reach us. From all these natural sources of radioactivity individuals may receive a total exposure in a lifetime of about ten roentgens equivalent.

Weapons

In recent years there has been a man made component added to the general exposure from natural sources of radioactivity. The sequence of nuclear detonations conducted in the course of the development of atomic weapons has resulted in the addition of substantial amounts of fission products to the general environment.

Through the action of stratospheric winds, this material has been more or less uniformly distributed over the face of the earth, with somewhat greater concentrations in the United States and generally with greater abundance in the Northern Hemisphere than in its Southern counterpart.[2] The mixture of fission products emits both gamma and beta radiations. It is estimated that from the fallout material thus far descended from earth there will be a total average lifetime exposure of about one-tenth of a roentgen equivalent.[3] This amounts to approximately one per cent of the lifetime exposure of people to natural radiation of the earth and cosmic sources.

Reactors

As nuclear reactors are constructed by private enterprise, there will be added to our responsibility a radioactive source of great potential danger. The potential harm is created by the large amount of radioactive fission products that accumulate in reactors under continuous operation. Nonetheless, the fact that reactors are potentially hazardous does not mean that they need to be so, or that we cannot learn to live with them in complete safety. Industry has learned how to control and live with many hazards.[4]

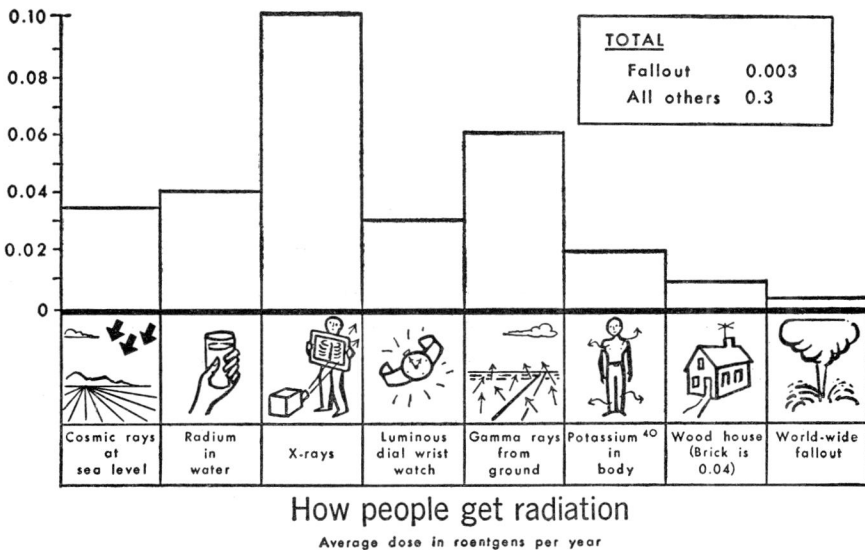

How people get radiation

Average dose in roentgens per year

Figure 58. (From Teller, E. and Latter, A. L., *Our Nuclear Future,* Criterion Books. New York, 1958.)

WHAT A NUCLEAR REACTOR (PILE) IS

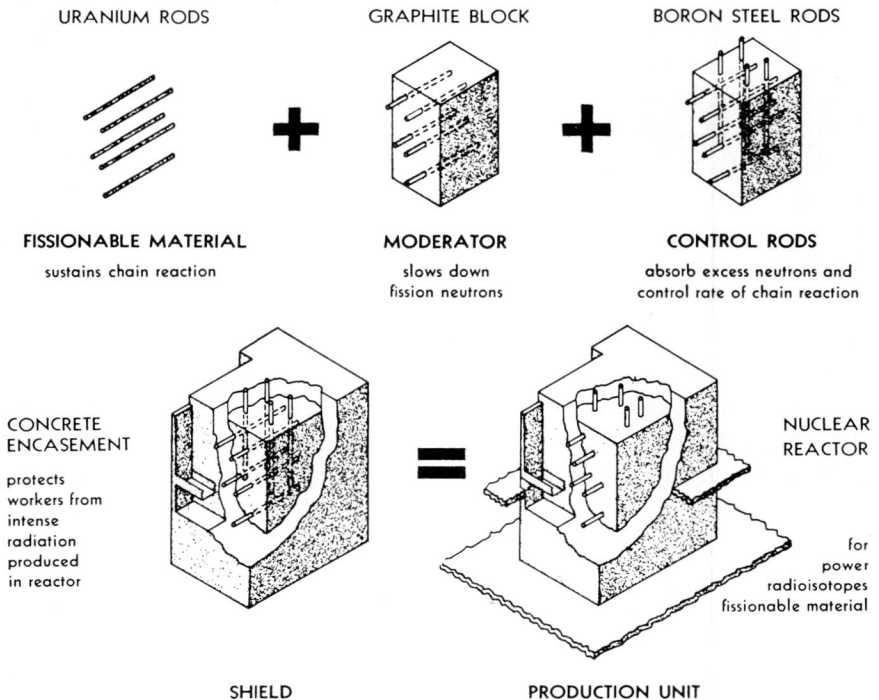

Figure 59. (From *You Can Understand The Atom*. U.S. Atomic Energy Commission.)

Medical Sources

A fifth source of radiation exposure is in the use of x-ray for various purposes. Essentially, these are diagnostic and therapeutic x-ray machines in hospitals and in offices of radiologists, physicians, dentists, chiropodists, chiropractors, and veterinarians. As far as the public is concerned, exposure to radiation is probably most common as a result of chest x-rays, dental x-rays, gastrointestinal series, and many other clinical procedures. Improperly shielded industrial x-ray equipment may cause exposure of operators; careless and incompetent operation of x-ray equipment may cause unnecessary exposure of the patient and of the operating technician. It has been estimated that the average individual exposure from such sources may amount to three or four roentgens during the reproductive lifetime.[5] Other common external sources include television tubes and watch dials.

MEASUREMENT OF RADIATION*

ROENTGEN OR R. Quantity or dose of x-rays and gamma rays. Exact definition based on ionization produced in air by x-rays or gamma ray.

ROENTGEN EQUIVALENT MAN OR REM. That quantity of any type ionizing radiation which, when absorbed by man, produces an effect equivalent to the absorption by man of one roentgen of x- or gamma-radiation.

CURIE OR C. A measure of the strength of the radioactive source in terms of atoms disintegrating per second.

RAD. A measure of the energy absorbed from radiation in a given amount of tissue. Roughly equivalent to a roentgen. (100 ergs absorbed per gram of tissue.)

HALF-LIFE. The time required for radioactive elements to lose one-half their activity. For example, the half-life of one ounce of cobalt-60 is 5.3 years. Therefore, one ounce of cobalt-60 after 5.3 years becomes one-half ounce; after 5.3 more years becomes one-quarter ounce; after 5.3 more years becomes one-eighth ounce, etc. The half-life is important to us because it tells us how much of a radioactive element will remain after a given time, and how active the radioactivity is at any moment. The rays and half-life of various radioactive elements are compared below:

ELEMENT	RAYS	HALF-LIFE
Phosphorus-32	Beta	14 days
Iodine-131	Beta, gamma	8 days
Sulfur-35	Beta	87 days
Cobalt-60	Beta, gamma	5.3 years
Carbon-14	Beta	5,000 years

The fact is that the shorter the half-life, the faster the decay, and the greater the intensity produced by decay. The formula is:

$$\text{Half-life} = \frac{1}{\text{intensity}}$$

ELEMENT	HALF-LIFE
Radon	4 days
Strontium-90	28 years
Radium	1,600 years
Uranium-238	10^9 years
Thorium	10^{14} years
Potassium	10^{20} years (in milk)

* For a more complete list of definitions and fundamentals of nuclear radiations refer to Appendix 6.

From the above list of elements, for example, we know that radon is the most dangerous. Internal and external human injury depends upon the half-life of the radioactive element.

Maximum Permissible Dose

The International Committee on Radiological Protection defined a maximal permissible weekly dose as a dose of radiation that, in the light of present knowledge, is not expected to cause appreciable bodily injury to any person at any time during his lifetime. This level has been steadily reduced, as shown below:

YEAR	MAXIMUM PERMISSIBLE DOSE
1928–1936	100 rads per year
1936–1947	35 rads per year
1948–1957	15 rads per year
1957–	5 rads per year

(It takes 50 normal chest x-rays per year to equal five rads.)

All recommendations as to permissible radiation exposures should be interpreted by recognizing the basic fact that any radiation exposure, except as required by medical necessity, is undesirable. There is a certain amount of background radiation present in our environment that is unavoidable. The only valid philosophy of radiation safety, based on present knowledge, is to reduce all radiation exposures above background levels to the lowest possible dose. Thus, maximum permissible exposures, such as those stated below, are to be used only as general guides. It should not be considered that these are tolerable exposures, but rather that they represent upper limits and should be reached only infrequently, if ever. The latest recommendations of the National Committee on Radiation Protection as to maximum permissible exposures are:

1. The maximum permissible accumulated dose, in rems, at any age, is equal to 5 times the number of years beyond age 18, providing no annual increment exceeds 15 rems. Thus the accumulated maximum permissible dose equals $5(N-18)$ rems where N is the age and greater than 18. This applies to all critical organs except the skin, for which the value is double.

2. The maximum permissible weekly whole-body dose is 0.3 rem. Should the maximum permissible weekly dose be exceeded, no more than 3.0 rems should be accumulated in 13 weeks.

One of the most fundamental and at the same time most difficult problems is the determination of the degree of hazard associated with any particular radiation factor, and achieving a consensus
as to what level of radiation should be considered acceptable in
our present-day society.

HEALTH ASPECTS

General Considerations

There are four major considerations that we must consider in
discussing the biological aspects of radiation. They include:

1. Type of ionization. For example, the alpha radiation, although possessed of considerable energy, is incapable of deep
penetration. In striking contrast, gamma radiation is capable of
deep penetration into tissues and is capable of traversing appreciable thickness of material. Between these two extremes with
respect to penetration, various energy levels of beta radiation are
to be found that have appreciable penetrating power in tissue,
although limited in depth of effective action.

	PENETRATION		IONIZATION
	Air	*Tissue*	
Alpha	$.1^1$	.01 centimeter	10,000
Beta	10^1	1.0 centimeter	100
Gamma	1,000	10.0 centimeter	1

2. Intensity or energy of ionizing influence. This depends upon
distance and amount and type of shielding between the source and
the person.

3. Duration or number of minutes or hours a person is exposed to radiation.

4. Area of the body radiated. As indicated in the following
discussion, proliferating cells are more sensitive to radioactivity.
The whole body exposure to radiation is appreciably different from
the irradiation of a single part. The tolerance of the entire individual to radiation is much less than that exhibited by any single
organ or component of the body. Furthermore, there seems to be a
great deal of variability among individuals to radiation.

INJURY BY IONIZATION OF WATER. While there are several different physical forms of nuclear radiation, they all have similar
biological effects. It appears that the chief mechanism of injury to
living cells is through the ionization of water, of which all living
tissues are largely composed. Other cell destruction theories in-

clude: (1) Radiation alters the permeability of cell membranes; (2) Radiation produces inherent toxic materials; (3) Radiation produces a change in intercellular relationships; (4) Radiation produces a disturbance of enzyme systems.

In a very real sense man is an aquatic animal. He not only is composed mostly of water, but he lives and continues to exist in an aqueous state, being dependent on foodstuffs that are themselves mostly water. Radiation, therefore, strikes at life through the medium of its most basic substance—water.[7] The ionization also creates a disturbance between the nucleus and cytoplasm of the cell.

In the interaction of ionizing radiation with water, several particularly toxic compounds are produced, which in turn have chemical effects upon the constituents of a living cell, especially upon the proteins. Detection of amino acids, building blocks of proteins, are noticed in the urine of a person exposed to too much radiation.

INFLUENCE OF NUMBER OF CELLS. Another principle involves the number of cells present in the organism. The more cells present, the less radiation is needed to kill the organism. For example:

ORGANISM	NUMBER OF ROENTGENS CAUSING DEATH
Mammals	200–1,000 roentgens
Frogs and goldfish	700 roentgens
Tortoise	1,500 roentgens
Snail	10,000 roentgens
Kissing bug	50,000 roentgens
Fruit fly	60,000 roentgens
Paramecium	300,000 roentgens
Virus	1,000,000 roentgens

The above chart indicates that some species can survive a radiation dose many times greater than that which would kill an elephant or man. Cells are most susceptible to radiation damage when they are in the process of dividing. Since many insects, unlike humans, undergo no cell division during much of their lives, they are more highly resistant to radiation.

INFLUENCE OF LEVEL OF OXYGEN. The level of oxygen within a cell or organism at the time of radiation is also important. For example, oxygen deficiency slows the kissing bug's cell division, and when it moults, the bug shows two to three times less radiation damage than bugs that are irradiated in normal air. This indicates that less cell oxygen produces less cell damage, or conversely, more cell oxygen produces more cell damage. Since cells in humans are continually dividing, man may never hope to achieve an insect's resistance.[8]

INFLUENCE OF CELL PROLIFERATION. Proliferating cells, or the cells that grow the fastest, are most sensitive to radioactivity. A scale of *decreasing* cell sensitivity includes:

1. Lymphoid tissue—most sensitive of all tissue
2. Bone marrow, leukocytes and other elements in the blood
   (a) immature cells more sensitive than mature cells
   (b) red blood cells least sensitive component
3. Gonad, ovary, pancreas, kidney and other epithelial cells
4. Blood vessels and other endothelial cells (peritoneal tissue)
5. Connective tissue
6. Muscles
7. Bone
8. Nerve.

Biologic Effects of Radiation

In the light of these general considerations and principles, we may consider two broad classes of biologic effects. The first of these has to do with the effects on the individual himself. These may be spoken of as the somatic effects in contrast to those which are manifested only in the children or grandchildren of the individuals exposed. The second effect is the genetic effect and results from the action of radiation on the germ cells of either the male or female.

SOMATIC EFFECTS. Somatically, certain types of disease tend to be associated with excessive radiation exposure. It must be pointed out, however, that there is no agreement regarding genetic or somatic damage. Many scientists believe that a radiation threshold exists for somatic effects, but that we have not yet exceeded this value. However, it is well known from animal experiments and observations on humans that exposure to radiation in sufficient amounts induces leukemia in susceptible individuals. The death rate from leukemia is about three times higher for all physicians than for the general population, and is considerably increased in physicians customarily exposed to radiation. The induction of bone tumors in humans by ingested radium has been clearly established.

Effect of Fallout. The fifteen-country United Nations Scientific committee on the Effects of Atomic Radiation, after studying world radiation for two and one-half years, reported in August, 1958. The report stated that, assuming the world population is

3,000,000,000, the current nuclear bomb fallout is estimated to account for between 400 to 2,000 leukemia cases per year, as compared with 15,000 from natural radiation. Science is not yet sure how much radiation is needed to produce leukemia. The United States National Academy of Sciences estimates the threshold as 40 roentgens. If this is true, and all the bomb tests had stopped in 1959, the ultimate total of fallout cases is estimated to be between 25,000 and 150,000.[9] It must be pointed out, however, that many scientists believe that fallout radioactivity has no practical importance compared with natural radiation, and that fallout does not constitute a danger to the health of mankind.

While debate rages in many parts of the world about radioactive fallout and its potential dangers, medical scientists are keeping a relatively unpublicized watch on a small group of natives from two Pacific atolls. These 82 Marshallese were living on Rongelap and Ailinginae in 1954 when an American nuclear device was exploded, accidently showering the natives with radioactive debris.

The *British Medical Journal* reports that no abnormalities have been found among children born after the mishap. Nine of the male children exposed to the fallout have lagged in growth. The boys, ranging in age from three to 15, show a mean deficiency in height of 2.1 inches and 7.2 pounds in weight, compared to a group of children on an atoll missed by the fallout. However, the "irradiated" girls of the islands do not show significant differences in size, and the investigators believe the boys' growth lag is probably due to other factors. They point out that boys may be less able than girls to withstand "unfavorable changes in environment." None of the fallout victims has died of radiation-linked ailments, but several years after the nuclear blast the natives still had traces of radioactivity in their bodies.

The study group has now entered the period of maximum risk from acute leukemia, although it is "quite possible, considering the rarity of the disease, that no actual cases will be observed." Failure to observe a case of acute leukemia among these fallout victims should not be considered evidence that a "threshold dose" can be inferred for radiation-induced leukemia. Some other possible radiation effects, such as tumors, may not show up for another six to eleven years.[10]

Effect on Life Span. A very important general manifestation of radiation with no specific pattern of disease is decreased life span, which is found to be quantitatively related to the total amount of radiation exposure.[5] The measure of this effect is an increased rate of general aging. The exposed population simply grows older at a rate greater than the population that has not been exposed. Evidence is accumulating to show that this is probably the most sensitive indicator of population injury that is available, and it is probable that studies of whole populations will demonstrate changes that would be imperceptible on the individual observation basis. Much remains to be learned, but from animal studies and careful observation of human experiences both in the United States and Japan, it appears that 100 rads of gamma radiation to the whole body may shorten life expectancy by as much as one half to two years. Similar proportionate shortening of life span appears to exist for many experimental animals as well. Other major somatic effects include retinal lesions, cataracts, and possible adverse effects on the pregnant mother's fetus.

GENETIC EFFECTS. In considering the question of genetic effects certain general scientific principles have been well established. In the case of gene mutations, it is believed by many competent geneticists that the number of induced mutations is proportional to the dose received by the gonads up to the time of reproduction, no matter how low the dose is and how it has been distributed with respect to time. Most radiation of this kind comes from the element cesium-137, which has been deposited in the ground and absorbed by the body. Assuming the same birth rate and the same estimated gonad dose of 0.1 roentgen in 30 years, the *estimated* world-wide increase of defective children is 2,500 to 13,000 per year.[11] This is the ultimate increase; this increase is estimated to occur if the additional 0.1 roentgen in 30 years persisted for a great many generations. Doubling the present human mutation rate would probably not lead to the race's extinction. But many scientists agree that any increase at all may lower the average of human intelligence and life expectancy. Some scientists believe, however, that random mutations, almost always harmful and never proceeding according to any plan, have nevertheless been responsible over the centuries for all the many magnificent living creatures that nature has produced, including the human species.

The mutations produced may lead to serious abnormalities in some cases or to trivial departures from the normal in others. Most modern geneticists look with concern on any appreciable increase in the frequency of mutations in man. Not enough is as yet known about human mutation frequency and the susceptibility to mutational change induced by radiation in the human species. There is general agreement among geneticists that radiation exposure should be kept to the lowest possible amount, although there is appreciable disagreement regarding the quantitative aspects of the ultimate effect upon the population.

Some scientists are certain that radiation from atomic tests will increase the chance of mutations by only a very small amount. These man-made mutations seem even less significant when compared with the high degree of natural radiation endured without noticeable harm by the world's mountain dwellers. For example, the people of Tibet have been exposed for generation after generation to the intense cosmic radiation which bombards their plateau through a relatively thin layer of atmosphere. Compared with people who live in low countries, the Tibetans have been exposed over the centuries to a much greater additional intensity of radiation than is caused by atomic tests. Yet, genetic differences have not been noticed in the humans of Tibet, or for that matter, in any other living species there.

Radiation Research

A great many varied and intensive research projects have been launched to determine the nature and effects of radiation. A few of the most important ones will be discussed. The Atomic Energy Commission has started on one of the most elaborate biological experiments ever conducted. At Iowa State College, about 6,000 pigs a year are being studied to determine the genetic effects of radiation. At the University of Wisconsin, a similar study is taking place with rats. At the University of California and the University of Iowa, strontium-90 is being fed to 400 dogs to determine its effect upon them. Even studies using human tissue cells are being considered. It is believed that these new Atomic Energy Commission studies will shed far more light, eventually, on the real effects of fallout.

Strontium-90

Strontium-90 is the most feared of all the fallout isotopes. The element, strontium, is relatively uncommon. It is the illegitimate, black-sheep step-brother of harmless strontium found naturally in rocks, soil, and water. In all the world and its atmosphere, there is but a single bucketful of strontium-90. But it is the most deadly bucketful of material in the history of man. Theoretically, at least, a concentrated teaspoonful could kill 30,000,000 people. Its most common use is for the rich red of its flame in fireworks and flares. Scientists detected it in laboratory analyses soon after they had split the first atom. But strontium-90 did not become a hazard until the United States tested the first H-bomb in the Pacific. The tremendous fireball of a hydrogen bomb can shoot strontium-90 into the stratosphere where it floats around the world before drifting to earth. By the year 1960, approximately 350 pounds of strontium-90 had been carried aloft by the churning hot gases of the mushroom explosions.

EFFECTS OF STRONTIUM-90 RADIATION. Approximately one-half the strontium-90 in the stratosphere drops to earth after a period of two years. It is found in all parts of the globe, but recent indications are that the heaviest amounts have fallen on the Northern part of the United States. The silver-white metallic material has no smell, no taste, and cannot be seen as it falls to earth. But this insidiously invisible powder is in the air, in the soil, in the oceans—everywhere. Settling in the soil and on plants, it enters the food supply of animals and men; it finds its way into their bones, where it may cause bone cancer or leukemia. Some of it is taken up chemically through the roots of plants to become part of grass or seed, and eventually part of the glass of milk or the bowl of rice. In the United States about 80 per cent of the minute quantity of strontium-90 that enters our bodies comes to us in our milk. In Japan more than two-thirds comes from rice. Unpolished whole wheat, unfiltered rain water, raw vegetables, and similar food items may also contribute a significant amount of strontium-90. Cows seem to do some filtering, and milk, for the calcium it gives, is lower in strontium-90 than cheese and vegetables. Japanese rice eaters are consuming a great deal more strontium-90 than American milk drinkers because their calcium-deficient soil draws in more strontium. Nevertheless, there is mounting evidence that the strontium-90 content in milk, wheat, and other foods is increasing at a dangerous rate. A study conducted by *Consumer Reports* in co-operation with the United States Public Health Service and the Atomic Energy Commission revealed that strontium-90 in the milk supplies is increasing in most cities, and that several cities are far above average.[12] Strontium-90 may also be absorbed by drinking a glass of water, by eating a slice of bread, or simply by breathing.

This isotope has a long half-life of 28 years, and the human body tends to mistake it for calcium, which it resembles chemically, and to build it into bone. As it disintegrates over the years, it may cause cancer by the effect of its radiation on tender living cells. The world average content of strontium-90 is estimated to be increasing in human bone about 30 per cent per year. The increase in young children, whose bones are growing actively, is estimated to be about 50 per cent. Although the amount of strontium-90 finding its way into human bones is apparently below the threshold of damage at the present time, many persons are concerned about increasing concentrations in the future.

TREATMENT FOR STRONTIUM-90 RADIATION INJURY. Biochemists at the Argonne National Laboratory are testing a chemical that flushes out strontium selectively and spares the body's calcium. Used so far only in rats, the chemical is a tasteless yellow dye, the rhodizonic salt of either sodium or potassium. Biochemists are confident that human subjects could take the chemical by mouth at the first sign of radio-strontium exposure. Other experiments indicate that tea may be an antidote for strontium-90; research has shown that tannic acid combines with strontium-90 to produce an insoluble oxide that can be passed out of the body.

Research projects have revealed that contamination of food crops from strontium-90 fallout can be reduced by simply adding lime to the soil. Plants growing in calcium poor soils are avid for strontium; however, if they receive enough crushed lime, containing 40 per cent calcium, they lose their appetite for strontium.

Other Fallout Products

The isotope carbon-14 is a normal component of the air and of our food. But it also is made in appreciable quantity by all nuclear weapons, fission or fusion, dirty or clean. These already have contributed a good deal of radioactive material to the air, enough to raise the amount present in living things by about one-third of 1 per cent. This isotope is very long-lived, having a half-life of 5,700 years. In the present generation, the effects of carbon-14 will be small, compared to the genetic and possible leukemia-inducing effects of the other components of fallout. But since it lasts such a long time, its cumulative genetic effect is about ten or 20 times greater than that of the other fallout components.

Another isotope, cesium-137, is copious in fallout. It can be detected from within the living body because, like potassium, it emits penetrating radiation. It bears much the same relation to the essential potassium that strontium bears to calcium. But it is a rather short-time resident of the body, staying there a matter of months, rather than the decades typical of strontium. The over-all effect of cesium is to increase the dose received from radiations like that of potassium by about 15 per cent. Cesium-137 spreads throughout the body and affects the reproductive tissue.

The possibility of damage by other fission-produced isotopes, not yet extensively studied, should not be forgotten. For example, plutonium-239 may be inhaled and strontium-89 is 160 times more plentiful than strontium-90 at the moment of blast.

X-RAYS—GOOD OR BAD?

Most authorities agree that any radiation is potentially danger-ous. Too much radiation at body sites can cause skin conditions resembling severe burns or local cancers. Widely distributed over the body, so that it penetrates much of the blood-forming marrow, excessive radiation can cause leukemia. If excessive radia-tion strikes the gonads, mutations in the genes may arise which, in turn, may mean deformities in the patient's descendants. Radiation experts claim that many physicians and dentists are not taking the precautions they should when they use x-ray apparatus. For example, some doctors have no idea as to how much radiation their machines are delivering. Others use outmoded equipment and fail to add readily available safeguards, while some recommend x-ray when other methods of diagnosis or treatment might be as effective or even more effective.

Few regulations on the operation of x-ray machines have been attempted. Handbooks are available, however, from the National Committe on Radiation Protection. Only six states have specific regulations governing all radiation hazards. In other states the rules are so full of loopholes that untrained or poorly trained persons can operate obsolete and defective machines with complete impunity. Most physicians, osteopaths, dentists, chiropractors, or naturopaths can obtain and use x-ray equipment for any examina-tion they may choose without any radiological training.

With radiation from industry and bomb fallout constantly increasing, it is now more important than ever for us to place sensible limits on what we receive from such controllable sources as medical x-rays. This does not mean that one chest x-ray or dental x-ray per year will harm us; it means that each x-ray study of each individual should be considered in terms of both its ad-vantages and its possible dangers. Physicians should maintain a cumulative record or history of all major x-ray studies or treatments each patient has had in the past.

Major x-ray sites, possibility of danger, and latest preventive measures include:

DENTAL. The American Dental Association maintains that no dental examination is complete unless the teeth are x-rayed. The Association points out, however, that a complete dental x-ray examination can be made with very low exposure of the face and negligible exposure to the gonads. The average dental x-ray now delivers five roentgens, but this is only to the jaw. The "scatter" radiation reaching the gonads from this is a mere .005 roentgens in a man and .001 roentgens in a woman. It would take 2,000 x-rays to deliver a presumably damaging ten roentgens to a man's gonads. Even so, the currently used five roentgen doses are unnecessary. The total radiation used in each exposure can be reduced to 0.1 roentgen by using higher voltages, better filters, lead diaphragm, faster films, and shorter exposures. Other techniques that will reduce exposure include tilting the chair, covering the patient's lap with a lead sheet or other protective device, and taking only a limited number of films. The National Bureau of Standards has developed another way to reduce x-ray exposures; a panoramic machine photographs the entire mouth with a single, sharply focused exposure, instead of 14 separate plates.

CHEST. The hazards of undiscovered lung diseases, such as tuberculosis, are far greater than the alleged hazard of the small amount of radiation required by annual chest x-rays. The amount of radiation required for an annual x-ray of the chest is considered by most experts to be well within the limits of safety. The conventional chest x-ray, taken at a six-foot range on a film 14 inches by 17 inches delivers 0.06 roentgens to 0.01 roentgens to the chest, and about 0.001 roentgens to the gonads. At the 24 inch range used in mass chest x-ray surveys, the dosages go as high as two roentgens to the chest, but the scatter to the gonads is scarcely increased. The Executive Committee of the American Trudeau Society recommends that tuberculin testing in infants, children, young adults, pre-natals, and young diabetics should be developed as a primary guide to tubercular contacts and as one case-finding method. X-ray of the chest for the detection of tuberculosis, could then be limited to those with a positive tuberculin test. Also, case-finding programs should be reassessed for those segments of the population most deserving of chest x-ray surveys or tuberculin testing.[13] More potent than the x-ray in fluoroscopy, in which the image is viewed instantaneously on a screen, takes longer, and may entail three to ten roentgens per minute to the chest and 0.1 to 0.4 roentgens per minute to the gonads.

PRE-NATAL. X-rays of pregnant women may endanger the fetus.[14] Recent studies have indicated that x-ray pelvimetries radiation reaching the gonads of the fetus may run as high as three roentgens; an equal amount may reach the ovaries of the mother. The amount of damage depends upon the time of pregnancy; the younger the fetus, the greater the possible damage. When there is specific need for x-ray pelvimetry, however, much can be done to reduce the exposure by technical methods.

FRACTURE DETECTION IN LIMBS. X-rays of limbs to detect possible fractures, or arthritic deposits in joints, usually require only short exposures. The radiation used is not enough to damage bone marrow, and is far enough from the gonads for safety.

THERAPEUTIC. X-rays which are used to treat diseases require hundreds of times the dosage needed for ordinary diagnostic work. For that reason there is an increasing tendency to use x-ray therapy only for cancer and other serious diseases. The following diseases and ailments may be treated more effectively and more safely with drugs and other methods: ringworm, acne, bursitis, enlarged thymus and sterility. Although the amounts of radiation required in medical treatment for cancer average much higher than those in diagnosis, they are generally safer. Treatment is usually given by a radiologist who uses elaborate shielding to protect parts of the body not intended to be irradiated. In some cases, radiologists take a calculated risk of damaging some healthy tissues for the sake of attacking the cancer and prolonging life.

FLUOROSCOPE. Fluoroscopy, in particular, is often done under conditions recognized as unsafe. Some fluoroscopic procedures subject the patient to many times the radiation exposure obtained from an x-ray. Furthermore, many physicians are careless about fluoroscopic techniques. For example, if a doctor wears special goggles for at least ten minutes in the examining room before the examination, he can see a good image on the screen with a relatively low intensity of x-ray. Other dangers include leaving the machine on too long, repeated examinations, no shielding devices, and no cone and filter on the machine.

Fluoroscopy for shoe fittings. Technical studies have demonstrated that a high percentage of shoe fitting fluoroscopes are frequently in poor condition and emit dangerous stray radiations. The use of fluoroscope exposes shoe sales personnel, customers, particularly children, and by-standers to a hazard that they do not recognize or appreciate, and that cannot be controlled effectively. For these reasons, the American Medical Association advocates the discontinuance of the use of fluoroscopes for shoe fitting. However, more than 10,000 shoe fitting fluoroscopes are currently being used by about 40,000 shoe salesmen with no professional training in the administration of radiation. Although Pennsylvania, Vermont, Ohio, New York, and California have taken legal steps to abolish the shoe fitting machine, in most localities shoe stores remain free to endanger the health of their patrons and future generations.

ROUTINE EXAMINATIONS. Few experts today recommend routine or periodic x-rays for the following: gastrointestinal series, genitourinary series, spine or backbone series, chest x-rays for children, or fluoroscopic examinations for well babies.

A great deal has been done to lessen the x-ray dangers. The American College of Radiology, for example, has prepared a detailed manual to guide physicians and dentists in the use of x-rays. The American Medical Association, American College of Radiology, and the United States Public Health Service have distributed a new film on radiation protection. Today, many hospitals and medical schools are training nurses, internes, and residents in x-ray procedures. Many colleges and universities are initiating courses designed to educate students in all aspects of radiation. In any procedure the danger increases with old-fashioned x-ray machines and inexperienced operators.

Doctor Wendell G. Scott, President of the American Roentgen Ray Society in 1958, listed five questions which a patient might ask his doctor in advance of x-ray studies:

1. Is the examination necessary?
2. What physician is to make the examination?
3. Has the examining physician, if other than a radiologist, received formal training in radiology? If so, how much, and will there be a written report of the examination acceptable to other physicians?
4. Is the technician who will assist the radiologist certified or qualified by formal training?
5. Would you choose your surgeon without asking similar questions?[15]

MEDICAL MANAGEMENT OF RADIATION INJURIES

Medical management begins with decontamination of all persons exposed to radioactive fallout to prevent cross contamination of hospitals and medical personnel; bathing, hair-clipping and changing clothes are basic methods. Then, first aid is administered and casualties are segregated according to their need for specialized care. The segregation methods employed by military forces in combat zones may be utilized. When casualty segregation is accomplished, there remains the task of treating a large variety of thermal, mechanical and radiation injuries. Food that is carried or packaged is safe to eat after the container has been washed. Water that has been in city mains will probably not be radioactive, but should be monitored.

Burn casualties of an atomic attack include those who sustain not only flash burns caused by the nuclear fireball, but also burns from fires ignited by the blast.[16] Major medical efforts should be directed to those burn patients who have a chance for survival. Local care of burned tissue is always important. The immediate problem is management of shock and loss of body fluids with transfusion of whole blood, plasma, and electrolytes. Antibiotic therapy and tetanus prophylaxis are also of prime importance.[17]

The atomic blast effect, collapse of buildings, and flying debris cause 60 per cent of all deaths occurring within the first 24 hours of a nuclear attack. Since any severe mechanical injury is invariably associated with some degree of shock, many lives can be saved if antishock measures are instituted immediately.[18] Emergency measures include controlling hemorrhage, maintaining adequate airway, conserving body warmth, relieving pain and anxiety, and restoring blood volume. Provided there are shortages of whole blood and blood-cell suspensions, these vital materials should be saved for patients who seem to have a chance of survival.

Acute Radiation Illness

The course of illness in acute radiation syndrome can be described from the case records of Japanese exposed to atomic bombings, where their injuries were uncomplicated by blast damage or flash burns. The sequence of symptoms among all exposed to heavy radiation was roughly the same, but the time intervals of various phases of the illness varied according to the severity of the exposure. Those who received around 400 roentgens or less developed additional symptoms—loss of hair and severe infections. The illness of a typical patient among the latter group goes through four phases:

PHASE *I*. Within an hour or so after exposure, the patient becomes nauseated, vomits, and suffers general prostration and weakness. Diarrhea may occur and his blood pressure may fall a little. In general, the heavier the dosage, the more ill the patient will be. This phase is quite similar to the "radiation sickness" suffered by patients treated intensively with x-ray or radium.

PHASE *II*. After the first onset of the illness, symptoms tend to disappear, and for a period of a few days to several weeks the patient feels less ill. For patients who have suffered the heaviest radiation, this period will be short. Reports have stated that Japanese injured by radiation alone were entirely without symptoms during this time, but the best information is that they were sick people who, because of the emergency, drove themselves to do what had to be done.

PHASE *III*. The illness reaches its height during this phase. Whether or not the patient survives depends on his ability to endure this acute stage. The patient becomes apathetic and develops a fever and rapid heart action. He becomes increasingly weak and loses weight. He loses his appetite, may become nauseated and suffer severe diarrhea which is sometimes bloody. Small hemorrhages may appear in the skin and the gums bleed. In severe cases, infected ulcers may spread throughout the mouth and alimentary tract. The hair may fall from the head and body about three weeks after exposure. The slightly injured recover quickly, but those who receive a heavier dose of radiation may continue gravely ill for weeks. The most severely injured may grow progressively worse over a period of weeks and finally succumb, or may die within a few days.

PHASE *IV*. Patients who survive enter a convalescence during which a feeling of weakness and fatigue are the outstanding symptoms. It may be months before the patients recover normal strength and weight. The skin hemorrhages disappear and the hair, if lost, gradually regrows. Usually within six months, the patient feels completely well. All usual methods of examination indicate that, by this time, the patient is normal. Nevertheless, it is too soon to say that survivors will not suffer further ill effects.[19]

Further Effects of Radiation Illness

Besides the symptoms described, the acute radiation illness includes damage that can be detected only by laboratory tests—changes in blood cells, in male sex organs, and in the functioning of other organs.

Several symptoms of the third, or acute, phase of the illness stem directly from injuries to certain elements in the blood. Infections and ulcerations arise because radiation destroys white blood cells that normally aid in combating bacteria. A few days after radiation exposure, the number of white cells declines and, in severe cases, the cells disappear almost entirely. The skin and gum hemorrhages are seemingly connected with a fall in the number of platelets in the blood, since these substances play a role in the clotting of the blood. Other causes, such as increase in an anti-clotting substance that resembles heparin, a normal blood chemical, also contribute. Platelets begin to decline only after an interval of weeks and, where the patient survives, reappear during convalescence. A third, and very serious, effect upon the blood, the decline in the number of red cells, causes anemia and contributes to the general weakness and debility in acute radiation illness. The decline in the number of red cells starts immediately after exposure and may continue for months.

Microscopic studies of tissue, amplified by more complete research with animals, indicate these blood changes are caused by radiation damage to the bone marrow and to the lymphoid tissue where these various cells are born. The injury to tissue, as well as the course of illness in the patient, can be traced to damage of the cells. Radiation causes the cells to swell, disorganizes their structure and prevents their reproducing. The stoppage of cell division occurs immediately after irradiation; structural changes appear more gradually. The most spectacular change is the collapse of certain parts of the cell, and the shrinkage of the nucleus followed by death and disintegration. The interruption of cell division is temporary, but when new cells begin again to divide they often show bizarre changes in their inner structure.

Hazards of Internal Radiation

Radioactive materials can enter the body through the mouth, through breathing, or through a wound. They are particularly destructive when retained in the body for some time. Alpha and beta particles, which can be stopped by the skin, meet no such barrier inside the body. If lodged there, materials that emit these particles can cause serious damage. In evaluating the radiation hazard from these sources, three main factors must be considered:

1. The chemical characteristics of a radioactive element are important, because they determine in what organ the material is likely to be deposited. Materials that behave like calcium chemically will be deposited in bone. Plutonium and strontium are two such elements.

2. If a material is taken in through the mouth, its solubility in body fluids is important. What chemical forms are we dealing with? How much is absorbed from the gastrointestinal tract? Fortunately, most of the fission products are quite insoluble and will not be absorbed in significant amounts. Compounds of strontium, barium, and iodine are the most soluble. Plutonium exists usually in the form of an oxide and only about 0.05 of 1 per cent of the amount ingested is fixed in the body. Swallowed materials must gain access to the circulating blood before they can be deposited in an organ. Thus, even in the stomach and intestines, they are for all practical purposes still outside the body as far as radioactive poisoning is concerned.

Once plutonium enters the blood stream, it may be carried to all parts of the body, and much of it is desposited in the liver, spleen, and bone. The most significant points of deposit, as far as serious injury is concerned, are close to the blood-forming tissue in the bone marrow. Here, because of the tremendous ionizing power of its alpha particles, plutonium is a constant source of injury to the adjacent tissues. If it remains in the body long enough, the injury will result in the formation of malignant tumors and severe anemia.

3. The length of time materials remain in the body depends upon their "biological half-life"—the time required by the body to lose one-half the radioactivity by decay and the body's regular processes of elimination. This varies from hours to years with the different elements. In the case of plutonium, the biological half-life is 50 years.[20]

Other substances that contribute to radiation from within the body include potassium-40, carbon-14, radium, and its radioactive decay products. Although carbon and potassium are necessary components of life, radium plays no known role in the life process. Radium is widely distributed in the soil and rocks; it is ingested or sometimes breathed into the lungs and concentrates in the bones. The element is present in very small amounts, but its activity can be more important than that of potassium-40 or carbon-14. Evident consequences of radium irritation have been seen in the form of bone and blood malignancies.

Treatment

Although no drugs have been developed that will quickly rid the body of radiation symptoms, treatment includes bed rest, sedation, restoration of nutritional, electrolyte, fluid and mineral balance, antibiotics, blood transfusions, antihistamines, vitamins, and other appropriate drugs.

RADIATION SAFETY PROGRAM

Seven major preventive measures are necessary to control community and personal radiation hazards and injury:

PERSONAL MONITORING. Sensitive machines or badges should be utilized by any agency or group working with radioactive materials. These sensitive machines detect the slightest traces of radioactive particles on the hands and feet, while the badges assure workers that they have not been exposed to more than the permissible dose allowed.

FILTER SYSTEM. Powerful ventilation and filter systems assure that no radioactive particles are allowed to enter the air either inside or outside plants in which radioactive materials are stored. Exhaust from the ventilation system is filtered to prevent the slightest possibility of contamination. Similar stringent methods are used to prevent radioisotopes in the sewage or water.

RADIOLOGICAL SURVEY. Samples of air, water, and soil at various points in the vicinity of radioactivity should be taken regularly to double check the fact that no radioactivity of any kind is being allowed to escape into the surrounding area. Highly trained radiation safety officers are a necessity. There is always the risk, even in peaceful uses, of an accident. However, experience thus far has been reassuring. The atomic energy industry, already employing hundreds of thousands of persons, is, on the record, the safest of all industries. Its accident rate, even in terms of nonradioactive accidents, is the lowest of any industry. The most serious accident thus far has been the explosion of a reactor in Idaho; there were three casualties.

PROTECTIVE CLOTHING. Personnel working with radioactive materials should be required to wear protective clothing. In addition, geiger and scintillation counters should be used to prevent personal contamination or inhalation of radioisotopes.

SHIELDING, RESTRICTION OF EXPOSURE TIME, DISTANCE FROM SOURCE, AND CONTAINMENT. These are very effective barriers against radiation injury. (See Figure 60.)

PREEMPLOYMENT PHYSICAL AND REGULAR MEDICAL EXAMINATIONS. Careful medical history for anemia and other underlying disease, blood counts, and physical examinations make it possible to choose a worker who is not unduly susceptible to radiation injury. Careful and continuous medical examinations, individual urine analysis, and periodic chest x-rays allow the discovery of early symptoms in personnel and thus prevent radiation damage.

RADIOACTIVE WASTE DISPOSAL. There is no satisfactory solution to radioactive waste disposal as yet. In 1959, the Atomic Energy Commission licensed the Navy's Military Sea Transportation Service to dump waste material, imbedded in concrete and steel containers, at selected points in both the Pacific and Atlantic. The oceans are used only for low-energy leftovers—radioactive rubber gloves, mops, rags, discarded laboratory equipment—but over the years an impressive amount of material has been dumped. The Military Sea Transportation Service joins the Coast Guard, other Navy units and seven private firms in the atomic garbage business; the others have already dumped some 30,000 steel and concrete packages into the Atlantic, and 24,000 into the Pacific.

The main criterion for selecting a dumping spot is depth, with 1,000 fathoms (6,000 feet) as a minimum. Diving tests show that most of the dangerous material remains sealed in the containers, but some leaks out, and might yet show up in seafood. Oceanographers and marine biologists are studying the effects wrought on the radioactive graveyards by such phenomena as bottom currents, movement of bottom sediment and the upwelling of bottom waters. The Atomic Energy Commission is also concerned about such future needs as a program of international coordination (Britain now pumps its low-energy atomic garbage through a pipe into the Irish Sea.) and the radioactivity that will remain in the oceans in the wake of nuclear-powered ships. One of the major objections to this method is that atomic wastes could possibly jeopardize the United States' multibillion dollar fishing industry.

High-energy waste material from nuclear reactors at Oak Ridge, Los Alamos and other atomic energy plants is too dangerous for sea disposal. Instead the United States has spent $120,000,000 to build vast, concrete-encased underground steel tanks, which hold a total of 65 million lethal gallons. The largest concentration is at the Atomic Energy Commission's Hanford Works at Richland, Washington, where tanks hold 80 per cent of the high-energy waste

WHAT RADIATION PROTECTION IS

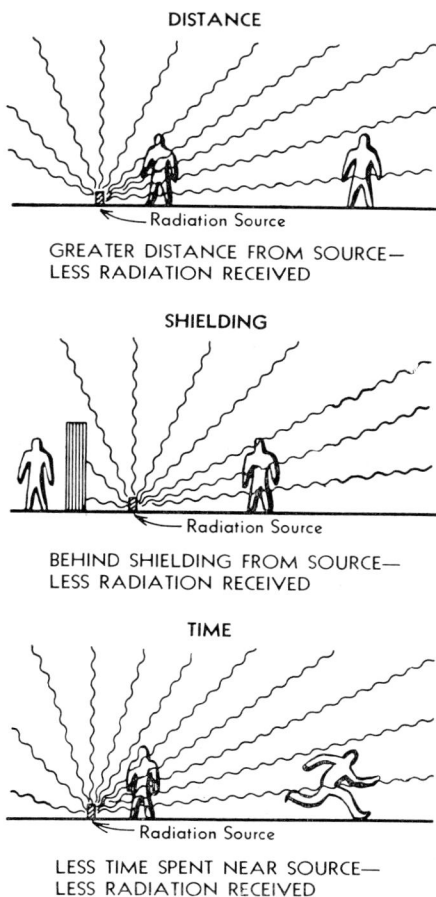

DISTANCE

Radiation Source

GREATER DISTANCE FROM SOURCE—
LESS RADIATION RECEIVED

SHIELDING

Radiation Source

BEHIND SHIELDING FROM SOURCE—
LESS RADIATION RECEIVED

TIME

Radiation Source

LESS TIME SPENT NEAR SOURCE—
LESS RADIATION RECEIVED

Figure 60. (From You Can Understand The Atom. U.S. Atomic Energy Commission.)

in the United States. It will remain dangerous at least until the year
2959. The government is spending $2,000,000 a year to maintain the
tanks. The maintenance cost, therefore, is approximately *two dollars*
per gallon. Even though the storage tanks are several feet thick,
the Atomic Energy Commission estimates their lifetime at only
30 years. In a thousand years, they may have to be replaced 30 or
more times. The problem is magnified when we consider that by the
year 2000, 15 times as many tanks will be required each year. This
means that atomic waste products will require 100,000 acres a year
as "burial grounds". One scientist commented, "The tombs of radioactive waste are becoming as elaborate and expensive as those for
the mummies of the Pharaohs."[23]

One way to dispose of atomic waste is to use it. By reprocessing, some of it can be turned into isotopes for use in medicine,
agriculture, and industry. A reprocessing plant is already set up at
Oak Ridge Atomic Energy Plant. The House Committee on Science
and Astronautics reported on another use for atomic wastes as
follows: inserted in modified grenades, leftovers from nuclear reactors could be lobbed across enemy lines. The small releasing
blast would do almost no damage to roads and real estate. But the
radioactivity would, within a reasonably short time, bring death
to every person within a wide area.

Community Programs

The local health department must provide the advice and
encouragement needed to conserve the public health. A radiological health team can be organized with existing staff members
and a modest budget.[24] The Atomic Energy Commission has in-
corporated in its program of isotope distribution strict regulations
governing utilization. But the rigid control system of the Atomic
Energy Commission governs only synthetic isotopes produced in
nuclear reactors. X-ray machines, fluoroscopes, and other equipment, naturally occurring radioactive materials, and isotopes from
nonreactor sources are not included within the purview of the
Atomic Energy Commission. Those sources that are controlled by
the Atomic Energy Commission are so numerous that the majority
of users are never visited by Commission representatives to see if
the requirements of safe use are met. A wide area of responsibility
exists here for state and local public health agencies. A typical
health department program plan for radiological health should
establish the following three major functions: (1) Determination

of the extent and character of the radiation problem; (2) Reduction of exposure to radiation by supervising installations and providing assistance to local health units which can perform this supervision when they are staffed to do so; (3) Evaluation studies to obtain new information and develop better methods of control by research.

Operational responsibilities under each of the above headings include one or more of the following:

1. To locate all detectable sources of ionizing radiation
2. To train personnel—you can seldom recruit them
3. To keep informed on new developments in the application of radiation in order to control new hazards that may be created
4. To determine the legislative and regulatory needs
5. To gain support of various professional societies and citizen groups for the program
6. To encourage self-discipline among personnel authorized to use radiation
7. To evaluate techniques and results in the control program.[25]

It seems very important for world, federal, state, and local authorities to cooperate, coordinate, review, and evaluate their findings fully before disseminating dubious information to the public. Continual disputes and contradictions lead to mass fear, insecurity, and bewilderment. Also, radiological health education is essential in public schools, colleges, and community groups. We must educate our present and future community and national leaders in the nature, uses, and dangers of radioactivity.

NUCLEAR TESTS—THE WORLD DEBATE

The fiery debate over whether or not the United States should halt nuclear tests has become one of the biggest issues ever to face the nation. On the one hand, the "stop-the-tests" group is headed by Cal Tech's Nobel prize-winning chemist Linus Pauling, who in 1957 presented to the United Nations a stop-the-tests petition signed by 9,235 United States and foreign scientists, including three dozen Nobel laureates. This group believes that many thousands of persons in the world will suffer agonizing death from bone cancer and leukemia, as well as marked changes in genetic patterns. On the other hand, the stoutest advocate of continued testing is the University of California's Hungarian-born nuclear physicist Edward Teller, famed as father of the hydrogen bomb. Dr. Teller's team includes Atomic Energy Commission's Willard Libby, a distinguished nuclear chemist who believes that the hazards from fallout are limited, and that nuclear tests are needed to lessen the thrust of nuclear war. Furthermore, this group believes that fallout radioactivity has no practical importance compared with natural radiation and man made sources. For example, a wrist watch with a luminous dial or x-rays for medical purposes subject us to much more radiation than fallout. However, both ranks agree that there is danger in the continued testing of nuclear weapons. Scientists disagree only as to the degree and depth of the danger. In one of Dr. Teller's most recent books, he sets forth the facts about radioactive fallout as he sees them and the reasons for going on with nuclear tests.[21]

A much heard argument against nuclear tests is that since H-bombs are already powerful beyond comprehension, it is useless to go on developing bigger and deadlier specimens. But Teller points out that the United States' purpose in testing nuclear weapons is not to make them bigger, but to make them smaller, more versatile and less dangerous to people outside the target area. Starting with the assumption that the West absolutely needs nuclear weapons to deter or defeat communist aggression, he holds that it would be "completely inexcusable" to fail to push ahead with development of "clean" nuclear weapons with little or no radioactive fall out.

As director of the Atomic Energy Commission's laboratory at Livermore, California, Teller is directly involved in the Atomic Energy Commission's clean-bomb project, and it is "well on the way toward success." The stop-the-tests camp sometimes talks as though atomic radiation is a new and unnatural hazard; Teller says radioactivity is a pervasive feature of man's environment. Human beings are exposed to an unending spray of radiation from cosmic rays and natural radioactive substances—radium, uranium, potassium-40, carbon-14, etc. Fallout radiation is no different in biological effects from this natural radiation, and is very much smaller in quantity.

Teller estimates that fallout at present levels might increase the number of leukemia and bone cancer cases by one-fifth of 1 per cent, but he adds that the increase "could be zero."

With regard to fallout and human heredity, Teller estimates that in the United States, fallout radiation capable of causing genetic mutations averages 1/500 of a roentgen a year, mostly from cesium-137. That is much less radiation than a human being is exposed to from wearing a luminous-dial wrist watch. As physicist

Teller figures it, the overall mutation-rate increase resulting from fallout is something like one-tenth of 1 per cent.

Cal Tech's Linus Pauling estimates the increase in mutation rates at only 1 per cent. A hazard increase of 1 per cent or less is hardly enough, in Teller's view, to explain the antitest fervor among thousands of his fellow scientists. "It seems probable," he writes, "that the root of the opposition to further tests is not connected with fallout. The real reason is the desire for disarmament and peace."

Edward Teller shares the desire for peace, but he doubts that halting tests would bring peace any nearer. He is convinced that the Russians would evade any no-test or disarmament agreement, unilateral or otherwise, and that absolutely foolproof detection of tests is impossible. Believing that the Russians could and would cheat on any disarmament promises, physicist Teller feels that United States weakness would invite communist aggression. "If we stay strong," he said recently, "then I believe we can have peace based on force. Peace based on force is not as good as peace based on agreement, but in the terrible world in which we live, it may be the only peace that we can have."[22]

To see fallout radiation in proper perspective it should be compared not only with other kinds of radiation but also with other dangers to health. Some estimates are, for example, that being 10 per cent overweight seems to reduce a person's life expectancy by 1.5 years; that the life-long habit of smoking one package of cigarettes a day cuts life by seven years; that living in the city instead of in the country reduces life expectancy by five years, and so on. On this statistical scale the reduction in life expectancy from world-wide fallout at present levels totals less than two days. Or, to put it another way, the world-wide fallout is as dangerous to human health as being one ounce overweight, or smoking one cigarette every two months. Another example exists in terms of automobile fatalities and injuries in the United States. Each year approximately 40,000 people are killed and 1,500,000 people are injured in auto accidents; over one-third of these are young people. Total accident costs involve $12,000,000,000 per year. While there is concern about this accident slaughter, it is evident that we consider the cost to be within reason for the comfort and convenience of the transportation furnished by the automobile.

Finally, two major arguments in favor of continued experimentation and development of nuclear weapons have been advanced by the Teller group. If we renounce nuclear weapons, they say, we open the door to aggression. If we fail to develop clean explosives, we expose people to disaster from radioactive fallout in any serious military conflict. The spectacular developments of the last centuries, in science, in technology, and in our everyday life have been produced by a spirit of adventure, by a fearless exploration of the unknown. When we talk about nuclear tests, Dr. Teller claims, we have in mind not only military preparedness but also the execution of experiments that will give us more insight into the forces of nature. Such insight has led and will lead to new possibilities of controlling nature.

CIVIL DEFENSE

Estimated Damage—Atomic Attack

In 1959, nuclear war experts were asked to estimate a "moderate-sized" war toll to the United States. The supposition was that the enemy had dropped 263 nuclear bombs, equivalent to 1.4 billion tons of TNT, on 70 key cities and 154 military bases. The estimated damage is outlined below:

1. The attack would kill 23,000,000 Americans and fatally injure another 25.9 million persons. It would also inflict nonfatal blast and burn injuries on 7,300,000 persons; 12.7 million persons would receive harmful radiation doses.

2. One ten-megaton blast, of the type likely to be used on the largest United States cities, would flatten all brick houses for a seven-mile radius and all frame houses within a nine-mile radius, would set fires and cause second-degree burns within a 25 mile radius, and would spread a cigar-shaped pattern of radioactive fallout 17 miles wide and 100 miles long. Assuming the enemy would use two ten-megaton bombs on each giant city, the death estimates for metropolitan areas include: 1,057,000 fatalities in Baltimore, or 79 per cent of the city's population; 2,136,000 fatalities in Boston, or 75 of that city's population; 6,098,000 fatalities in New York, or 47 per cent of that city's population.

3. The attack would destroy, badly damage, or irradiate 22.5 million homes, or approximately half the total number of homes in the United States.

4. Unrestricted consumption of exposed foodstuffs and crops would seriously threaten the lives of all survivors. The milk and water supplies would be dangerously contaminated.

The scientists and experts concluded, however, that the nation could and would survive, and the extent of survival would depend directly on the number of preparations made in advance. Inexpensive but effective civil defense precautions would save millions of lives.[29]

Civil Defense Program

Although civil defense has made progress during the last decade, there still remains a great deal of confusion, controversy, indifference, and doubt among the general public. The United States war plan assumes that the nation will suffer the first blow in any major nuclear war. Defense experts count on the expectation that the nation will not only survive the first onslaught, but will have the military strength to launch a massive counter-strike, and the morale to put the nation back on its feet. Yet, despite the urgent recommendations of major investigation groups and most civil defense experts, not a single city or state in the nation has a realistic nuclear bomb shelter system that on a national scale could save many millions of lives and perhaps make the difference between defeat and survival. Home front defenses are not ready for a massive nuclear attack, and there are no guarantees that they ever will be ready. Most people are not interested in warning signals, first aid kits, or bomb shelters.

United States Congressional members, who are national leaders and who control national funds, are partially responsible for the indifference and controversy in civil defense planning. These Congressional doubts about civil defense are reflected in the reduced civil defense budget requests. For example, from 1949 to 1958 civil defense officials requested a total appropriation of $2,176,000,353; Congress appropriated $492,276 or 23 per cent of the request. In 1959, a substantial increase in appropriations, totaling $15,000,000 made the civil defense future look somewhat brighter. Congressional controversy and indecision about civil defense are partially due to the fact that under the changing menace of atomic bombs, then hydrogen bombs, and now missiles, the planning emphasis has also dramatically changed. For example, protection emphasis changed from mass shelter programs to evacuation; at present, defense plans include both methods.

There is a great deal of controversy and confusion between the Federal Office of Civil and Defense Mobilization and the House Government Operations Committee concerning the quality of planning and the type of action that should be taken. For instance, the

Federal Office of Civil and Defense Mobilization (OCDM) urges evacuation of cities if there is enough warning; the House Committee says this will not work. Both agencies agree that there must be shelters to protect people against radioactive fallout. The OCDM, however, has ruled out any massive, federally financed shelter construction program; they believe it is up to each individual to build his own shelter. Vigorously dissenting, the House Committee argues that unless the federal government accepts the major responsibility for planning, financing, and building atomic shelters, the country will have no effective civil defense program. At any rate, the OCDM states that if every American family built its own basement shelter, atom deaths would be reduced by 12,000,000 persons and injuries reduced to another 12,000,000 persons. The government could save a high percentage of United States citizens from blast and fallout by spending $5,000,000,000 to $20,000,000,000 on federal shelters. At the present time, however, Congress is unwilling and the administration does not seem very interested. In 1959, the House Appropriations Committee refused President Eisenhower's request for funds to build an underground shelter for key government agencies in case of nuclear assault. The estimated cost was $2,700,000.

In 1959, New York's Governor Nelson Rockefeller became the first elected official in the United States to support a compulsory state-wide fallout shelter program. Rockefeller announced he would urge the state legislature to support the recommendations of his Special Task Force on Protection From Radioactive Fallout. The recommendations were:

1. A campaign to tell New York's 16,000,000 citizens about fallout dangers and what can be done about them.

2. A state law making fallout shelters mandatory in all new buildings, including private homes, and requiring owners of existing buildings to provide fallout protection for their occupants by a specified future date.

3. A state program to develop an inexpensive survival kit, including a water container (ten gallons per person), a two-week supply of dehydrated food, candles, a battery-powered radio, and a toilet container. The task force also suggested the development of an inexpensive, accurate, simple radiation detection device. Radiation cannot be seen, touched, tasted or felt, and if people in shelters had no reliable way of testing whether or not radiation had fallen to endurable levels outside, fear and doubt could shatter their morale and impair the nation's capacity to rebound.

The New York task force, made up of nine state officials, based its recommendations on two fundamental facts:

1. In a nuclear attack upon United States cities, fallout radiation could cause three or four times as many deaths as the blast and heat from exploding nuclear warheads.

2. Inexpensive fallout shelters would provide a very high degree of protection against fallout radiation.

In spite of shortcomings and handicaps, civil defense throughout the nation has made enough progress so that many millions of casualties would be prevented. For example, the Office of Civil and Defense Mobilization estimates that with three hours' warning, evacuation could reduce immediate casualties 47 per cent. In critical target zones, OCDM says blast shelters could reduce casualties 37 per cent. Improvised fallout shelters, perhaps in basements, could lower the death total 15 per cent. Perhaps the greatest challenge, however, is persuading and educating people that survival is a starkly personal responsibility they must accept and meet.

Six Steps For Survival

Civil defense authorities recommend the following six steps for survival:

1. Prepare your family for emergency. Stock home shelters

Loose, light-colored clothing affords better protection against thermal radiation from nuclear weapons than does dark, tightly fitting attire. Arrows indicate how various types of clothing reflect radiation.

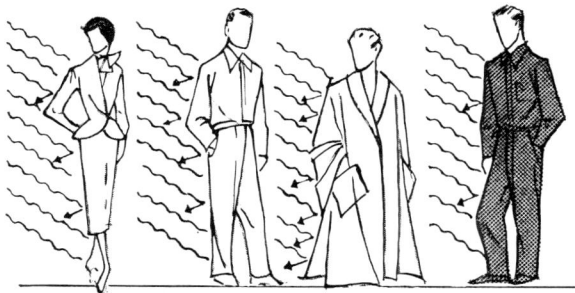

Steel, concrete, earth, and water provide different degrees of protection against radioactive substances. Equivalent effectiveness of these materials is represented by thicknesses shown. (After Stein and Warren)

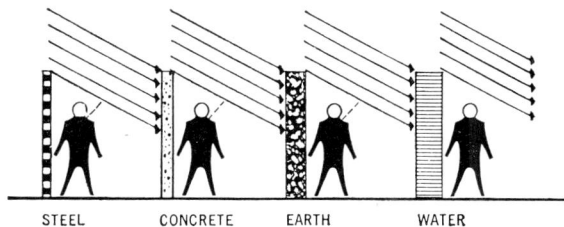

STEEL   CONCRETE   EARTH   WATER

Figure 61. (Modified from Stein, J. J., Warren, S. L., *Medical Problems of Atomic Attack.* California Medicine, 83:271, 1955.)

with a two-week supply of food and water, flashlight, battery-operated radio, can opener, first-aid supplies, and emergency cooking and sanitation facilities. Family members should have received Red Cross first-aid and home nursing courses.

2. Build a home shelter. The best protection against radioactive fallout is an outdoor shelter covered by at least three feet of earth, and with a suitable device to filter out dust. A basement shelter offers good protection. Learn the basic principles of "duck and cover" and seek the best available shelter.

3. Learn the civil defense public action signals: *Alert signal*—a steady blast of three to five minutes meaning that attack is probable. *Take cover signal*—a wailing tone, or a series of short blasts of three-minute duration.

4. Learn and follow evacuation principles in your area. This includes school, home, and office. Learn your community's plan for emergency action.

5. Learn the facts about radioactive fallout. Check with your local college, health department, or civil defense office.

6. Know the Conelrad stations—640 and 1240 on your radio dial. At the first indication of enemy bombers approaching the United States, all television and FM radio stations will go off the air. All standard AM stations will likewise be silent. The Conelrad stations, 640 and 1240, are the surest and fastest means of getting emergency information and instructions. These numbers should be marked on the radio dial.

PEACEFUL USES OF ATOMIC ENERGY

THE INDUSTRIAL ATOM. American industry has been alert to the opportunities for using radioisotopes. Today, more than 3,000 companies are using them in their production and research. In some cases, use of the isotope is resulting in new and better products. In other applications, the quality or shape of the products you buy are not changed, but production techniques are improved, enabling industry to save vast amounts of money—a saving that can be passed along to the consumer. It is estimated, in fact, that radioisotopes are already reducing industrial production costs by $150,000,000 annually. As new uses for the radioisotope in industry are discovered continually, this figure is certain to increase.

By using the radioisotope, manufacturers are developing a whole host of new and improved products. Here are a few examples:

BETTER PAINT. Manufacturers are studying the moisture resistance of paint by dipping samples in water tagged with hot hydrogen atoms. The amount of seepage can thus be accurately measured.

STRONGER PLASTICS. Radiation helps achieve material with greater strength and heat resistance than would otherwise be possible.

BETTER TIRES. A radioactive chemical is added when the tire is made. Then, with a Geiger counter, the wear on the tire is measured as it occurs.

BETTER TOOTHPASTE. The abrasive qualities of new toothpastes can be checked to protect you against loss of your own valuable enamel.

BETTER SOAPS AND DETERGENTS. Clothes are being deliberately soiled with dirt containing radioisotope tracers. After washing, a radiation detector checks the clothing to see how thoroughly the soap tested has removed the dirt.

BETTER MOTOR OIL. Engine parts such as pistons and piston rings can be made radioactive. After a brief test run, the amount of radioactivity in the engine oil is measured. Metal particles that have been worn away are revealed, and the effectiveness of the oil is accurately determined.

Industry is using radioisotopes in countless ways. They are used, for example, to measure and locate all sorts of things that otherwise could not be seen. In oil pipelines, scrapers sent through the lines to clean off obstructions are tagged with hot atoms. If they get stuck, a Geiger counter outside the pipe can easily spot the location. Radioactive detectors check whether or not food containers have been properly filled; they measure the thickness of sheet materials such as paper, plastic, rubber, or textiles. Friction and wear on machine tool parts can be accurately measured by radioisotopes. So sensitive are they that it is possible to detect the transfer of only one one-hundred billionth of an ounce of metal worn off the cutting surface.

These are but a few of the ways in which industry is utilizing the radioisotope in its never-ending quest for ways of doing old jobs better, or for doing jobs that previously could not be done at all. Top scientists and engineers in industry, government and universities are engaged in constant research to find new industrial uses for the constructive atom. For example, a major oil company is using radioactive cobalt pipe in an effort to find streamlined processes for the refinement and production of all kinds of petroleum products; the food industry is experimenting with radiation and its application to the preservation of meat and vegetables.[26]

The Medical Atom

Doctors say that through the use of atomic energy, medical knowledge has been advanced at least 25 years and that atomic energy is the greatest boon to medical science since the invention of the microscope and the discovery of germs. It is estimated that through the use of atomic energy in the field of medicine, more lives have been saved in recent years than were lost at Hiroshima and Nagasaki.

With radioisotopes used as tracers, doctors are learning much about how the body absorbs nutrients. Vitamins, minerals, sugars and salt can be tagged with radioisotopes to learn where they go, and how they are utilized. Many mysteries of the human machine are at least being solved, and the solutions are leading to the development of better therapeutic treatments.

Atomic energy also contributes to the science of medicine in the diagnosis of specific ailments in individual patients. In the more than 870 hospitals that now have atomic equipment, an estimated half-million persons have been given radioisotopes for diagnostic purposes during the past nine years.

Atomic energy is being used in the production of pharmaceuticals. Certain drugs, including penicillin and streptomycin, can be sterilized by radiation from isotopes. In addition, bandages, gauzes, sutures, and other medical aids are being subjected to radiation before packaging.

These accomplishments in relieving suffering and saving lives only foreshadows the ultimate possibilities for the widespread use of atomic energy in the medical field. The manner and speed with which additional medical discoveries can be shared with all mankind will be an important demonstration of America's constructive leadership in the world.[27]

The Agricultural Atom

The frontiers of farm science and land development must be pushed forward at an ever increasing rate to provide for world population growth and to improve living standards. Food production is not increasing as fast as population demands. World population is increasing at the rate of about 1 per cent or over 30,000,000 persons per year. Reliable estimates indicate that over half of the more than 3,000,000,000 people in the world today do not get enough to eat. To keep food production in pace there must be ever increasing production from the land and this advance must be based upon the work of plant and animal scientists.

All over the country, agricultural research is being stimulated through the use of radioactive and stable isotopes. These new tools are unlocking the secrets of the growth of plants and animals and the scourges that injure or destroy them. Most of these isotope uses are related to the fate of metabolites and nonmetabolites in plant and animal systems. The major applications of radioisotopes to agricultural problems have been concerned with soils and fertilizers, photosynthesis, entomology, and animal and plant nutrition.

A few of the aids to better farming brought about by the use of radioisotopes are listed here:

Important questions about livestock nutrition are being answered by atomic tracers. For instance, dairy cattle are being given small doses of radioisotopes in order to determine mineral requirements.

Techniques for feeding growing plants are also being improved, because radioactive tracers have definitely proved that

CLINICAL USES OF ATOMIC ENERGY

GOLD (AU 198)	decrease pleural effusions due to carcinoma . treat prostatic cancer
PHOSPHORUS (P 32)	treat polycythemia vera, certain leukemias . locate intraorbital tumors
COBALT (CO 60)	test for intrinsic factor in pernicious anemia . treat internal cancer
SODIUM (NA 24)	determine adequacy of blood supply in pedicle skin grafts . treat leukemias
BORON (B 10)	treat glioblastoma multiforme
IODINE (I 131)	diagnose and treat thyroid disorders . treat angina pectoris (certain cases)
IRON (FE 59)	study erythropoiesis in bone marrow
CHROMIUM (CR 51)	determine red cell mass
ARSENIC (AS 74)	locate brain tumors
STRONTIUM (SR 89, 90)	treat benign growths of sclera
IRIDIUM (IR 192)	treat cancer of larynx
YTTRIUM (Y 90)	decrease pleural effusions due to carcinoma

Figure 62. (Modified from *The Practitioner In The Atomic Age.* Therapeutic Notes, Parke, Davis & Co., *64*:4, Jan., 1957, page 4.)

fertilizers may be absorbed through the leaves of some plants, as well as through their roots.

Agricultural scientists are learning how to apply radiation to living cells in order to change their hereditary characteristics. New types of plants, and heartier plants, more resistant to blight and disease, are being developed.

Better insecticides and fungicides are being marketed as a result of research with radioisotopes. Plant disease now costs $3,000,000,000 a year, so the opportunity for great savings is apparent.[28]

The Power Atom

The power atom can be used to generate electricity. Today, most electric power is produced by steam turbine generators—huge machines driven by steam from boilers in which coal, oil, or natural gas is burned. In making atomic-electric power, the boiler with its conventional fuel is replaced by an atomic reactor; this is, essentially, nothing more than a chamber in which uranium atoms are being split. As the atoms split, they produce heat; the heat is used to make steam for the turbines.

The nation's future need for electric power is tremendous. To supply electricity for our homes and factories, it is estimated that America's power-generating capacity will have to be quadrupled by 1975. With television, air conditioning and other electric equipment, each home in America now uses an average of 2,500 kilowatt hours of electricity per year. Ten years from now, each home may use twice this amount. The consumption of electricity is increasing in our factories, too. In 1945, each American worker had approximately 10,000 kilowatt hours of electricity to help him in his job; now he has about 30,000 kilowatt hours. Ten years from now he will probably use three times this amount to operate labor saving, automatic equipment. Thus, the importance of atomic-electric power is the assurance that we will have enough electric power for our future needs. One pound of uranium is potentially capable of lighting the city of Chicago for one full day, or your home for 9,000 years.

QUESTIONS FOR REVIEW

1. List and briefly discuss the four types of ionizing radiation.
2. List and briefly discuss the sources of radiation.
3. What are the four major considerations involved in the biological aspects of radiation? Discuss.

4. Discuss the possible somatic and genetic effects of radiation.
5. Why is strontium-90 the most feared of all fallout isotopes?
6. Are X-rays necessary? Discuss.
7. List and briefly discuss the seven major preventive measures necessary to control community and personal radiation hazards and injury.
8. (a) List the major functions and activities of a radiological health division of a local health department,
   (b) State health department,
   (c) United States Public Health Service.
9. Briefly list and discuss major peaceful uses of atomic energy.
10. "Why should I build a fallout shelter? There won't be any survivors anyhow." Discuss this statement.
11. List the six steps for survival recommended by civil defense authorities.

REFERENCES

1. Cowan, F. P.: *Everyday Radiation*. Physics Today, 5:18–20, 1952.
2. Eisenbud, Merril, and Harley, John H.: *Radioactive Fallout in the United States*. Science, 121:677–80, 1955.
3. Commission on Atomic Energy: *Health and Safety Problems and Weather Effects Associated with Atomic Explosion*. Washington, D.C., U.S. Printing Office, 1955.
4. Davis, W. K.: *Industrial Power Reactors and Their Location*. Chicago, American Medical Association, 1955.
5. National Academy of Sciences: *The Biological Effects of Atomic Radiation*. Washington, D.C., National Academy of Sciences, 1956.
6. Stone, Robert S.: *The Concept of a Maximum Permissable Exposure*. Radiology, 41:7, 1952.
7. Bugher, John C.: *Radiation and Human Health*. Am. J. Pub. Health, 47: 682–87, 1957.
8. Alexander, Peter: *Atomic Radiation and Life*. England, Pelican-Penguin Books, 1957, Page 85.
9. United Nations Scientific Committee on the Effects of Atomic Radiation: *Report on Effect of Fallout on Leukemia*. Time, August 25, 1958, Page 37.
10. Editorial: Four Years After the Fallout. Today's Health, 36:50, 1958.
11. Advisory Committee on Biology and Medicine to the Atomic Energy Commission: *Part II—Statement on Radioactive Fallout*. California's Health, 15:112–17, 1958.
12. Consumer Reports: *The Milk All of Us Drink—and Fallout*. Mount Vernon, N.Y., March 1959, Pages 102–11.
13. National Tuberculosis Association: *National Tuberculosis Bulletin*. Washington, D.C., December, 1957.
14. Report of 58th Annual Meeting of the American Roentgen Society: *Radiological Health*. Pub. Health Rep., 72:1113–20, 1957.
15. Ibid., Page 1113.
16. Armstrong, G. E., et al.: *Radiation Survival*. U.S. Armed Forces M. J., 7:320, 1956.
17. Casberg, M. A.: *Emergency Treatment of Burns in Mass Casualties*. California Med., 83:289, 1955.
18. Regan, J. F.: *Proper Handling of Mass Casualties during a Major Disaster*. California Med., 83:282, 1955.
19. Department of Defense and Atomic Energy Commission: *Medical Aspects of Atomic Weapons*. Washington, D.C., U.S. Government Printing Office, 1950, Pages 13–14.

20. Ibid., Pages 20, 21.
21. Teller, Edward, and Latter, Albert L.: *Our Nuclear Future*. New York, Criterion Books, Inc., 1958.
22. *Nuclear Tests: World Debate*. Time, April 7, 1958, Page 16.
23. Calder, Ritchie: *Burying Live Atoms Is As Expensive as Burying Dead Pharaohs*. World Health, *12*:11, 1959.
24. Bergma, D.: *Radiological Health Service in New Jersey*. Pub. Health Rep., *70: 778–81*.
25. Hilleboe, Herman E., and Rihm, Alexander: *Program Planning for Radiological Health*. Am. J. Pub. Health, *48*:967, 1958.
26. Atomic Energy Commission: *Uses of Isotopes in Industry and in Physical and Chemical Research*, Washington, D. C., U.S. Government Printing Office, 1956.
27. Atomic Energy Commission: *Uses of Isotopes in Medical Research, Diagnosis and Therapy*. Washington, D.C., U.S. Government Printing Office, 1956.
28. Atomic Energy Commission: *Uses of Isotopes in Agricultural Studies*. Washington, D.C., U.S. Government Printing Office, 1956.
29. *The Atom*. Time, July 6, 1959, Page 14.

SUGGESTED READING

American Public Health Association: *Public Exposure to Ionizing Radiations*. New York, Public Health Association, 1958.

A United Nations Document, Vol. 10 & 11. *Peaceful Uses of Atomic Energy*. New York, Columbia University Press, 1956.

Bylinsky, Gene: *Atoms and Agriculture*. The Wall Street Journal, Oct. 27, 1960, Pages 1, 15.

Glasstone, Samuel: *Sourcebook on Atomic Energy*. New Jersey, D. Von Nostrand Co., Inc., 1950.

Hilleboe, Herman E., and Larimore, Granville W.: *Preventive Medicine, Principles of Prevention in the Occurrence and Progression of Disease*. Philadelphia, W. B. Saunders Company, 1959.

Hilleboe, Herman, M.D., and Rihm, Alexander, Jr.: *Program Planning for Radi ological Health*. Am. J. Pub. Health, *48*:965–70, 1958.

Kinsman, Simon, et al.: *Radiological Health Handbook*. U.S. Public Health Service, Washington, D.C., 1957.

Report of the U.S. National Academy of Sciences on *Biological Effects of Atomic Radiation*. Washington, D.C., National Research Council, 1956.

Report of the United Nations Scientific Committee on *the Effects of Atomic Radiation*. United Nations Secretariat, New York, 1958.

Sacks, Jacob: *The Atom at Work*. New York, The Ronald Press Co., 1956.

Schrick, Ray: *Atoms and Safety*. The Wall Street Journal, Nov. 7, 1960, Pages 1–14.

Schubert, Jack, and Lapp, Ralph E.: *Radiation: What it Is and How it Affects You*. New York, The Viking Press, 1958.

Scientific American Book: *Atomic Power*. New York, Simon & Schuster Co., 1955.

Stahl, W. R., Sullivan, R. R., and Erickson, H. M.: *Oregon's Radiological Health Program*. Pub. Health Rep., *75*: 331–36, 1960.

U.S. Atomic Energy Commission: *Semi-Annual Reports of*. Washington, D.C., U.S. Government Printing Office.

United States Dept. of Defense: *The Effects of Nuclear Weapons*. Washington, D.C., U.S. Government Printing Office, 1957.

Chapter XII

Space Health

THE POWER and pace of technology in man's new world have brought man to the brink of his greatest technological accomplishment. He is now ready to rocket himself into the endless emptiness of outer space. This can be expected in the United States or Russia well within a decade, barely 70 years after the first airplane was flown.

Many obstacles confront scientists, engineers, and physicians as they prepare ships and men for space flight. Space ships must be impervious to intense heat and cosmic rays. Interplanetary trips demand a light, longlasting fuel and precise navigational systems. The space pilot needs protective clothing and a self-contained, self-replenishing environment. For example, five pounds of common pond algae growing in a tank of sewage will give off enough oxygen for one man's needs. Pumped and dried, this plant can be made into food pills. Furthermore, the pilot and crew will have to be psychologically prepared to cope with such depressing phenomena as isolation, confinement, boredom, and weightlessness. Most of these obstacles, however, have been surmounted.

263

Space research is teaching man new concepts, methods, and ideas, and has unveiled new and challenging horizons. Research in the area of weightlessness, for example, may teach us entirely new methods of movement and orientation. The basic research involved in space medicine will affect each individual in the nation. Intensive investigations are uncovering solutions to basic past and present problems, such as radiation, many aspects of physiology, mental health, genetics, biochemistry, nutrition, and safety. It also increases the opportunity for scientists, sociologists, anthropologists, psychologists, physicians, and others to join hands in the promotion of physical, social, and emotional well-being throughout the world.

Clothing

The space pilot will be encased from head to foot in a suit of many layers. One part will keep the blood from rushing to his head or his feet under peak gravitational forces during blast-off and re-entry. Another layer (actually two layers of clear plastic, with nonoverlapping holes for air to get in and out) will cool him. An insulating layer will prevent his being burned in the inferno of atmospheric friction, both outbound and inbound. Above 63,000 feet the body's blood boils, and the air is like a vacuum for a pilot who might bail out. Another layer of the space suit, with airtight linkage to the pilot's plastic-visored helmet, will maintain a comfortable atmospheric pressure, even if his space cabin should be punctured. This may serve also as an immersion suit in case he lands in the ocean. The suit will be air tight, water tight, and lightweight. The wearer of the suit will be quite comfortable at 67 degrees below zero—a temperature which may be found on the moon.*

Atmosphere

The space capsule, like the pressure suit within it, will be pressurized at about seven and one half pounds per square inch—the pressure normally found at 18,000 feet. Instead of ordinary air (21 per cent oxygen), the space capsule will be filled with an artificial atmosphere containing at least 40 per cent oxygen, to give the spaceman the same quantity of oxygen he would enjoy at sea level. During launching and reentry, the space pilot will have his pressure suit inflated. In relaxed, straightaway flight, he will be able to

* *Outward Bound.* Time, May 26, 1958, Page 77.

deflate his suit, open his visor and rely on cabin air. The air will be filtered, probably through lithium hydride, to remove carbon dioxide and excess water vapor from breath and sweat. It will also be cooled and deodorized.

A valuable lesson has been learned from the Indians at Morococha, a mining town in Peru's central Andean highlands. At 14,900 feet elevation, Morococha has an average atmospheric pressure slightly more than half that at sea level. But its barrel-chested natives, after generations of exposures to perpetual oxygen shortage,

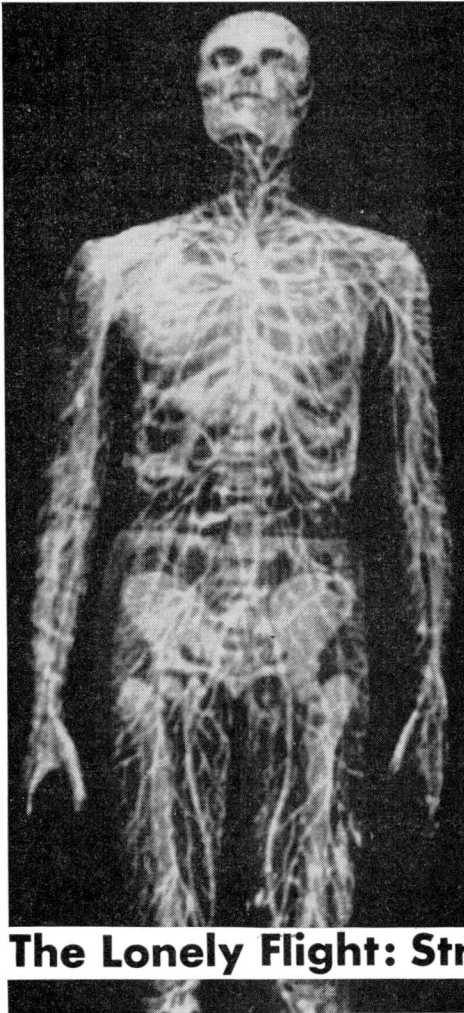

5. Outer space: On long, lonely voyages man will undergo severe psychological stresses of isolation, detachment, confinement.

↑

4. In space: Condition of zero gravity. Body becomes weightless, loses orientation. Nervous system and stomach affected.

↑

3. Above atmosphere: Solar radiation in the form of cosmic, ultraviolet, and X rays bombards tissues and reproductive cells.

↑

2. Lower atmosphere: Even here, without pressurized suit or cabin, blood begins to boil. Oxygen supply necessary.

↑

1. Take-off: Crushing force of rocket acceleration multiplies body weight, impairs circulation. Vision and movement hampered.

↑

The Lonely Flight: Stresses and Strains

Figure 63. (From *Man In Space*, Newsweek, Feb. 3, 1958.)

have a lung structure and blood pattern especially adapted to extract full value from the last available atom of oxygen. They even go to 16,000 feet to relax by playing a murderously fast game of soccer. Key questions for the Air Force researchers were: (1) Would this adaptation help a spaceman survive if he accidentally lost his oxygen supply? and (2) can people from other areas achieve the high Andean's resistance to oxygen deprivation in a matter of weeks instead of centuries? Investigations revealed that a space-man, or astronaut, having temporary trouble would be able to func-tion effectively far longer and thus perhaps save his life, if he had the high Andean's altitude endurance.[1]

Weightlessness

In dozens of military and civilian laboratories across the nation, researchers are working to perfect ways of keeping a human being alive and functioning efficiently when he soars into space. None of their problems is as intangible as weightlessness, the gravity-free state that will envelop man when he orbits around the earth or reaches for the moon and planets. This is because in the earth's atmosphere and gravity belt, this unearthly state can be created only for a fraction of a minute at a time.

Time's Medicine Editor Gilbert Cant went weightless in one of the fast jet fighters of the Air Force. His account follows:

> At 500 knots the F-100F Super Sabre pulled out of its dive and rocketed upward. Up went the needle on the accelerometer or "g meter," which gauges the piling up of gravity forces. In a "g suit" hooked up to an automatic air-compressor system, I felt a giant's fist pressing into my belly, two pairs of giant hands around my thighs and calves, to retard the flow of blood to the feet and reduce the risk of blackout. Belatedly I remembered to try the "M-1 maneuver"—tensing the abdominal muscles to reduce the blood drainage still more. The g-meter needle crept up past 2 to 3 and on to 4. My normal 145 lbs. now weighed 580: I felt compressed, depressed. Even the light rubber ball of the pneumatic re-lease for my camera shutter, held in my hand, seemed unbearably heavy. With the eyeballs tugged downward, with eyelids feeling like rusty iron curtains, it was an intense effort to peek "up" to keep watching the meters. As we approached the peak of our climb, the relentless 4-g pressure was lifted and suddenly we slipped through a man-made loophole in the law of gravity: we weighed nothing at all. . . .[2]

Weightlessness is reached when an object's outward speed or cen-trifugal force exactly balances and cancels out the downward pull of gravity exerted by the earth. For a brief instant, a state of near zero gravity may be experienced when springing from a diving board, driving fast over a sudden dip in the road, or going over the top of a roller coaster. Breathing, digestion, and blood circulation seem to present no apparent problems; a man can inhale and swallow while hanging upside down from a trapeze bar. However, the acceleration pressure of eight times the pull of gravity may make breathing difficult. The spaceman may strain his respiratory muscles in order to overcome the crushing force, and breathing may become irregular. His heart size may double, and the instruments before his eyes may fade from view. There is some evidence that weightlessness produces mental confusion and air sickness, or more properly, space sickness. Without gravity pull, body sense organs will continually pass false information to the brain. A fear of falling, and in some cases actual terror, have been observed in tests. The eyes will have to provide a sense of balance by feeding the brain visual clues for orientation.

Scientists are concerned about the development of minor physiologic disturbances that, if cumulative or irritating, may cause or enhance psychiatric symptoms when the weightless state becomes longer. We can best investigate this by utilizing our rocket capabilities to establish biological laboratories in the sky. There is now a statistically significant basis for the assumption that man can handle the zero gravity situation for short periods of time. The final answer concerning longer periods, however, can only be found in a manned orbiting vehicle. It is up to the ingenuity of the engineer to invent magnetic and other kinds of devices that may provide a make-believe gravity.

Elusive, intangible, and therefore frightening, is the weightlessness, or zero-g state that the pilot will experience in orbital flight

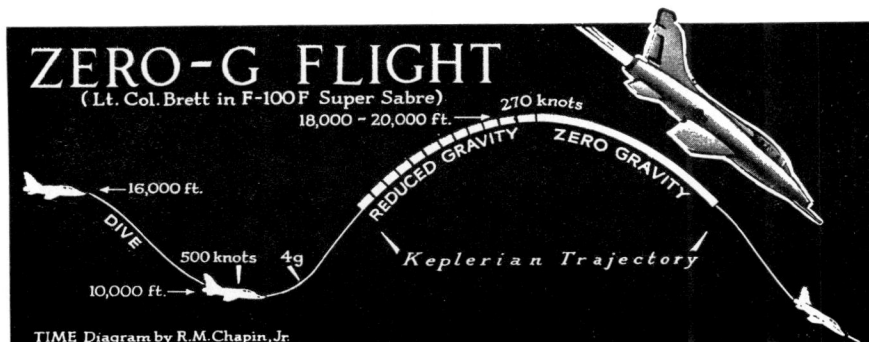

Figure 64. At 50,000 feet, man is the same physiologically as he would be on the moon. (From *How to Go Weightless*. *Time*, June 9, 1958, page 55.)

or true space travel. Quick movement of an arm in this state would spin him around or hurl him against the wall. Major Herbert Stallings of the Randolph Air Force Base believes that weightlessness will actually help the space pilot. He feels that a man can probably get as much rest from four hours of weightless sleep as he can from eight hours on a feather bed because there are no pressure points. He also finds weightlessness exhilarating, and notes that the maneuvers he now has to execute while flying a jet in this state are much more difficult than a space pilot will have in straightaway flight. But of 115 volunteers who have flown with Major Stallings, one-third suffered nausea, vomiting or vertigo to the point of incapacity. Air Force physiologists foresee possible grave difficulties for both the circulatory and respiratory systems under long exposure to gravity-free conditions.*

G Forces

The human body can stand travel at any rate of speed provided that it is constant. A too-abrupt change in speed or direction is what hurts. Standard of measurement for such changes is the g (from gravity), which is equal to the acceleration produced by the earth's pull at sea level. Unprotected and in normal sitting position, the body cannot stand more than about three and one-half g's for more than about 15 seconds. Semisupine, even without a pressure suit, it can stand six g's for four and one-half minutes, as much as 12 g's for only six seconds. But in blast-off or reentry, g forces build up; not only is speed sharply increased or decreased, but the rate of change is itself increased. When the ship accelerates, pull increases much as a motorist experiences slightly when a sudden start pushes him back in his seat.

To find out how many g's man can endure, Colonel John Paul Stapp hurtled through a succession of harrowing rides on a rocket sled at Halloman Air Force Base, New Mexico. As he accelerated to a speed of 632 miles per hour and came to a dead stop, Stapp took forces as high as 40 g's for one-fifth of a second. In the process he also suffered broken ribs, a torn retina, and several hemorrhages; but when he was through, he had demonstrated that man can tolerate the massive g forces of a space-bound rocket. With present-day rocket fuels, peaks of eight or nine g's might last as long as three minutes; tests show man can cope with these peaks best if he is protected by a special pressurized g-suit and lies prone,

* *Outward Bound.* Time, May 26, 1958, Page 77.

so that his head and heart are level. In this position blackouts caused by blood draining from the head, or redouts caused by blood pooling in the skull, are effectively avoided. But during these moments only one or two major decisions may be expected of him. For example, if the spaceman's rocket falters on the launching pad, or vibrates too much and coagulates body fluids in the first few seconds of powered flight, the passenger must be able to hit an ejection switch that would explosively, but safely, throw him clear of the vehicle.

Man can stand the addition of one g every four and one-half seconds for only 54 seconds up to a maximum of 12 g's. Fortunately, from Dr. Stapp's work and other tests, researchers at Wright Air Force Base have found that a man quickly recovers his ability to withstand a new g onslaught. After first-stage burnout of a three-stage rocket, a man coasts for several seconds at high but steady speed; when the second stage blasts off, he can take it, and his body is also ready for the acceleration of the final blast. On reentry, the g forces caused by deceleration are likely to be far more perilous. Impact of hitting even the thinnest outer layer of the atmosphere head-on at 18,000 miles per hour is like driving a car through a blast furnace against a cliff at 60 miles per hour. To slow down, the pilot may have to glide in at an angle of no more than four degrees, then return to cool off as soon as he has slowed down a bit. He may have to repeat this a dozen or more times, taking terrific buffeting in the process. Only after he has slowed down to about 3,000 miles per hour will the pilot be able to set his air brake and open a stainless steel parachute. The shock that this produces may be the worst of all. Sustained g effects from a multi-stage rocket's typical three-peak acceleration is being conclusively tested by a new rocket sled track at the Holloman Air Force Base. Stretching seven miles across New Mexico's Tularosa Valley, the track is the longest known in the world and will permit accelerations to 200 g's.*

Temperature

Experiments with grounded space capsules reveal that the average man functions best when temperatures are maintained between 50 and 70 degrees Fahrenheit, and humidity is kept from 40 to 60 per cent. Carbon dioxide must be present in the air because the gas stimulates brain breathing centers, but must be carefully controlled to prevent more than two per cent in the air. The ter-

* Ibid., Page 77.

rific heat built up in the shell of the space cabin after blast-off will soon be lost by radiation; on reentry it will be a continuing problem. In orbital flight, dodging in and out of the earth's shadow, with the capsule's insulating wall and the pilot's private, form-fitting air conditioning, this problem should be overcome. Flying to the moon or beyond, one side of the capsule will overheat, while the other will fall to the far-below-freezing temperatures of the void. It may be necessary to rotate the ship slowly. Still, data from the space ship Explorer I showed a comfortable inside temperature of from 50 to 85 degress. *

Food and Drink

Although food and vitamin pills can be stored in the space ship, a proposal has been made to provide each space ship crew member with a forty-gallon mixture of water, bacteria, and two strains of algae. The mixture can provide all the oxygen and fresh drinking water needed for a space trip of indefinite length. The mixture can also provide much of the crew's daily protein food requirements, and can consume all the ship's human waste products. The basic life cycles of photosynthesis and oxidation can exist indefinitely in a closed system. In the space ship's system, the bacteria would convert organic waste materials into carbon dioxide and water; the algae would use the carbon dioxide and some of the water to produce oxygen and more algae. The crew members could drink the water, breathe the oxygen, eat the extra algae in the form of protein-rich pills, and consume a few extra nutrients as well. The interposition of an animal such as a goat, slug, snail, or some other animal which eats algae directly would yield animal protein for the space crew. Urine may be double distilled to yield pure water; 10 per cent of a man's own water can be recovered daily.

It is thought that the man in space will eat highly concentrated, nourishing pastes, squeezing them into his mouth from plastic containers that will stay depressed when squeezed. Though he will be sitting still, exerting himself hardly at all with no gravity or friction to overcome, the Air Force estimates he will need 3,000 to 3,400 calories a day. If fliers' appetites increase with altitude, as some have reported, the only explanation is nervous tension.

Drinking is more difficult. Some of the space passengers trying to drink from a plastic cup have succeeded only in soaking their suits, or having the water pour up into their nasal passages and

* *Outward Bound.* Time, May 26, 1958, Page 77.

sinuses. The answer to this problem seems to be elastic containers, with polyethylene tubes for the pilot to suck the liquids out. Only after food has reached the stomach can the muscles in the digestive tract be relied on to keep things moving.

Elimination

The muscles and nerves controlling elimination should function normally even in long g-free flights. The space pilot will urinate into a vessel similar to those in air-bound military planes today. Defecation is more of a problem. For a weekend trip, the pilot will be preconditioned by eating a low-residue diet (no bulky leaf vegetables, peas, corn or beans, or fat). For longer space voyages, lasting weeks, months or years, all the difficulties of food, drink and elimination are increased. Weight is the first foe of the rocketeer trying to get a manned capsule into space, so everything that can possibly be saved and reused must be conserved. Therefore, in addition to recycling his oxygen supply (perhaps with elaborate photolysis, to break down the accumulating carbon dioxide), the space pilot will have to recycle his body wastes. Extraction of palatable water, though still not perfected, might be practical for space flight if the equipment weight were reduced. One suggestion for maintaining a near-perpetual cycle of food is to use the pilot's wastes as food for algae, which will convert them into something edible; algae will also consume carbon dioxide and make oxygen. Another foreseen possibility is offering the spaceman a diet of sugar water, enriched with vitamins, minerals and protein factors and thickened with shredded paper towel.

Cosmic Radiation

One of the most serious dangers facing the spaceman is solar radiation, particularly the cosmic ray particles thrown off by giant solar storms. Terrestial man is protected to a great degree from cosmic radiation by the atmosphere and magnetic fields around the earth that screen out and deflect the shower of particles. Swirling storms of atomic particles in space cause mutations in bread mold, and will probably have the same effect in humans if they strike the genes in the reproductive systems. In order to test the effects of radiation in space, selected members of the plant and animal kingdom were placed in the Able-Baker monkey-Jupiter space ship in 1959. Members included tubes containing living onion tissue, yeast cells, corn and mustard seeds, fruit flies, human blood, and the eggs and sperm of sea urchins. Some of the eggs and sperm were arranged to be mixed during flight, thus causing the first conception of earthly life in space for later study. Yeast, a single-celled plant, is ideal for radiation studies because it multiplies rapidly, yet uses oxygen as human cells do. Yeast cells double by simple cell division once every two hours at 86 degrees Fahrenheit. The packet of 200 corn seeds were of a genetic strain known as heterozygous green-yellow. The leaves of this corn get their characteristic coloring from chromosomes in the seed, just as a child gets eye color from its parents. From laboratory experiments, it is known that radiation produces changes in these seed chromosomes, which show up as a pale yellowness in the leaves. By planting the seeds bombarded during the flight, geneticists can see how pale and yellow the leaves become, and in turn reconstruct the intensity of the less cosmic rays. Other good candidates for research data include the mouse, pig, and monkey. The mouse is small and sturdy and has skin that permits easy attachment of electrodes for recording effects of blast-off and radiation in orbit. Furthermore, mice breed rapidly, are easy to handle, and inexpensive to feed and house. The pig is second in intelligence only to primates and has an endocrine system similar to man. The monkey is tough, resident, and ingenious, and is similar to man in anatomical make-up and emotional response. Chimpanzees, however, will probably be the last step before man enters space.

The most recent important development in the field of radiation and space is from Dr. James Van Allen's report that the radiation belt does not die off evenly.[3] Beyond it are irregular bursts of radiation that may be clouds of electrons and protons arriving fresh from the sun. An inner radiation belt occurs at approximately 600 miles from the earth, and a second large doughnut-shaped radiation belt occurs at approximately 8,000 miles from the earth. Such invisible clouds in space may prove serious hazards for deep space voyagers. However, one preventive measure would include avoiding the solar storms which occur in predictable eleven-year cycles.

Isolation

A. Scott Crossfield,, the man scheduled to be the first to journey into space 100 miles or more above the earth in a rocket-powered X-15, commented: "Aeromedical problems in orbit are, in order of importance, boredom, weightlessness, radiation, and then some of the difficulties of detachment. The boredom thing is serious. It is nature that a pilot literally goes to sleep at the switch when he has nothing to do. Demanding tasks enhance his entire performance."[4]

Loneliness is an appalling depressant. Although Rear Admiral Richard E. Byrd had navy training and lofty motivation, a six-month Antarctic night threw him into depression. Studies of airmen and other volunteers in such settings have shown that a man studying a dimly lit instrument panel or radarscope in darkness and total silence soon begins to see things that are not there. Psychologists agree that the space pilot must have an abundant "sensory input" as well as work to do. He must be able to talk to the ground whenever he is awake and ask himself such questions as, "Where am I? How am I doing?", and get reassuring answers. He must have music wherever he goes, and perhaps a television screen on which he can see where he is in relation to the earth.

Exposure to "everyday life" in space over a period of one to several weeks or even months, in an orbital test bed is an important factor in conditioning a space crew for prolonged absence from earth. Perhaps providing submarine condition periods for duty, recreation, and sleep would be effective. Submarine crews change duty every four hours, and this may be best for space crews, too.

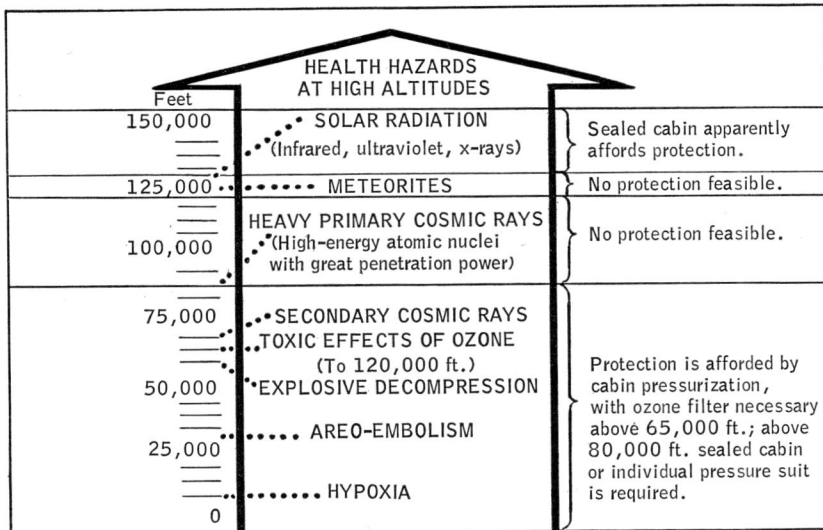

Figure 65. After Graybiel, A., *Future Trends In Aviation Medicine*. (Modified from Therapeutic Notes, Parke, Davis & Co.)

WHAT MAKES A GOOD SPACEMAN?

Candidates nominated by various psychologists for mankind's first space journey include Buddhist monks who are less time-oriented than Western man; midgets who take up less space; women for fortitude; personality deviates who often enjoy their hallucinations; and happily married couples. However, Dr. Hubertus Strughold, father of space medicine, and other experts agree that the following qualifications are necessary: a superb physical specimen; a mature man, well adjusted to life on earth, with a keen appreciation of his own importance and identity; highly motivated, experienced jet pilot, steady hand; high IQ; steady judgment; and a personality to adapt to loneliness. The space mission needs the strongly motivated team player who is also sufficiently self-assured and experienced in peril to act effectively on a solo mission, when he can rely only upon himself and his ship. Such versatile men best survived the shipwrecks of World War II and the prison camps of Korea.

Seven men have been chosen to test for the first time whether or not a human can be shot beyond the atmosphere to orbit the earth from 125 miles up, at 18,000 miles per hour and return safely to tell about it. One will try first. If he survives, the other six will follow his trail; if he fails, the other six will be there to carry on. These seven men are five feet, eleven inches tall or less, which will enable them to squeeze into the space capsule. Their ages range from 32 to 37. This is old enough to have the required engineering background and experience in the air, and young and fit enough to explore the unknown. Each man was born in a small town, is married, a father, and an active sportsman; each expressed an intimate love for the skies and an abiding faith in the heavens.

The seven astronauts of Project Mercury were screened by the most searching tests man could devise and machines could execute. The Air Force, navy, and marines selected the nation's 110 most likely military test pilots who had at least 1,500 flight hours. Punch card selectors pared the list to 69 men of optimum size, health, and intelligence. Finalists were jolted, spun, vibrated, crushed, chilled, and roasted in physical and psychological tests simulating the stresses of space flight. Each man hiked a treadmill elevated one degree per minute, and pedaled increasing amounts of weight on a bike-like device. Each was whirled three and one-half minutes in a centrifuge speeding at various angles that simulated pressures up to 12 times the pull of gravity; placed for one hour in a pressure chamber at a simulated altitude of 65,000 feet; then placed in a heat chamber of 130 degrees Fahrenheit for two hours. Each was bombared with piercing noises and incredibly high frequency sounds; each was shut into a dark, soundproof room for three hours to measure his adaptability to isolation. Before, during and after these tests the men were given the most thorough physical examinations ever devised.*

There are many motives for the push into space. Satellites can serve as communication relays, act as aids for navigation, and observe enemy territory. The most simple and basic motivation into space is man's enduring and insatiable drive to explore and know his environment. It is supreme adventure for man's spirit as well as his rockets. The stars and the moon have long been symbols of a remote and indifferent universe, a reproach to man's insignificance. Now man, for the first time, is challenging the planets themselves.

QUESTIONS FOR REVIEW

1. Why should we be concerned about space health?
2. What are some examples of weightlessness that we experience routinely?
3. What makes a good spaceman?
4. Briefly discuss each of the following space health problems:
   (a) temperature
   (b) food and drink
   (c) elimination
   (d) cosmic radiation
   (e) isolation
5. List five sources of space health information.
6. What are the implications of space health in the schools? Public health departments?
7. How can we help prepare future astronauts?
8. Explain the following statement: "Man's push into space is simply an extension of his desire to climb a tree or a mountain."
9. "It would be of more value and less money to our nation at this time to explore the oceans instead of space." Discuss this statement.

REFERENCES

1. *Way Station to Space.* Time, November, 24, 1958, Page 77.
2. *How To Go Weightless.* Time, June 9, 1958, Page 55.
3. *Reach into Space.* Time, May 4, 1959, Pages 64–70.
4. Golin, Milton: *The Moon Is Old Hat.* J.A.M.A., *169:*492, 1959.

SUGGESTED READING

Bakulev, A.: *Destination—Space.* USSR, Illustrated Monthly, Washington, D.C., 1960.

* *Space.* Time, April 20, 1959, Pages 17, 19.

Bibliography of Space Medicine, U.S. Dept. of Health, Education and Welfare, Public Health Service, PHS Publication No. 617, Government Printing Office, Washington, D.C., 1958.

Davis, T. R. A.: *Man Alive In Outer Space.* Atlantic Monthly, 205:39–44, 1960.

Flickinger, D. D.: *From Outer Space: New Concepts in Medicine.* Today's Health, 37:50–55, 1959.

MacGuire, H. C.: *Space Medicine Is Coming Down to Earth.* Reader's Digest, 75:57–60, 1959.

Chapter XIII

Organization and
Administration of Official
and Voluntary Health Agencies

THE CONSTITUTION as originally adopted in 1788 made no direct
reference to public health. Public health had not become as significant a national need as other more pressing problems, and thus
public health became a responsibility of the individual states. Fear
of importation of disease prompted state legislatures to draft and
adopt minimum health codes and establish state health departments. These state laws were soon expanded to provide for local
ordinances pertaining to community health and sanitation, and this
precipitated the birth of county and city health departments.

Public health workers have witnessed rapid growing, complex,
health organizations striving to keep pace with rapid growing,
complex societies. Public financial support has been growing
steadily with increased understanding of how public health services
actually save the tax payers' money as well as their lives. Unfortu-

277

nately, many areas still lack the services of a health department. Since public health can move no faster than the public allows, education has always been basic to all public health work. While the health departments have responsibility for enforcement of a great many laws and regulations, compulsion has never been their most important method of protecting the health of the public. The ultimate responsibility for community health, therefore, rests with the interested people of the community.

Local Health Department Organization

Health departments continue to emphasize their two major objectives—preventing disease and prolonging life. The organization of local health departments varies in complexity and in number of staff but Figure 66 represents a typical, large county health department program and service.

The staff, in general, consists of well trained, professional persons. The health officer and his physicians usually hold M.D. degrees plus a Masters of Public Health. Special academic preparation is also required of the public health nurse, public health laboratory technician, dentist, sanitarian, industrial hygienist, statistician, chemist, health educator, social worker, and many others. For recommended qualifications for public health personnel, see *Administration of Public Health Services* by R. B. Freeman and E. M. Holmes.[1] The following professional schools of public health offer various degrees in the field:

School of Public Health
University of California
Berkeley 4, California

School of Public Health and Administrative Medicine
Columbia University, 600 West 168th Street
New York 32, New York

School of Public Health
Harvard University, 55 Shattuck Street
Boston 15, Massachusetts

School of Hygiene and Public Health
Johns Hopkins University, 615 N. Wolfe Street
Baltimore 5, Maryland

School of Public Health
University of Michigan
Ann Arbor, Michigan

School of Public Health
University of Minnesota
Minneapolis 14, Minnesota

School of Public Health
University of North Carolina
Chapel Hill, North Carolina

School of Public Health
University of Pittsburgh
Pittsburgh, Pennsylvania

School of Public Health
University of Puerto Rico
San Juan, Puerto Rico

School of Public Health
Department of Tropical Medicine and Public Health
Tulane University, New Orleans 12, Louisiana

Yale University, Department of Public Health
111 Cedar Street, New Haven 11, Connecticut

SERVICES OF THE LOCAL HEALTH DEPARTMENT. The activities of a local health department are varied and interrelated, but they still include the following six broad categories that are essential: health education, sanitation, disease control, maternal and child health, vital statistics, and laboratory facilities. Each of these areas will be discussed below.

Vital Statistics. Two major services, vital registration and statistical tabulation, are performed by this division. All births and deaths occurring in the health department jurisdiction are registered and routed to the county recorder and state health department. The statistics division also receives records and tabulates reports of communicable diseases. From records of such vital events, analyses are made of trends and changes in the over-all public health situation. With this information, the health department is able to measure progress and to plan its work efficiently and realistically. Although all states have adopted regulations relating to the immediate reporting of certain communicable diseases to the health department, it is quite evident that this is not the case in most situations, and therefore, local and state statistics are only as reliable as the reporting person or agency. The statistics division also records health department activities, issues certified copies of births and deaths, and keeps private physicians and the public informed of changes in the health status.

Disease Control. Immunization, sanitation, and *health education* are key words in disease control. Immunizations against diphtheria, tetanus, pertussis, poliomyelitis, and smallpox are given to preschool and school-age children who have not been immunized by their family physician. These immunizations are recorded in the student's cumulative health record. The United States Public Health Service recommended immunization schedule follows:

Table 14.   Recommended Immunization Schedule[2]

	ESSENTIAL SHOTS	
DISEASE	TIME OF INOCULATION	BOOSTERS
Diphtheria Whooping Cough Tetanus	As early as 2 months of age. Series: 3 injections one month apart.	One at 1 yr. of age, one entering school. Tetanus every 4 years.
Polio	After 2 mo. Series: injections a month apart. A fourth 7–12 mo. later. (Sometimes combined with above 3.)	One shot upon entering school.
Smallpox	Vaccination. After 3 mo. and before 1 yr. of age.	Revaccination before entering school. Booster every 3 yrs. for repeated travel.
	RECOMMENDED SHOTS	
Influenza	Any age past 3 mo. Series: 2 shots one mo. apart for person exposed to flu in their work.	Annually for persons exposed or endangered.
German Measles	Series: 1 shot of gamma globulin for pregnant women exposed to German Measles in first 4 mo. of pregnancy.	None unless exposed in another pregnancy.
Infectious Hepatitis	One shot of gamma globulin if recommended by physician for persons exposed.	None
Typhoid	After 3 mo. Series: 3 shots one to four weeks apart. For persons taking trips where water supply is questionable.	One shot every three years if visiting frequently or living in typhoid area.
Tuberculosis	After 3 mo. Series: 1 shot BCG vaccine for selected persons unavoidably exposed to continuous contact with T.B.	As recommended by the family physician.
Rabies	Any age. Series: Up to 14 injections after being bitten by an animal rabied or suspected of being rabid.	None
Yellow Fever	After age 6 mo. Series: 1 shot if going to yellow fever area.	Booster, if remaining in a yellow fever area for prolonged period.
Cholera	After age 6 mo. Series: 2 shots 7 to 10 days apart if traveling to cholera area.	Booster 4 to 6 mo. apart if living in cholera area. After 4 years repeat immunization.

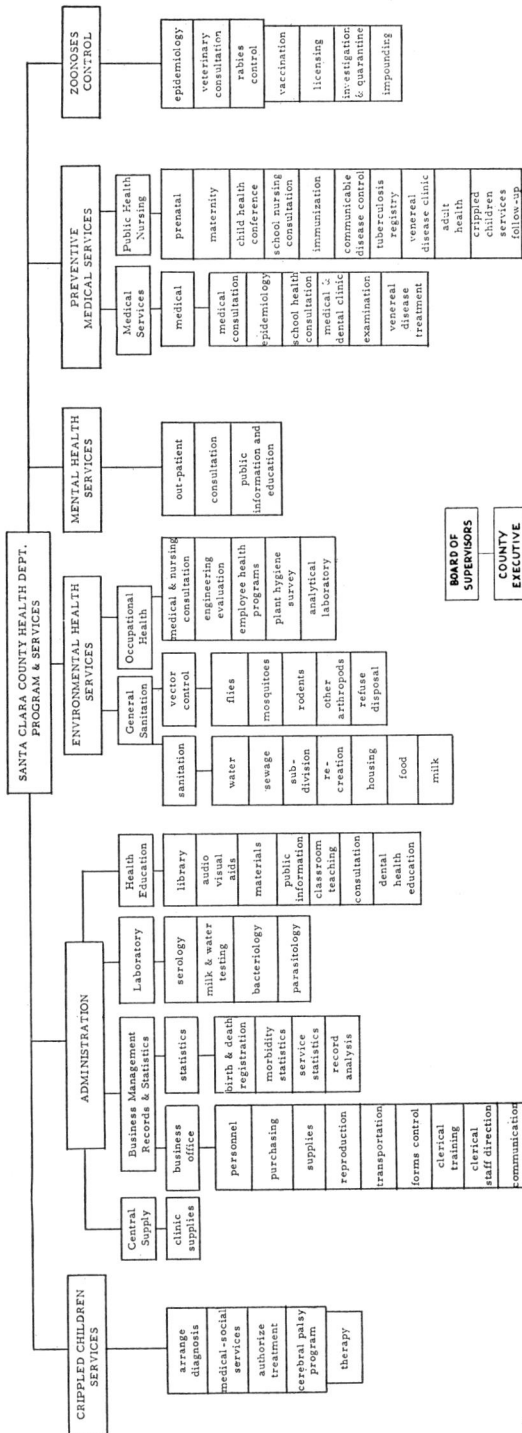

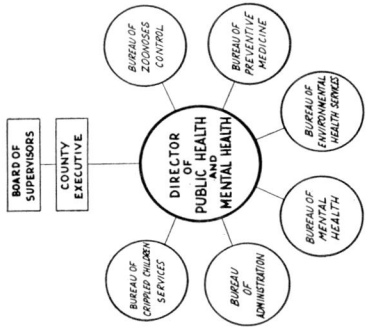

Figure 66. Program and services of the Santa Clara County Health Department, Calif.

281

Sanitarians work for the suppression of disease transmission by controlling potential sources of disease through the regular supervision of food establishments, water and milk supplies, sewage disposal systems, and insect and vector control.

The health department provides both treatment and education in its venereal disease clinic. Visits include those people who have been referred to the clinic by their family physician and others who come voluntarily for diagnosis or treatment. Contacts of venereal disease patients are investigated to prevent further spread of the disease. Premarital and prenatal examinations are also available.

Community protection against tuberculosis is accomplished by case finding, referral to diagnostic and treatment services, and nursing supervision of cases and contacts. Records of all known cases of tuberculosis within the county are recorded and filed in the Tuberculosis Case Registry, which is the key to the control program. The registry is used by private physicians, the tuberculosis association, local sanitarians, and public health nurses to coordinate case finding, treatment, and home care of patients.

Health education is stressed by each member of a local health department in an effort to prevent disease. For example, the sanitation division of most local health departments conducts training classes regarding the proper handling of food. Upon completion of this course by restaurant employers and employees, each class member receives a card that recognizes his training.

Sanitation. The varied activities of the sanitation division include provisions for the safety of public water, air, and milk supplies; safe and adequate disposal of wastes; sanitary supervision and assistance to food establishments; study of new subdivision proposals and community developments; mosquito, vector, and rodent control services; auto court, motel and trailer camp sanitation; consultation to schools for sanitation and safety; recreational sanitation; and investigation of citizens' complaints and abatement of public health nuisances.

Prevention of the spread of water-borne diseases necessitates inspection and survey of water systems, and collection of water samples for analysis in the public health laboratory. Periodic inspection of swimming pools insures both water purity and pool safety, thereby protecting swimmers from disease and injury. Plans for proposed new public pools must have health department approval prior to construction.

Sanitary supervision of dairies, creameries, milk distribution plants, and equipment insures clean, pure milk and milk products. Counsel and assistance is provided to milk producers and processors.

Animal disease control services include the inspection of live-stock to prevent the transmission of tuberculosis, undulant fever (brucellosis) and other diseases to humans. Milk and meat super-vision may be conducted by representatives from the Department of Agriculture in some communities.

The rabies control program is maintained primarily to avoid the possibility of humans becoming infected with this disease and to protect dogs from the threat of rabies. The mandatory vaccination and licensing of dogs; control of stray animals and investigation of animal bite cases; and the isolation of known or suspected rabid animals minimize the danger of rabies outbreaks and are within the jurisdiction of the health department.

The ultimate goal of the sewage disposal program is the com-plete sewering of urbanized residential areas throughout the local or county area. The sanitation division assists in the promotion and construction of sanitary sewers. The division has established standard methods for the construction of septic tank sewage disposal systems for use in areas where sewers are not available.

The rapid population increase and resultant growth of new resi-dential areas in many counties require the study of each proposed subdivision to insure adequate supplies of potable water; the safe disposal of sewage and other wastes; and protection from such nuisance or disease carriers as flies, mosquitoes, and rodents. Builders of new residences are required to obtain approval for underground disposal of sewage. Sanitarians aid the builder by performing scientifically engineered soil studies and by indicating best con-struction principles.

The objective of the vector control program is to reduce and eliminate sources of insects and rodents on private and public premises. This is accomplished by education, persuasion, and co-operation; spraying and elimination of breeding places are routinely conducted.

Periodic supervision and consultation to operators of food establishments require a great amount of the sanitarian's time. Guidance and education of the operators have replaced reprisals and legal action in the vast majority of instances. Refer to Appendix 5 for a typical sanitation inspection sheet.

Public Health Nursing.   The public health nurse gives, arranges for, or teaches nursing care; plans for coordinated medical services for individuals and families under her care; appraises individual and family health needs; provides health counseling; consults with and refers families to appropriate personnel within the health department, school or other community services; and organizes community groups for health purposes. Her activities include educational and demonstrational work in the home, clinic, school, community, or health center. In all phases of the work, emphasis is placed on the prevention of disease, the promotion of health, and rehabilitation of patients.

Laboratory. The facilities of the public health laboratory are used by private physicians and health department personnel to assist them in diagnosing, treating, and controlling communicable diseases. Examinations performed in the laboratory each year include serological tests for syphilis; bacteriological examinations for diagnosis of typhoid and paratyphoid fevers, diphtheria, streptococcal infections, bacillary dysentery, parasitic infections and ringworm; analysis of water samples taken by health department sanitarians; and testing of milk samples for total bacterial count, amount of butter fat and nonfat solids, presence of coliform organisms and the completion of pasteurization.

Occupational Health. This is a comparatively new service offered by few local health departments. The division of occupational health is designed to conserve and promote the health of employed personnel; to prevent the occurrence of disease or injury from occupational sources through control over the industrial environment; and to restore health and earning capacity to injured or ill workers. Members of this team also promote occupational health services in industries with established medical programs by consultation, survey, investigation and analysis of health hazards, and educational programs in all phases of occupational health. Another aspect of the program is that of air pollution control. This is concerned with the reduction of air pollution from existing industrial and nonindustrial sources; with the review of plans for new industries, and the analysis of the atmosphere to determine the amounts and kinds of pollutants in the air.

Crippled Children Services. The purpose of the program is *to arrange for* diagnostic examinations and treatment for physically handicapped children residing in the county who are unable to afford the entire cost of care. By definition, a physically handicapped child is a person under 21 years of age, who does not have complete use or control of his body or limbs because of physical defects.

These may have been caused from congenital anomalies or acquired through diseases or accidents.

Some samples of handicapping conditions that are acceptable for care under the program are:

1. Orthopedic—club foot, congenital hip, scoliosis
2. Plastic—cleft palate and lip, disfigurements due to burns
3. Orthodontic—severe malocclusion, deformities accompanying cleft palate
4. Eye—strabismus, cataracts
5. Ear—conditions leading to loss of hearing
6. Rheumatic or congenital heart disease if surgery is indicated
7. Rheumatic fever
8. Cerebral palsy
9. Other disabling or disfiguring deformities such as skin, urological, neurological.

Diagnosis and treatment are provided by qualified specialists in private practice.

To receive services the child must have an eligible condition and the family must be unable to afford the entire cost of private care. Financial eligibility is determined by a medical social worker who balances the total resources of the family against the total needs. Psychiatric counseling is given to help the family meet the special problems often arising from the crippling condition.

Maternal and Child Health. Pediatric services are provided at clinics called "child-health conferences" or "well-baby clinics" for those who are financially unable to obtain the care privately or are referred by their private physician. The conference includes a health examination of the child as well as parent counseling. It must be pointed out here that faithful volunteers offer their time and assistance to help make these clinics successful. Arrangements are also made for home visits for demonstration of such procedures as bathing the baby or making a formula. It must be realized, however, that regular medical supervision by the family's own physician is the best kind of care for children and adults. The family physician, knowing the child in health, will be better able to care for him in illness.

Expectant-parent classes are conducted to teach the elements of good maternal health and care of the new-born infant. Prenatal visits are made by the public health nurse to assist the expectant mother in making preparations for the prenatal care of the child, to interpret and implement the physician's instructions, and to keep the physician informed of any apparent abnormality.

The health department is also responsible for the promotion, implementation, and enforcement of legislation dealing with premarital and prenatal examination requirements. These may include serologic tests for syphilis, tuberculin skin tests, and chest x-rays.

Health Education. The local health department's long range objectives through education include:

1. A community that accepts responsibility for its health
2. A community informed of its health status, i.e.,
    a. Morbidity and mortality
    b. Individual measures for the prevention and control of health problems
    c. Availability of community facilities and services for the prevention and control of health problems
    d. The program and services of the health department.
3. A community participating in coordinated planning and programming for:
    a. Appraisal of community facilities and services
    b. Utilization of existing community facilities and services
    c. Provision of additional needed community facilities and services.
4. A community composed of individuals motivated to observe the personal practices conducive to physical, mental and emotional health.

The health education division is the focal point of the wide variety of educational programs carried out by the health department in an effort to accomplish the educational objectives. The division assists in the educational work of the department; provides educational materials; disseminates reliable health information to the public through newspaper, radio and television; advises on the use of educational methods pertinent to public health programs; and assists in community health education programs sponsored by the department or other community agency. Educational materials not available from other sources are prepared or assembled in the health education workshop. These include films, slides, exhibits, pamphlets, posters and other teaching aids for use in conjunction with the educational programs carried out in schools, homes, industries, communities and professional groups.

The health education movement has progressed into many foreign countries. Of the 44 countries that are cooperating through the International Cooperation Administration 36 have requested assistance in health education. In each of these countries, individuals have been selected by their government and have been sent to the United States for training in public and school health education.

THE HEALTH DEPARTMENT AND THE SCHOOL HEALTH PROGRAM.

The primary responsibility for the health of children rests with the parents or guardians, who are obligated to provide adequate medical and dental care, and such home conditions as are conducive to good health. As the children mature, however, they should assume more responsibility for their individual health. The local board of education and the local health department coordinate and cooperate to give aid and seek correction of physical and emotional problems through family physicians and other appropriate agencies. The health department contributes to the school health program by periodically appraising the health of school children, providing health education services, and supervising the sanitary facilities of the school.

Many schools cooperate with members of the health department in an effort to appraise the health of certain students who have been referred by the teacher. Screening in the school health program is a preliminary examination by fairly simple and routine procedures for the purpose of identifying those children in need of further examination or diagnosis by qualified specialists. In this way, many disorders can be prevented, and defects can be corrected. Screening tests most commonly performed by teachers and nurses include growth and development measurements, and vision and hearing testing. The school physician, who may or may not be a member of the health department, gives periodic health appraisals to students who have been referred by the teacher or nurse, new students, prekindergarten children and those who will engage in competitive athletics. Immunizations are also provided for those students who so desire, and who have obtained parental permission. Observations, deviations, and corrections are carefully noted on the students' cumulative health record. Consultation, referral to the family physician or specialist, and follow-up are necessary adjuncts to the program. Health department officials suggest that regular medical supervision by the family's own physician is preferred.

The school health program helps prevent communicable disease; helps find and correct physical and emotional problems; helps prepare for emergency or disaster situations; helps lay the foundation for sound health knowledge, attitudes, and habits; and helps promote the physical, social, and emotional well-being of the students. Emphasis must be placed upon community coordination and cooperation, as indicated by Figure 67.

A CONCEPT OF A SCHOOL HEALTH PROGRAM

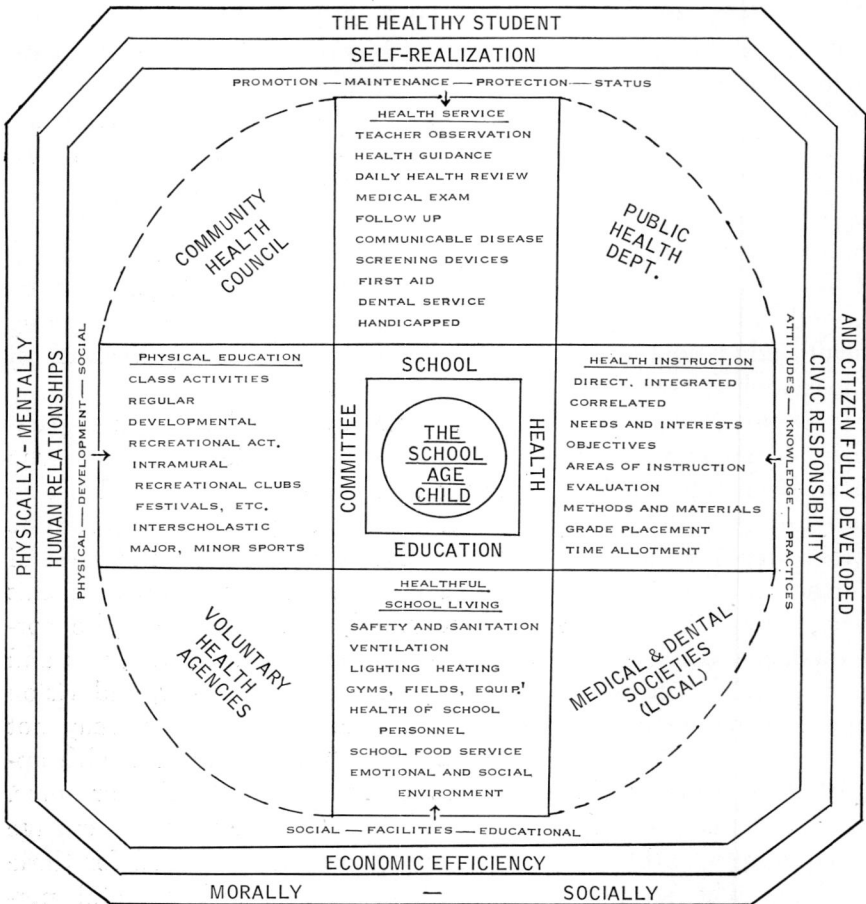

Outer Frame:	The Ultimate Aim
Second Frame:	The Purposes of Education
Inner Frame:	Immediate and Intermediate Goals
Squares:	Divisions of the Program -- Activities & Functions
Inter-Squares:	Community Agencies & Societies -- Coordinating Body
Central Square	School Health Committee -- Coordinating Body
Central Circle:	The Total Program Designed for the Healthful Living of the School-Age Child

Figure 67. (From L. J. Sparks, *The School Health Program,* Unpublished syllabus, Willamette University, 1939.)

PROBLEMS CONFRONTING LOCAL HEALTH DEPARTMENTS. There are many problems confronting local health departments. A few include a scarcity of qualified personnel; opposition by certain groups; inadequate salaries, facilities, and buildings; overlapping of services in the city and county; administrative line relationship between city council or county board of supervisors and the health officer; and in many instances, health workers are "afraid of stepping on someone's toes!" There seems to be a dichotomy between being a public servant and at the same time trying to promote community health by enforcing state and local laws.

Health department workers must actively participate and demonstrate leadership in the community health councils. In this way all health agencies and interested persons can define health problems and objectives and cooperate more effectively in an effort to solve community health problems. Community health workers must constantly review and evaluate the changing problems and needs in a rapidly changing society.

The State Health Department

A state health department is organized on basically the same pattern as a local health department. The responsibilities of the state health department are contained in concise sections of the health and safety codes of the states. From these stem a myriad of laws, rules and regulations which mold the activities, functions, responsibilities, programs and projects of the department.

In brief, the state health department is generally responsible for: examination into the causes of communicable disease in man and domestic animals; investigation of the sources of morbidity and mortality; investigation of the effects of localities, employments, conditions and circumstances on public health; licensing of hospitals and nursing homes; detection and prevention of adulteration of food and drugs; examination for and the prevention of pollution of public water and ice supplies; and preparation and distribution, at cost, of antitoxins, vaccines, and other approved biologic products for the control or prevention of communicable diseases. The department may advise all local health authorities, and, when in its judgment the public health is menaced, it controls and regulates their action.

The department encourages and stimulates local health departments to meet the public health needs of the areas that they serve. Direct public health service to the people of the state is provided by local public health departments; the state department provides only direct service that cannot be provided locally. The state department strives to help maintain superior local health services by providing:

1. Leadership in assisting communities without full time health departments to recognize their public health needs

2. Financial aid in the establishment and strengthening of local health services, including the provision of staff and other resources
3. Provision of educational opportunities for staffs of local health departments
4. Establishment of standards of service and personnel
5. Coordination of the total public health program within the state and of local, state and federal programs.

The California State Health Department, for example, is guided in its activities by a ten-member State Board of Public Health, of which the director acts as executive officer in addition to his duties as administrative head of the Department. The Board is composed of seven physicians, including the director, one dentist, and two lay members. Members are appointed by the governor for four-year terms, so staggered that there are always some experienced members to give continuity to policy. The Board functions as a policy-making, regulatory, judicial and licensing body.

To carry out these many activities and administrative responsibilities, the Department has been organized into eight divisions with supervision of 25 bureaus, services and laboratories. In addition, there are several special study projects administratively attached to Department units. (See Figure 68.)

The Health Department Versus Blindness

Many health departments throughout the United States are undertaking special projects in an effort to prevent blindness in children and adults. The problem is magnified when we consider an increased aged population with corresponding increased blindness due to chronic conditions such as diabetes, cancer, and hypertension. However, early detection of certain eye conditions can prevent blindness. For example, glaucoma, which is most frequent among middle age persons, is second only to cataract as a cause of blindness, and accounts for about 14 per cent of adult blindness in the United States. Glaucoma, often called "tunnel vision," is a condition of increased fluid pressure within the eye which causes atrophy of the optic nerve and results in gradual loss of vision. Symptoms include blurred vision, headache, eye pain, and nausea; if detected early enough the disease can be cured. Community screening programs and education can prevent blindness from glaucoma.

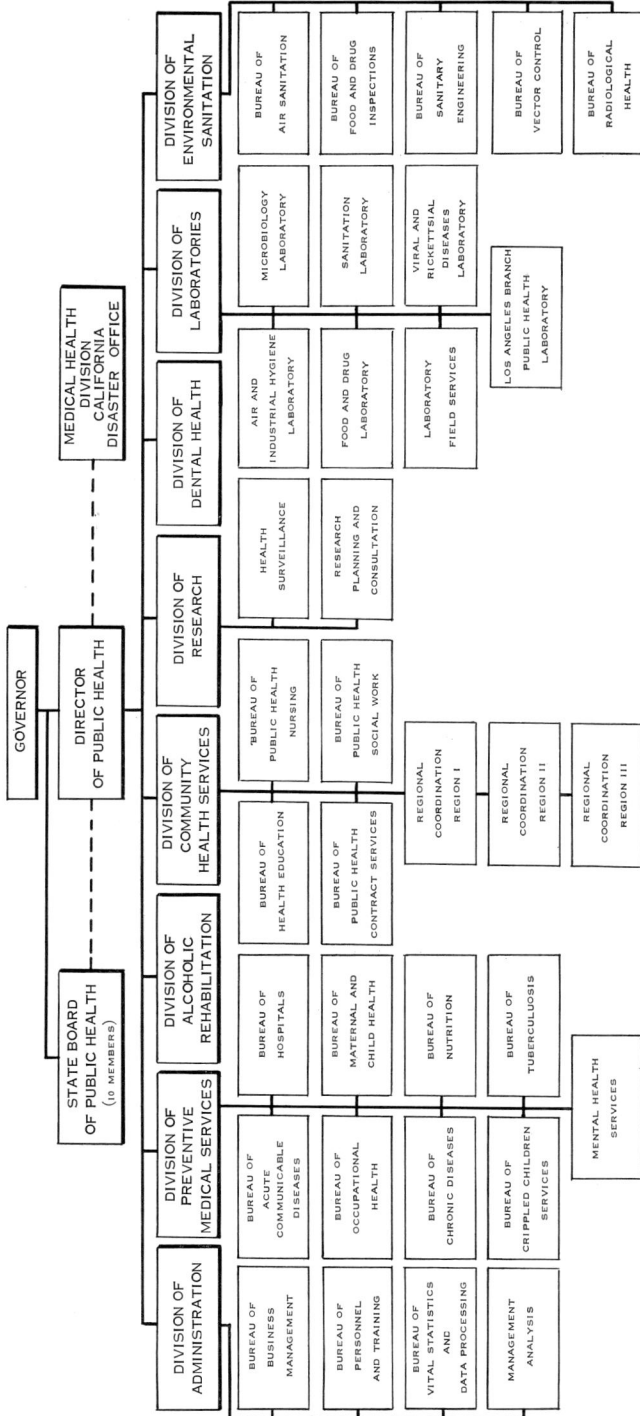

STATE OF CALIFORNIA, DEPARTMENT OF PUBLIC HEALTH

Figure 68. Organization chart for California State Health Department.

291

Amblyopia, also known as "lazy eye" or "one-eye vision," is a condition of vision dimness leading to blindness and is most common among children. In most cases, if this condition is not discovered by the time the child is six years old, he will lose the sight of one eye. This can prevented by preschool and primary vision screening programs.

The importance of vision defects in relation to public health is illustrated by the fact that World War II Selective Service rejections for visual defects ranked second; vision defects also rate high as a cause of rejection for industrial employment today. Furthermore, the problem is magnified when we consider administrative costs of state welfare aid to the blind, loss of productivity, taxes, and loss of purchasing power. Since early detection is the key to the prevention of blindness among adults and children, new ways must be found to reach these groups through education and case-finding.

Financial Support of Local and State Health Services

The financing of local health services has always been a critical matter in developing community health programs. With the increasing competition for tax funds, and with the uncertainties of the future role of federal grant-in-aid, financing is currently more critical than in the past. It is important that both citizens and public officials learn more about the intricacies of the local tax situation in relation to public health.

The provision of community health services in the United States today is a cooperative project with responsibility shared by federal, state, and local units of government. As a result of these combined efforts, 90 per cent of the country's total population now resides in areas with some form of organized health services. However, there is a lag between the development of new public health practices and their application in state and local health departments. This situation is partially caused by lack of funds necessary to establish new programs.

The national government is concerned with the public's health because disease moves freely and frequently from one state to another, and the strength of the nation is dependent upon the health and productive capacity of its people. The federal government contributes to public health in the form of assistance to states. In general, federal grants make up the highest proportion of total expenditures in states with small total population, and in those states with low per capita income. Even with extensive aid from federal sources, however, low income states still devote a larger share of their own resources to health than do the wealthier states. Generally, the federal government gives the most assistance to those states that: (1) frequently have the greatest health problems; (2) have the least financial resources; (3) and are putting forth the greatest effort in public health in relation to their own financial capacity.[3] Two constituents of the United States Department of Health, Education, and Welfare make grants-in-aid to the states for health purposes. These are the Public Health Service and The Children's Bureau of the Social Security Administration.

Federal health grants to states were first instituted in 1918 when funds were appropriated to the Public Health Service for venereal disease control services. Grants-in-aid for the protection of the health of mothers and children were initially provided through the Children's Bureau in the Sheppard-Towner Act of 1921. The provisions of this act expired in 1925. The Social Security Act of 1935 promoted the expansion of public health programs throughout

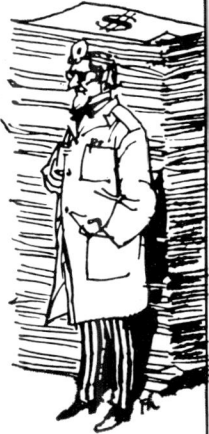

WHERE GOVERNMENT'S HEALTH BILLIONS GO

In year starting July 1, 1960 federal agencies will spend —

$904 million for: Promotion of public health (National Institutes of Health, U. S. Public Health Service, etc.).

$1 billion for: Veterans' hospitals (care of patients and construction of new hospitals).

$900 million for: Armed forces' "Medicare" and other programs.

$250 million for: Public-assistance grants for medical care.

$335 million for: Health and medical activities of State Department, Atomic Energy Commission, National Science Foundation, other agencies.

Total "health" expenditures under present law: **$3.4 billion a year**

Figure 69. (From *U. S. Budget Bureau estimates.* U. S. News & World Report, April, 1960, page 74.)

Table 15. *Federal Appropriations for Grants-In-Aid to States for Public Health Services—Selected Fiscal Years, 1936–1956[1] (in millions of dollars)*

TYPE OF GRANT	1936	1945	1948	1950	1951	1954	1955	1956 (Estimate)[2]
All grants (exclusive of construction and EMIC)	$6.1	$30.3	$57.5	$63.4	$63.6	$45.6	$46.0	$45.7
Public Health Service	3.3	21.6	39.0	44.9	40.4	22.8	23.2	22.9
General health	3.3	11.0	11.2	14.2	13.5	10.1	9.7	9.7
Venereal disease[3]	...	9.2	15.5	13.1	10.7	2.2	0.7	0.7
Tuberculosis control	...	1.4	6.8	6.8	6.4	4.3	4.5	4.5
Mental health	...	...	3.0	3.5	3.2	2.3	2.3	3.0
Cancer control[4]	...	...	2.5	3.5	3.2	2.2	2.3	2.3
Heart disease control	...	...	...	2.0	1.7	1.1	1.1	1.1
Industrial waste studies	...	...	...	1.0	1.0	...	...	1.0
Alaska disease and sanitation	...	...	...	0.8	0.7	0.6	0.6	0.6
Survey and planning	...	...	...	....	...	...	2.0[5]	....
(Construction)[6]	...	...	(75.0)	(150.0)	(85.0)	(65.0)	(96.0)	(125.0)
Children's Bureau	2.8	8.7	18.5	18.5	23.2	22.8	22.8	22.8
Maternal and child health	1.6	5.8	11.0	11.0	13.2	11.9	11.9	11.9
Crippled children	1.2	2.9	7.5	7.5	10.0	10.9	10.9	10.9
(EMIC)	...	(45.0)	(3.0)[7]	....	...	...	...	....

1. First year in which a specific type of grant is shown reflects date money was first available for this grant, except for the grant for venereal disease, available in 1939; for Emergency Maternity and Infant Care available in 1943; the grant for hospital survey and planning, available from 1947 to July, 1953; and the Alaska grant, which first became available in 1949. Grants in 1936, available February, 1936; initial tuberculosis grant, available May, 1945.
2. As included in the President's budget.
3. Amounts for 1948–1951 include funds allocated on the basis of the formula and funds for special projects; amounts for 1954–1956 include special projects only. Data for 1954 excludes $1,335,410 of grant funds covering supplies and assignment of personnel furnished in lieu of cash.
4. Does not include amounts for special control projects to public and nonprofit institutions as follows: 1948–1950—$1,000,000 each year; 1951—$949,000; 1954–1955 —$1,100,000 each year.
5. Available until spent for medical facilities survey and planning.
6. Amounts for 1948–1954 are for hospital construction; for 1955, $75,000,000 for hospital construction, $21,000,000 for medical facilities; and for 1956, $65,000,000 for hospital construction, $60,000,000 for medical facilities.
7. These funds were appropriated to cover the two fiscal years 1948 and 1949 with the proviso that the money was to be used for liquidation of the program.

[1] Haldeman, J. C., "Financing Local Health Services," American Journal, Public Health, Vol. 45, No. 8, August, 1955, p. 969.

the nation. Under this Act, general health grants, which support basic state and local public health services, and special grants for maternal and child health and crippled children services, were inaugurated. Since that time, grants have been extended to cover a much larger range, including hospital construction. (See Table 15.) Congress passed the Hospital Survey and Construction (Hill-Burton) Act in 1946. Since then it has been amended to permit federal assistance in the construction of health centers, nursing homes, and many other types of health facilities. Federal contributions are matched by from one third to two thirds of state and local funds. Although state and local health department appropriations for health services have been steadily increasing, federal grants to states have decreased, as Table 15 indicates. Reasons for this are: increases in state and local appropriations; reduction in federal funds; and keen competition with other governmental functions for the tax dollar.

Local health departments are usually supported by a tax levy on the assessed valuation of taxable property, personal income, sales tax, business and industry taxes, and other sources. However, it is a very difficult problem to provide adequate public health services in those rural areas so sparsely populated that they cannot support independent local health departments. In an effort to solve this problem, many state health departments furnish special services in such areas. California has enacted legislation with provisions for a county with a population of less than 40,000 to enter into a contract with the State Department of Public Health for public health services. However, the county board of supervisors must request the contract and appropriate at least 55 cents per capita for their total population. This contract plan stimulates local interest, responsibility, and fosters autonomy.

State funds are allocated to assist local health departments for a wide variety of public health purposes. In addition to subsidizing local health departments, states make grants for mosquito abatement, for construction of hospital and health centers, for care of crippled children, for community mental health programs, and for support of tuberculosis sanatoriums. (See Figure 70.)

Many new health services and programs must be provided to care for current public health problems. Local governments and citizens must understand and support financially the increased costs necessary to provide superior health services. In addition, the state and federal government must continue to provide stronger

WHERE IT COMES FROM —

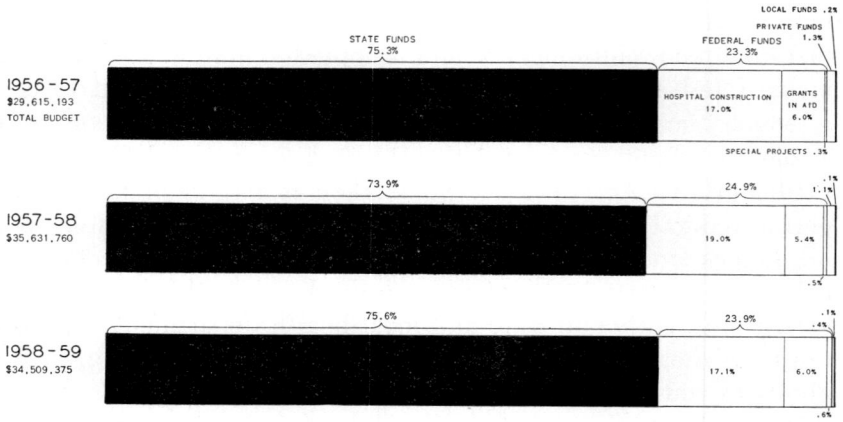

WHERE IT GOES —

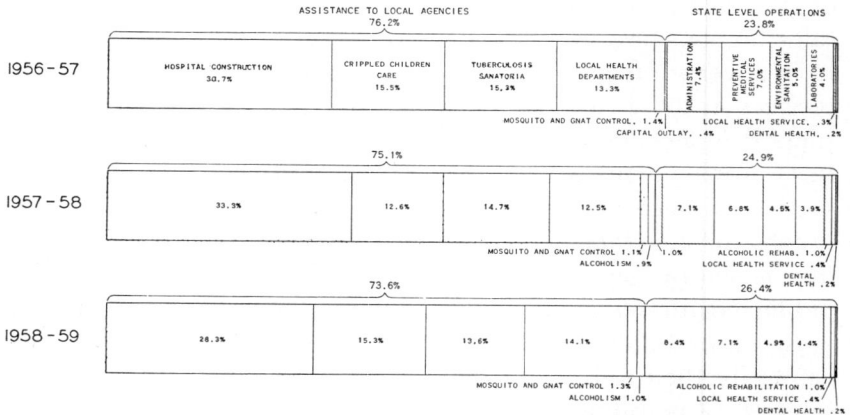

Figure 70. State funds received by the state health department are earmarked for distribution to local health agencies. (From *Public Health in California, 1956–1959, a Triennial Report.* California's Health, *17:* 71, September 15, 1959.)

leadership and greater financial support to encourage and assist in the development and improvement of local services.

Department of Health, Education and Welfare

This Department of the federal government was established in 1953 and consists of six major branches: (1) Office of Education, (2) Food and Drug Administration, (3) U. S. Public Health Service, (4) St. Elizabeth's Hospital, (5) Social Security Administration, and (6) Office of Vocational Rehabilitation.

Figure 71 shows the organization of the Department with the various subdivisions. This agency was created for the purpose of organizing the various health and welfare agencies of the government under one administrative unit and thus promote better coordination and efficiency in serving the health and welfare of the citizens of the country.

UNITED STATES PUBLIC HEALTH SERVICE. The Public Health Service originated in the congressional Act of 1798 sponsored by Alexander Hamilton, Secretary of the Treasury. It was designed for "sick and disabled seamen." Major functions of the Public Health Service are concentrated in research, demonstrations, quarantine, and consultation to state and local health departments, and foreign countries. Major health interests and services are shown in Figure 71.

Other activities of the Public Health Service are: (1) the operation of 26 hospitals, including two for narcotics, two for tuberculosis, one for Hansen's Disease (leprosy), and two for neuropsychiatric problems; (2) research in health conducted at the National Institutes of Health at Bethesda, Maryland; (3) training grants to educational institutions in the health sciences; (4) fellowship grants; (5) assisting states in their public health education program; (6) supervisory control and licensure of the manufacturers of biological products used in the prevention and treatment of disease; (7) the publication of vital statistics pertinent to the public health programs; (8) supervision of St. Elizabeth's Hospital for the treatment of mentally ill beneficiaries of federal employees.

Responsibilities of the Public Health Service also involve safeguarding the health of inmates of federal prisons, personnel of Coast Guard stations, residents of Indian reservations, users of and visitors to the national parks and monuments, projects of the Bureau of Reclamation, and the extensive recreational areas in the national forests. Other important environmental Public Health Service research centers include the Industrial Hygiene Laboratory in Atlanta, Georgia, the Environmental Health Center in Cincinnati, Ohio, and the Communicable Disease Center in Atlanta, Georgia.

The United States Public Health Service is administered by the Surgeon General who is appointed by the President of the United States. The Surgeon General also plans and conducts an annual conference of state and territorial health officers and other special committees and conferences as needed.[4]

THE CHILDREN'S BUREAU. This Bureau was established in 1912 as a branch of the Labor Department but is now a division of the

DEPARTMENT OF HEALTH, EDUCATION AND WELFARE

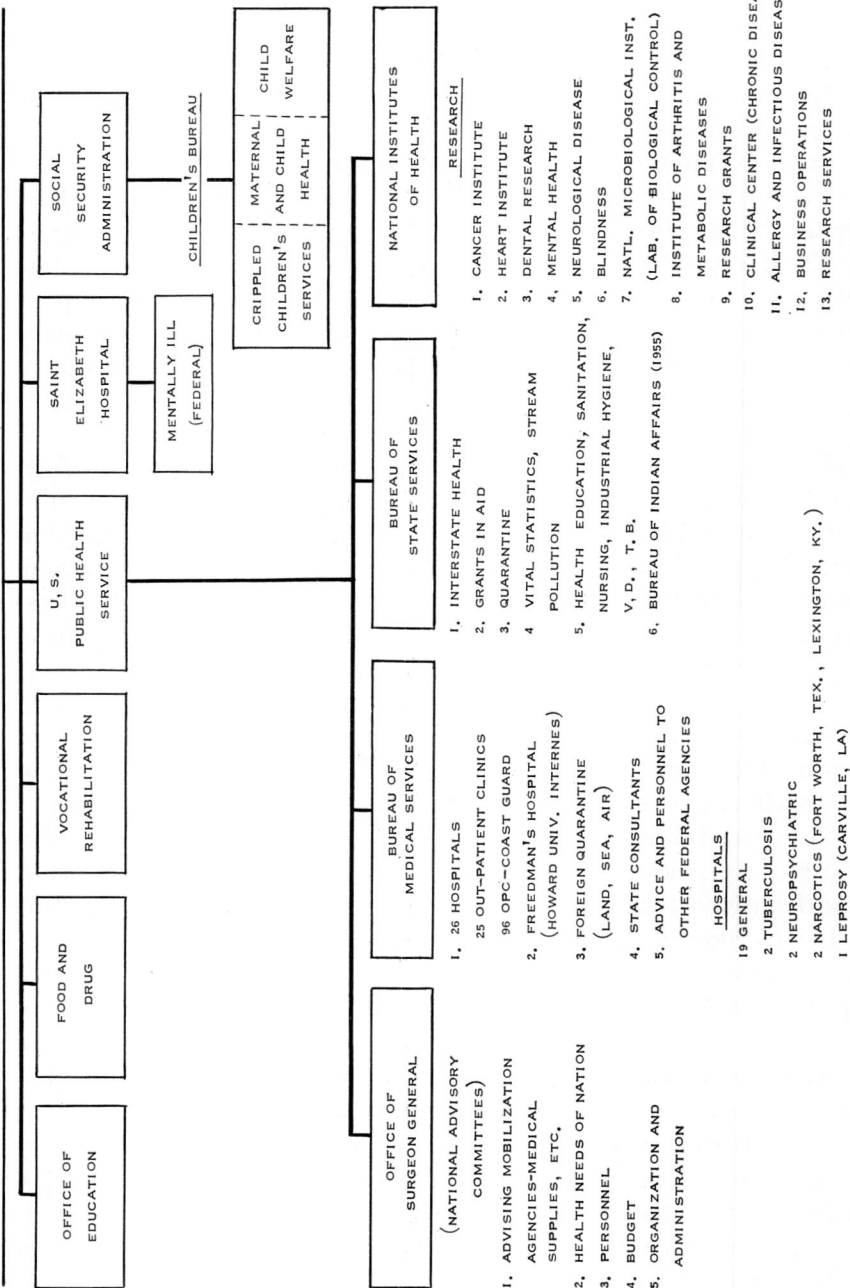

OFFICE OF EDUCATION

FOOD AND DRUG

VOCATIONAL REHABILITATION

U. S. PUBLIC HEALTH SERVICE

SAINT ELIZABETH HOSPITAL

MENTALLY ILL (FEDERAL)

SOCIAL SECURITY ADMINISTRATION

CHILDREN'S BUREAU

| CRIPPLED CHILDREN'S SERVICES | MATERNAL AND CHILD HEALTH | CHILD WELFARE |

NATIONAL INSTITUTES OF HEALTH

RESEARCH

1. CANCER INSTITUTE
2. HEART INSTITUTE
3. DENTAL RESEARCH
4. MENTAL HEALTH
5. NEUROLOGICAL DISEASE
6. BLINDNESS
7. NATL. MICROBIOLOGICAL INST. (LAB. OF BIOLOGICAL CONTROL)
8. INSTITUTE OF ARTHRITIS AND METABOLIC DISEASES
9. RESEARCH GRANTS
10. CLINICAL CENTER (CHRONIC DISEASES)
11. ALLERGY AND INFECTIOUS DISEASES
12. BUSINESS OPERATIONS
13. RESEARCH SERVICES

OFFICE OF SURGEON GENERAL

(NATIONAL ADVISORY COMMITTEES)

1. ADVISING MOBILIZATION AGENCIES-MEDICAL SUPPLIES, ETC.
2. HEALTH NEEDS OF NATION
3. PERSONNEL
4. BUDGET
5. ORGANIZATION AND ADMINISTRATION

BUREAU OF MEDICAL SERVICES

1. 26 HOSPITALS
   25 OUT-PATIENT CLINICS
   96 OPC–COAST GUARD
2. FREEDMAN'S HOSPITAL (HOWARD UNIV., INTERNES)
3. FOREIGN QUARANTINE (LAND, SEA, AIR)
4. STATE CONSULTANTS
5. ADVICE AND PERSONNEL TO OTHER FEDERAL AGENCIES

HOSPITALS

19 GENERAL
2 TUBERCULOSIS
2 NEUROPSYCHIATRIC
2 NARCOTICS (FORT WORTH, TEX., LEXINGTON, KY.)
1 LEPROSY (CARVILLE, LA)

BUREAU OF STATE SERVICES

1. INTERSTATE HEALTH
2. GRANTS IN AID
3. QUARANTINE
4. VITAL STATISTICS, STREAM POLLUTION
5. HEALTH EDUCATION, SANITATION, NURSING, INDUSTRIAL HYGIENE, V., D., T. B.
6. BUREAU OF INDIAN AFFAIRS (1955)

Figure 71. Organization of the U. S. Department of Health, Education and Welfare.

Social Security Administration of the Department of Health, Education and Welfare. Some of the activities of the Bureau include: (1) allocation of grants to the states for the promotion of maternal and child health; (2) allocation of grants to the states for crippled children and child welfare services; (3) allocation of research grants; (4) distribution of educational material relating to maternal and child health; (5) promotion of the White House conferences on children and youth held at ten-year intervals since 1908; (6) conducting surveys and studies relating to child health problems; (7) allocating financial aid for specialized training projects; (8) cooperating and working with official and nonofficial organizations and institutions; (9) serving as a center for the development of standards of care and protection for children in the United States.

Food and Drug Administration

This Division was founded in 1906 and deals with the enforcement of interstate commerce involving misbranding, mislabeling, or adulteration of foods, insecticides, drugs, cosmetics, and health devices and materials. The current law, the Federal Food, Drug and Cosmetic Act of 1938, which gives the FDA authority to remove any harmful food, drug, or cosmetic from the market, also has a number of special sections for dealing with specific types of potentially dangerous chemicals; various amendments have been added since that time. With the increasing number of foods, drugs, and cosmetics, the work of this Division becomes increasingly complex and important. Purity of these products is essential to health since many products can deteriorate or be contaminated in ways that would be injurious or fatal to the user. This Department has protected the health of our citizens for many years.

Some of the important provisions of the Act of 1938 are: (1) prohibition of false and misleading claims on drugs that may lead the public to rely upon ineffective products rather than seek competent medical care; (2) supervision of commercial food labeling and package contents so that consumers will receive the nutritional values they have the right to expect; (3) maintenance of high standards for pasteurized milk and pure cheese; (4) testing and certification of coal-tar colors to insure their harmlessness and suitability for use in food, drugs, and cosmetics; (5) testing and certification of insulin vital to health because of the necessity for precise dosage in the use of insulin; (6) testing and certification of new drugs in order to guarantee safety and effectiveness to the manufacturer, physician, consumer, and patient; (7) enforcement of programs to prevent illegal sale of prescription drugs by pharmacists and others, with emphasis upon habit-forming drugs as barbiturates and amphetamines; (8) enforcement of the Caustic Poison Act which requires labels and antidotes on certain household chemicals; (9) research and study of the new health problems such as the health effects of sterilization of foods by radiation, of potent drugs in livestock feeding, of increased use of chemical additives in commercial food processing, and the use of antibiotics as food preservatives.

Advances in food and drug chemistry have made the work of the Division more complex and difficult. For example, over 5,000 chemicals are used in the processing, storing, and handling of today's food. Although most chemicals are probably harmless, many others may be cumulative in their affect, and over a period of months or years may cause tissue damage and death. Illegal quantities of such contaminants as DDT, penicillin, hormones, and pesticides are found in food and milk, even though their presence in food supplies is restricted by law. New federal and state laws are being adopted, however, which require manufacturers to prove that the many chemicals used in the growth and processing of today's food are safe for human consumption. Even so, the only way to prove chemicals safe is to prove by laboratory experiment that they are unsafe, and many tests are insufficiently reliable.

It is evident that the major problems of the FDA are inspection and enforcement of regulations. The Division's inspection staff, however, is limited to less than 500 men, and laboratory facilities for testing crop samples are inadequate. Although the FDA's 1961 budget for enforcement alone is only $16,852,000, this sum compares favorably with the Public Health Service's annual allotment for air pollution research and control, which has never exceeded $6,000,000. The FDA has done a commendable job in proposing and administering important new consumer-protection legislation and deserves the continued support of the public.

Other Federal Agencies Engaged in Health Work

Since public health involves disease prevention and prolonging life, and since health is defined as the social, mental, emotional and physical well-being of individuals, it is not suprising that many agencies of the federal government are involved in some aspect of health. For example, the United States Office of Education, which is a branch of the Department of Health, Education and Welfare, promotes health, safety, physical education, and recreation programs and services for the public schools throughout the United States. It also contributes information to the school health service program and the school lunch program. All the divisions of the Department of Health, Education and Welfare are linked with health in some way. In general, the federal government is most concerned with interstate health protection and prevention of disease from abroad.

Various public health programs and services are offered by all federal departments. For instance, many branches of the Department of Agriculture, which functions to serve the farmer and the agriculture industry, either directly or indirectly contribute greatly to the knowledge of health and the prevention of disease. One branch of this Department, the Agricultural Research Administration, directs and coordinates the physical and biological research programs of the Department. Research activities in human nutrition, animal diseases, insecticides, control of insects affecting man and animals, antibiotics and serums for the control of animal diseases, and rural family housing programs. All have a direct bearing on health, medical knowledge of disease, and health practices.

A few other federal departments interested in public health include: the Department of Commerce, collecting and publishing basic statistics that are used widely in planning public health programs; the Department of Defense, responsible for medical care programs of military personnel and their dependents; the Department of the Interior, supervising health programs in the territories of the United States, and various branches in this Department include the Bureau of Mines, which prevents health hazards and promotes safety, The Fish and Wildlife Service, which promotes programs for the destruction of rodents and elimination of stream pollution, and the National Park Service which insures recreational sanitation; The Department of Justice providing medical, psychiatric, dental, and nursing services to inmates of federal penal institutions; Department of Labor coordinating enforcement of wages, hours, child labor, and safety and health laws; Department of State supervising all international health programs; and the Department of the Treasury enlisting the Bureau of Narcotics to investigate and detect violations of narcotic and related laws. These are only a few of the many agencies which contribute to the prevention of disease and prolonging of life. For a more complete list of agencies engaged in public health, refer to *Guide to Health Organization in the United States,* Public Health Service Publication 196, by J. W. Mountin and E. Flook.[5]

World Health Organization

The creation of the World Health Organization, WHO, in 1948, was the culmination of a long series of efforts made over the centuries to prevent the spread of disease from one continent to another and to achieve international cooperation for better health throughout the world. The organization occupies the status of a specialized agency in the framework of the United Nations. It is not necessary, however, for a country to be a member of the United Nations to be a member of WHO.

The World Health Organization with headquarters in Geneva, Switzerland, derives its authority from the 98 member states that have ratified its Constitution since 1948. A director general is in charge of a staff of about 1000 professionals of 54 nationalities. (See Figure 72 for the organizational structure of WHO.) WHO's budget, contributed by member states, was about $18,000,000 in 1960. WHO works with national health services to prevent infectious diseases and to train health workers. It gives technical assistance to improve sanitary conditions in over 100 countries, warns of outbreaks of epidemic disease, promotes and coordinates research, recommends international standards for drugs and vaccines, and is the world clearing house for medical and scientific information.

CENTRAL TECHNICAL SERVICES. These form the basis of international health activities, and benefit all countries. Some of these services were taken from earlier international health organizations and have since been developed and extended by WHO. They include: epidemiological intelligence and quarantine, health statistics, standardization of therapeutic substances, and atomic energy and health.

Epidemiological Intelligence and Quarantine. The adoption of the International Sanitary Regulations (1952), which replaced 13 out-of-date conventions, is an important accomplishment of WHO. International Sanitary Regulations apply to land, sea, and air traffic throughout the world. They provide the maximum protection against epidemics with minimum interference in international transport and travel.

The Epidemiological Intelligence Service collects information

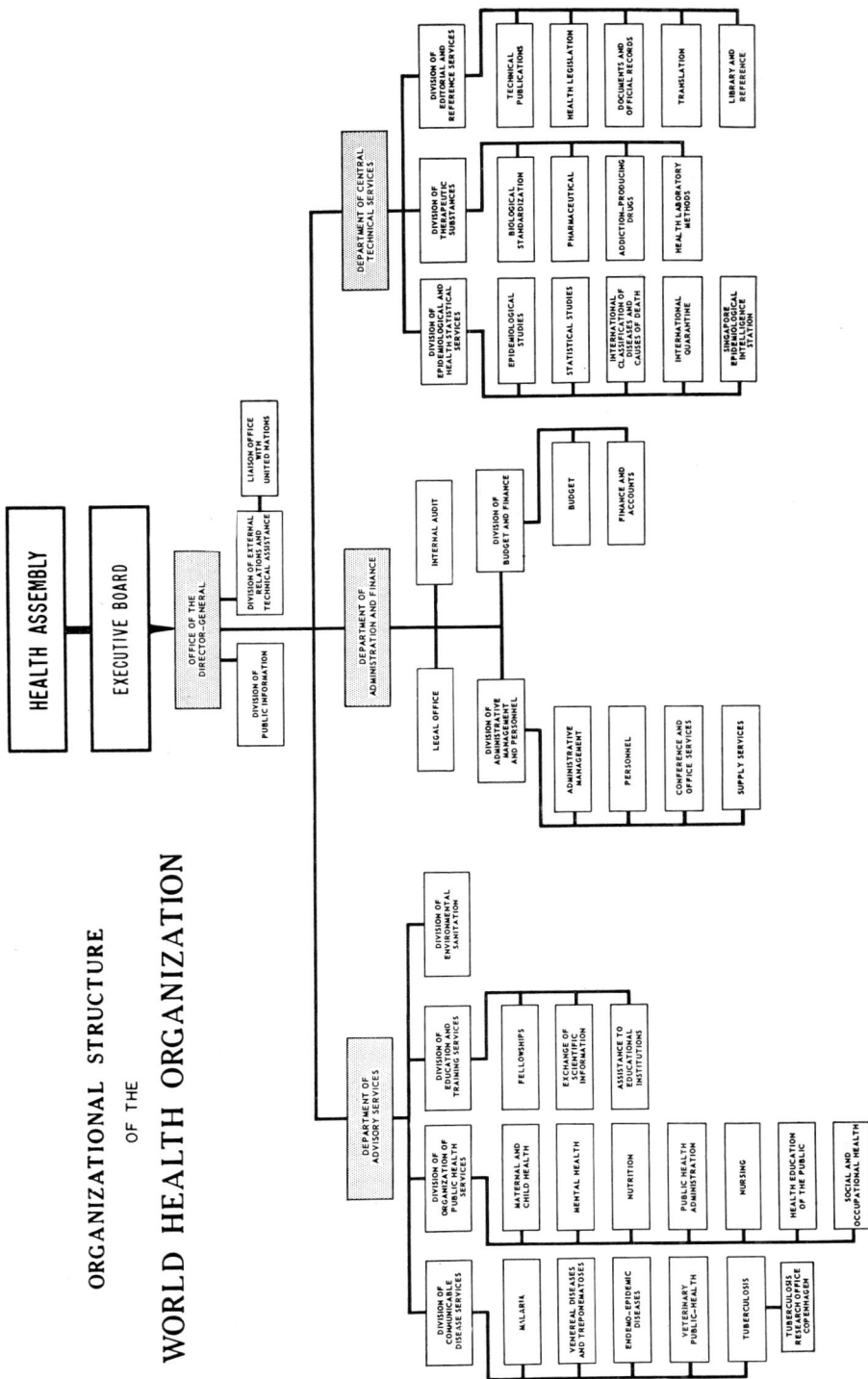

ORGANIZATIONAL STRUCTURE
OF THE
WORLD HEALTH ORGANIZATION

Figure 72. (Courtesy Office of Public Information, Pan American Sanitary Bureau. Regional Office of the World Health Organization, Washington, D.C.)

about the occurrence of disease anywhere in the world, and broaacasts information daily over an international radio network to health authorities, ports, airports and ships at sea.

International Health Statistics. International health legislation, promulgated by the World Health Assembly, provides for uniform health statistics of diseases and causes of death, thereby making it possible to evaluate health problems more accurately and, therefore, to adopt more effective public health measures. The list established by WHO comprises 999 categories of diseases, injuries and causes of death.

Standardization of Therapeutic Substances. Another important work of WHO is to recommend international standards for therapeutic substances. WHO has published the first International Pharmacopoeia that contains recommended specifications for use of drugs in all countries. WHO participates in international efforts for the control of drug addiction, and studies new synthetic drugs suspected of causing addiction.

Atomic Energy and Health. The World Health Organization has been instructed by its member states to study the health problems that arise from the use of atomic energy. Although the peaceful application of atomic energy will improve living conditions, it also threatens the health of workers in atomic establishments and the general public; the amount of background radiation increases with the development of this source of power. Radioactive wastes, if not carefully disposed of, may pollute the air, soil and water, and radiation may even have harmful effects on the heredity of the human race. In order to provide protection against these dangers, WHO, in cooperation with the atomic energy industry, has been requested to collect information and to advise governments and public health agencies regarding these dangers.

Health Laboratory Methods. WHO helps to establish public health laboratories; promotes simplification and standardization of techniques and diagnostic methods; and coordinates research on various laboratory investigations, including the potential dangers of chemical additives to food.

Publication and Documentation. WHO collects documentation on problems relating to health. It produces a considerable number of technical publications in the fields of health and medicine. A number of films are also available. For further information, write: World Health Organization, 1501 New Hampshire Avenue, N. W., Washington 6, D. C.

WHO VERSUS ANOPHELES. Malaria has been a menace to

man's health and economic development. Today's prevalence and mortality due to malaria have been greatly reduced and illustrate the effectiveness of the World Health Organization. WHO and other international agencies, plus 60 governments have joined hands and invested five million dollars in an effort to drastically reduce and possibly eliminate malaria by 1970. For example, in India, the world's greatest malaria reservoir, farm workers lost 170 million man-days a year, and many areas suffered semi-starvation because of the ravages of the disease. The direct death toll was a million dollars a year, and even the poorest Indian paid at least ten rupees (one rupee = 18 cents) a year for nostrums. Already, with partial control programs, India has reduced malaria cases from 75 million to 20 million, and the death toll from one million persons each year to two hundred thousand, at a cost less than one half a rupee per Indian.

Public health workers are counting and spraying houses, and educating the public from Thailand to Trinidad. The program has been underway in Mexico, Central America, coastal Ecuador and Peru, Formosa, Swaziland, Ceylon, Northern Venzuela, several Caribbean Islands, parts of Argentina, Turkey, Iraq, Iran, Afghanistan, Burma, and the Philippines. WHO and other international agencies pay one-fifth of the costs, the United States pays another fifth through economic aid programs, and the participating governments add the remaining three-fifths. Nevertheless, the work ahead is tremendous; by latest estimates, two-fifths of the world population are subject to the disease. Each year two hundred million persons suffer from malaria, and two and one half million die from it. Even with new drugs and insecticides, the female Anopheles mosquito has proved to be a formidable foe. The attack must be speeded because some of the mosquitoes develop resistance to the various insecticides, and thereafter thrive in its presence. Spraying must be periodic, and antimalarial preventive drugs must be added to the salt supply in some areas.

Since eradication is neither possible nor desirable unless it is achieved at reasonable cost and within a limited time, most governments have adopted a positive but doubtful attitude. Past successes, however, give us some indication of future expectations.

The Voluntary Health Agencies

The voluntary health agencies are supported by funds from public subscription, such as The Cancer Crusade, Christmas Seal Sale, March of Dimes, Heart Fund, and others. Funds are budgeted

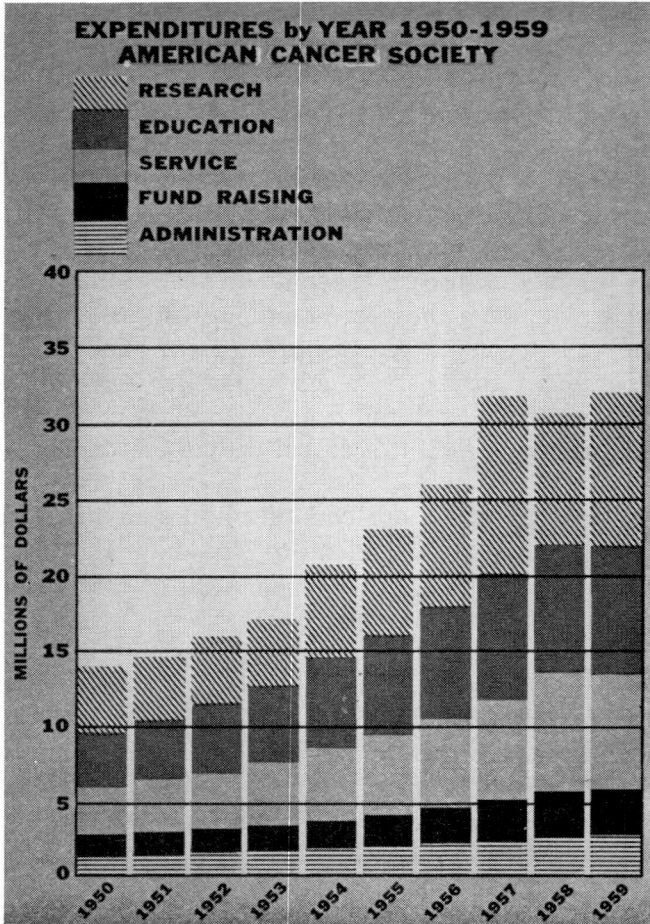

Figure 73. (From *Background For Hope,* courtesy American Cancer Society.)

according to needs. For example, local cancer societies allocate about 37 per cent of their funds to the national research and education program, 60 per cent remains in the local divisions to support local education and service programs, and 3 per cent is devoted to national grants and fellowships. (See Figure 73 for national office expenditures.) The first voluntary health agency was the National Tuberculosis Association which had its beginning in Philadelphia in 1892.

Most of the major voluntary health agencies have a major, national administrative office that is responsible for supervising and guiding the activities, functions, responsibilities, programs, and projects of its state officers. The state office, in turn, aids the local offices. The local society is usually administered by a salaried executive secretary who efficiently organizes a board of directors that represent the entire county. One major committee of each agency is the health education committee. The function and selection of committee members for a typical local Tuberculosis and Health Association follow:

A HEALTH EDUCATION COMMITTEE FOR A LOCAL TUBERCULOSIS AND HEALTH ASSOCIATION

Functions
1. Assist in planning and implementing a health education program based on needs
2. Support and interpret the health education program to the public
3. Reflect public opinion, bring problems to attention of committee
4. Give skilled advice on health education techniques.

Group composition
It should be:
—representative of groups within the community (the "consumers," the "what-the-people-want" group)
—representative of persons who can give skilled advice on health education techniques (the "producers," the "how-to-do-it" folks).
The chairman of the health education committee could well be a member of the board of directors.

Selection of members
Members could be selected from the following:

Education	Director of health education, state department of education (for state association) School administrator P.T.A. representative Health educator in health department College person interested in health education Adult education or night school teacher Classroom teachers.
Physicians	The health officer A physician interested in health education A physician from the tuberculosis hospital A school physician.
Social and Nursing Service	Public health nurse Representative of welfare department.
Community Relations	Newspaper editor or reporter Representative from radio or TV station Representatives of various religious faiths Representative of service club Representative of Y.M.C.A. or similar organizations.
Business	Representative of labor and management.
Industry	Representative of management
Agriculture	Representative of farm group: Farm Bureau, Grange, Home Extension Service.
Special Groups	Foreign language groups Groups with high tuberculosis prevalence.

Other members could be selected on the basis of association program, to represent such areas as nutrition, and social hygiene. The membership of the committee should come from the board of directors, the membership of the tuberculosis association and the general public.

Services provided by these agencies include education, service, and research. Each agency stresses prevention through health education, and disseminates health information through films, pamphlets, television, radio, exhibits, and other media. The National Tuberculosis and Health Association, The American Heart Association, and The American Cancer Society, in particular, have trained, professional, qualified public health educators on their staffs who assist individuals, schools, and community agencies and organizations in understanding and adopting preventive health measures.

Services offered by the voluntary agencies include such activities as first aid, water safety, and prenatal classes offered by the American Red Cross; bandages, friendly home visits, limited aid to needy patients, and tumor clinics offered by the American Cancer Society; chest X-rays, counseling to patient and his family offered by the Tuberculosis and Health Association; sheltered workshops, rehabilitation clinics, weight control programs, and nutrition counseling offered by the American Heart Association. It must be pointed out here that volunteer lay-workers, physicians, and other professional persons, give their time and support to all of these agencies, and many agencies frankly admit that effectiveness would decrease rapidly without volunteers.

The research aspect of the voluntary program is most rewarding and dramatic, as evidenced by the discovery of the Salk poliomyelitis vaccine. Dr. Jonas Salk and others were working under a research grant sponsored by the National Foundation for Poliomyelitis (now called The National Foundation). This agency is now directing its efforts toward viruses, congenital malformations, and arthritis. Thousands of public health research grants are awarded to individuals, schools, colleges, and universities by voluntary agencies each year. The American Heart Association as well as many other voluntary agencies, also offer undergraduate and graduate scholarships to motivate and encourage students to work in the public health field. Scholarships are available to physicians, nurses, educators, and other interested professional persons. For further information, contact your local voluntary health agency.

The Professional Organizations

Many professional agencies are organized on a national, state, or local basis, and furnish a wide variety of information and service. These organizations are financially supported by professional membership fees, donations, professional magazine sales, educational materials, and books. Each of these organizations is usually staffed by specialists in their particular field.

These organizations help develop new methods and materials, conduct studies and research, promote professional standards, and publish educational journals and data. A few such professional organizations are:

American Association for Health, Physical Education, and Recreation, a Department of the National Education Association.
American Association of School Administrators, a department of the National Education Association.
American Council on Education, 744 Jackson Place, Washington, D.C.
American Dental Association, 222 East Superior St., Chicago 11, Ill.
American Medical Association, 535 N. Dearborn St., Chicago 10, Ill.
American Public Health Association, 1790 Broadway, New York 19, N.Y.
American School Health Association, Room 617, 228 North LaSalle St., Chicago, Ill.
American Social Hygiene Association, 1790 Broadway, New York 19, N.Y.
Association for Childhood Education, International, 1200 15th St., N.W. Washington 5, D.C.
National Committee for Mental Hygiene, 1790 Broadway, New York 19, N.Y.
National Council on Family Relations, 1126 East 59th St., Chicago 37, Ill.
National Council on Schoolhouse Construction, George Peabody College for Teachers, Nashville 4, Tenn.
National Education Association, 1201 16th St., N.W., Washington 6, D.C.
National Safety Council, 425 N. Michigan Ave., Chicago 11, Ill.
National Society for the Prevention of Blindness, 1790 Broadway, New York 19, N.Y.
National Society for the Study of Education, 5835 Kimbark Ave., Chicago 37, Ill.
National Society of State Directors of Health, Physical Education, and Recreation, State Department of Education, Los Angeles, Cal.

QUESTIONS FOR REVIEW

1. Define public health; health.
2. List and briefly discuss the six basic services of a local health department.
3. "Since we have state health departments, it is not necessary to have local health departments." Comment upon this statement.
4. What factors led to the creation of your state health department? Local health department?
5. Briefly discuss the significance of the following acts in relation to public health:
   (a) Sheppard-Towner Act
   (b) Hill-Burton Act
   (c) Social Security Act, Title V and VI
   (d) Marine Hospital Service Act
   (e) National Quarantine Act

6. Draw and label the organization and administration of your state health department.
   (a) How is it financed?
   (b) Briefly describe the major services and functions of each of the divisions.
7. Draw and label the organization and administration of the Department of Health, Education, and Welfare.
8. Identify the following:

   (a) M. P. H.   (e) C. C. S.
   (b) Dr. P. H.   (f) W. H. O.
   (c) R. S.   (g) M. C. H.
   (d) P. H. N.

9. Briefly discuss the services of the World Health Organization.
10. List five major voluntary health agencies in your community. What do these agencies have in common? What services does each agency offer?
11. "We must gear our public health programs and services to the changing community problems." Briefly discuss this statement.
12. "Each member of the health department staff is a health educator." Briefly discuss this statement.

REFERENCES

1. Freeman, R. B., and Holmes, E. M.: *Administration of Public Health Services.* Philadelphia, W. B. Saunders Co., 1960, Pages 478–83.
2. U.S. Public Health Service: *Communicable Disease Center, Atlanta, Georgia.* Washington, D.C., U.S. Government Printing Office, 1960.
3. Haldeman, J. C.: *Financing Local Health Services.* Am. J. Pub. Health, 45:970, 1955.
4. Freeman, R. B., and Holmes, E. M.: *Administration of Public Health Services.* Philadelphia, W. B. Saunders Co., 1960, Pages 471–76.
5. Mountin, J. W., and Flook, E.: *Guide to Health Organization in the United States.* Washington, D.C., U.S. Government Printing Office, 1951.

SUGGESTED READING

American Public Health Association: *Proposed Report on Educational and Other Qualifications and Functions of Public Health Educators.* Am. Pub. Health, 47:112–119, 1957.
American Public Health Association: *The Local Health Department—Services and Responsibilities.* Am. J. Pub. Health, 41:302–307, 1951.
American Public Health Association: *Where Are We Going in Public Health?* Am. J. Pub. Health, 46:1–19, 1956.
Bachman, George W., et al.: *Health Resources in the United States.* Washington, D. C., Brookings Institution, 1952.
Burney, Leroy E., Surgeon General: *The Importance of WHO to Americans.* Pub. Health Rep., 73:4, 1958.
Carter, R.: *The Race for Your Charity Dollar.* Good Housekeeping, November, 1959.
Emerson, Haven, and Luginbuhl, Martha: *1200 Local Public Health Departments for the United States.* Am. J. Pub. Health, 35:898–904, 1945.
Freeman, R. B., and Holmes, E. M.: Administration of Public Health Services. Philadelphia, W. B. Saunders Co., 1960.
Hanlon, John J.: *A Bookshelf on International Health.* Am. J. Pub. Health, 48:4, 1958.

Hanlon, John J.: *Principles of Public Health Administration.* St. Louis, The C. V. Mosby Company, 1955.

International Health—A Symposium. Am. J. Pub Health, *41*:1455–1482, 1951.

Maas, P.: *Where Does Your Charity Dollar Go?* Look, *24*:40–46, 1960.

Maxcy, K. F., Editor: *Rosenau Preventive Medicine and Hygiene,* 7th Ed. New York, Appleton-Century-Crofts, 1951.

Morgan, Murray: *Doctors to the World.* New York, Viking Press, 1958.

Mountin, J. W., and Flook, E.: *Guide to Health Organization in the U.S.* U.S. Public Health Service, Washington, D.C., 1951.

Mustard, Harry S.: *An Introduction to Public Health.* New York, The Macmillan Company, 1954.

Philip, J. R., and Merrill, M. W.: *A Pattern for State-Local Relations in Public Health.* Am. J. Pub. Health, *46*:1505–512, 1956.

Pollack, Jack Harrison: *The Shame of Our Local Health Departments.* Colliers, *123*:32–34, 1949.

Simmons, James S. M. D.: *Global Epidemiology.* Philadelphia, J. B. Lippincott Co., 1944.

World Health Organization: *Report of the 11th World Health Assembly.* Geneva, World Health Organization, 1958.

Smillie, Wilson C.: *Preventive Medicine and Public Health.* New York, The Macmillan Company, 1955.

Smillie, Wilson C.: *Public Health Administration in the United States.* New York, The Macmillan Company, 1948.

Strode, George K., M. D.: *Yellow Fever.* New York, McGraw-Hill and Co., 1951.

United States Public Health Service: *The Public Health Service Today.* Washington, D.C., U.S. Government Printing Office, 1955.

Woodcock, Leonard: *Where Are We Going in Public Health?* Am. J. Pub. Health, *46*:278–82, 1956.

Appendices

Small Rural
Community Health Council

CONSTITUTION FOR THE HAMILTON (N.Y.) HEALTH COUNCIL

Approved May 8, 1950

I. **Name**

This organization shall be known as *The Hamilton Health Council.*

II. **Objectives**

1. To assist, whenever necessary, any type of health and safety program in the area.
2. To co-ordinate, as far as possible, the work of all organizations concerned with public health.
3. To stimulate interest and educate the public in health problems and their solution.
4. To study health needs and develop a community health program relative to those needs.

III. **Membership**

All persons living in the area covered by the Public Health Nurse shall be considered non-voting members.

The voting membership shall consist of one representative from each organization in the area interested in health activities and ten members at large (to be chosen by committee on membership).

IV. Officers

1. *Chairman*–whose duties shall be to preside over all regular and special meetings of the council and to appoint all standing and special committees from the entire membership as soon as possible after election.
2. *Vice-Chairman*–whose duties shall be to take over all responsibilities of the chairman during his or her absence and to act as program chairman.
3. *Secretary*–whose duties shall be to keep a record of attendance and work done by the council and to have charge of the council's correspondence.
4. *Treasurer*–whose duties shall be to receive and keep an account of all funds received and expended by the council and to file a complete financial report at the end of the council year and turn over all records and unexpended funds to successor.

These officers shall be elected each year by a majority vote of the voting members present at the annual meeting. Each officer may be re-elected for two succeeding years.

V. Funds

The funds for the council shall be raised by soliciting all persons in the area through the Community Chest.

VI. Proceedings

1. Meetings–The regular meetings of the council shall be held on the second Monday of October, January, March and May. Special meetings may be called by the chairman. The time and place of the meeting shall be announced by the chairman. At the March meeting, the chairman shall appoint a nominating committee of at least two members. The May meeting shall be the annual meeting at which time the election of officers shall take place.
2. One third of the voting members present at any meeting called by individual, written or telephoned notice shall constitute a quorum.
3. The order of business shall be:
   a. Call to order
   b. Reading of minutes of previous meeting
   c. Treasurer's report
   d. Committee reports
   e. Unfinished business
   f. New business
   g. Adjournment

VII. Standing Committees (with exception of executive committee, can be chosen from nonvoting membership)

Executive–to perform all functions of the council between meetings, including authorization of expenditure of funds. This committee shall consist of the officers of the council and one other member appointed by the chairman.

Survey–to learn needs and to recommend major projects for emphasis and to keep file up to date.

Publicity–to plan regular newspaper publicity of the council's activities and to assist the Public Health Nurse and other committees to inform the public of the work being done.

Program–to work up and carry out appropriate program for year.

Educational–to stimulate interest in individual and community health and arrange for group education, health library, mental hygiene, etc.

Service–to assist with clinics, classes in home nursing, first aid, etc. Help with school projects. Become acquainted with work of the Public Health Nurse and know her needs. Coordinate the Visiting Ladies program, etc.

VIII. Amendment

This constitution may be amended by a majority vote of the voting members present at any meeting called by written or telephoned notice to members.

What Bylaws Should Contain

Membership Provisions
    Who can be a member,
    Types of membership,
    Methods of admitting new members,
    Method of dropping members,
    What constitutes "good standing"?

Officers
    Duties and powers,
    Provision for filling unexpired terms,
    Rules for election,
    Procedure for recall.

Dues
    Amount: annual membership,
    When payable,
    Initiation fees,
    To whom all dues are payable.

Amendments to Constitution and Bylaws
    Notice to membership of proposed amendments,
    Type of notice required,
    Vote required to effect amendment,
    Procedure for proposing an amendment: petition, motion.

Meetings

    Types: regular and special,

    Procedure for calling special meetings,

    Quorum (designate a percentage of the membership),

    Parliamentary authority,

    Provision for notification of membership if no regular meeting date is established,

    Who shall preside at special meetings?

Board of Directors

    Eligibility for membership to board,

    Duties,

    Frequency of meetings,

    Delegation of authority to act between regular meetings of the organization,

    Who is delegated to speak for the organization in emergencies,

    What constitutes a quorum (usually majority of members),

    How to recall members,

    Authority to hire salaried staff.

Standing Committees

    Names (Finance, Membership, Constitution, Bylaws, etc.),

    How selected or elected,

    Term of office,

    Quorum (usually majority of members),

    Meetings (number and how called).

Appendix III

Sample Questionnaire

HEALTH SURVEY QUESTIONNAIRE
CONFIDENTIAL – Clinton County Health Council

Town or Township _____

Enumerator _____

FAMILY ROSTER (Give numbers according to years of age)

	Under 1 Year	1-5	6-15	16 or Over
1. Number in family – Now living in home - - - - - - - - - - - - -				

2. Immunization Status:

(a) What members have been vaccinated against smallpox - - _____ ____ ____ _____

(b) Number vaccinated in last 5 years for smallpox - - - - - - _____ ____ ____ _____

(c) Number who have received diphtheria shots - - - - - - - - _____ ____ ____ _____

(d) Number who have received tetanus shots - - - - - - - - - _____ ____ ____ _____

(e) Number who have received whooping cough shots - - - - - _____ ____ ____ _____

(f) Number who have received poliomyletis shots - - - - - - - _____ ____ ____ _____

3. Number in family who during the last 12 months have had: Diphtheria ____; Scarlet Fever____; Whooping Cough ___ .

4. Number in immediate family now living who have or have had: Tuberculosis ___; Diabetes___; Undulant Fever___ ; A Heart Attack ___; Polio___; Rheumatic Fever___; Typhoid Fever___; Cancer, of stomach ___; of male organs___; of female organs ___ ; of breast ___; or other___ ;

5. Estimate number of days during the last year members of family were sick in bed at home___; at hospital ___. (Do not include pregnancy or colds.)

6. Number of hospitalized illnesses in family in last 12 months ___. (Do not include pregnancy.)

7. Approximate number of visits in family to or by doctor the last 12 months. (Do not include pregnancy or visits for babies under 1 year of age.)

8. Were the eyes of school-age children (6-15) in the family checked in the past 2 years?____. How many in the family in this age group were found defective? ___ . How many of these defects were corrected?___ .

9. Has there ever been any history of tuberculosis in the family?___. How many have had a chest X-ray in the last year?___. Do you know how to get a free chest X-ray?___.

10. How many of your family visited a dentist for a dental checkup in the last year?___.

11. Do you keep cows?___. If so: Have your cows been Bangs tested within the past year?___. Have your cows been T.B. tested within the past year?____. Is your source of milk raw or pasteurized?___.

12. Drinking water supply: City___ ; or private___; Spring___; Cistern___; a well ___; drilled or dug ___?
Has your water supply been tested? Yes___; No___; When___; If not, would you like to have it tested?___ . Do you have running water in the house? Yes___ ; No___ .

13. Toilet Disposal: City sewer:___; Septic Tank___; Cesspool___; Privy Pit___; Surface Privy___; Other___ .

14. Do you have prepaid Hospitalization Insurance? Yes___; No___.

FILL IN THE LAST TWO ONLY IF IT APPLIES IN THE LAST 6 YEARS:

15. Total number of pregnancies of mother:
(a) Number of live babies born at regular or 9 months time___.
(b) Number of live babies born before time___.
(c) Number of babies born dead or miscarried___.
(d) At what time in last pregnancy did mother go to doctor for the first time: (estimate first, second, fourth month)___.
(e) How many times did mother visit doctor during last pregnancy (approx.)?___.
(f) Did mother go to doctor for examination after delivery (last pregnancy) Yes___ ; No___.

16. How many times did the doctor see the baby from birth to 1 year of age for sickness?___; for health supervision (while well)? ___.
(Indicate as once per month, once every two months, or one time every six months;) Last pregnancy only).[1]

[1] Clinton County Health Survey, pamphlet published by The Clinton County Health Council, 1950.

A Check List On

Community Health Resources

1. Does your city or county have a full-time health department?
2. Is your health department budget about the minimum standard for basic services?
3. What were your city or county death rates from the following communicable diseases last year?: diphtheria, typhoid fever, tuberculosis. What were the rates of infant and maternal mortality?
4. What were the five leading causes of death in your city or county last year?
5. Is the number of public health sanitarians in your city or county health department less than the generally recognized standard?
6. Is the total number of public health nurses in your city or county less than the generally recognized standards?
7. Are there adequate public health laboratory facilities easily available to the physicians of your city or county for the diagnosis of communicable disease?
8. Is the tuberculosis case-finding program in your city or county considered an effective one?
9. Has your city or county had within the last five years a chest x-ray program in which persons 15 years of age and over had a chance to be x-rayed free?

10. Is it possible to hospitalize promptly (within two months) all cases of tuberculosis that are recommended for hospitalization?

11. Within your city or county, are clinic facilities for prenatal advice and care provided either by the hospitals or by the health department?

12. Within your city or county, are there child-health conferences for well-babies and young children provided by the health department or otherwise?

13. Has a substantial percentage of the babies under two years of age in your city or county been immunized against diphtheria, poliomyelitis, whooping cough, tetanus, and smallpox?

14. Are supplementary immunization and vaccination provided for children on entering school?

15. Is there provision through the health department at the schools for the examinations of school children who are referred by the teachers and nurses?

16. Are special educational facilities available for children who have cerebral palsy, hearing defects, or vision defects?

Appendix V

Health Department Inspection Forms

SALT LAKE CITY BOARD OF HEALTH

DIVISION OF FOOD AND SANITARY ENGINEERING

INSPECTION FORM FOR EATING AND DRINKING ESTABLISHMENTS

Sources		Type ....
Milk, cream		Number served
Cream-filled pastries		daily ....
Meats		Any kitchen maintained
Shellfish		elsewhere? ....

Name .... Address ....

SIR: An inspection of your premises has this day been made, and you are notified of the defects marked below with a cross (x). Violation of the same item on two successive inspections requires immediate degrading[1] or suspension of permit. All menu cards or boards shall display grade[1] .... notice.

Item No.[2]

(1) **Floors.**—Easily cleanable construction, smooth, good repair (   ); clean (   ); cleaned only after closing or between meals (   ), by dustless methods (   ) .... (   )

(2) **Walls and ceilings.**—All: clean, good repair (   ); kitchen: light color (   ), walls smooth, washable to level of splash (   ) .... (   )

(3) **Doors and windows.**—Outer openings with effective screens and outward-opening, self-closing doors, or fly-repellent fans, or flies absent .... (   )

(4) **Lighting.**—Natural or artificial light equivalent to 10 foot-candles on working surfaces (except in dining room), 4 in storage rooms .... (   )

324

(5) **Ventilation.**—All rooms (except cold storage) reasonably free of odors and condensation . . . . ( )
(6) **Toilet facilities.**—Comply with plumbing code ( ); adequate, conveniently located for employees ( ); good repair, clean, no flies ( ); well lighted, outside ventilation ( ); in new establishments, no direct opening ( ); self-closing doors ( ); washing sign for employees ( ); privies, if used, comply State standards ( ) . . . . ( )
(7) **Water supply.**—Running water accessible as required ( ); supply adequate ( ); safe, complies State standards ( ) . . . . ( )
(8) **Lavatory facilities.**—Adequate, convenient ( ); hot and cold running water ( ); soap ( ); approved sanitary towels ( ); hands washed after toilet ( ) . . . . ( )
(9) **Construction of utensils and equipment.**—Easily cleanable construction, self draining, no corrosion, good repair, no chipped enamel ware, no chipped or cracked dishes, no open seams, no tin cans, no cadmium or lead utensils ( ) . . . . ( )
(10a) **Cleaning of equipment.**—Clean cases, counters, tables, back bars, shelves, fountains, ice containers, cream dispensers, bottle cabinets, beer cabinets, refrigerators, meat blocks, coffee urns, mixing machines, malted milk dispenser, stoves, hoods, exhaust fans, disher well, extractors ( ); clean cloths used by employees ( ) . . . . ( )
(10b) **Cleaning of utensils.**—Single service cups, plates, straws, caps, used only once, milk bottles, eating and drinking utensils thoroughly cleaned after each use, other utensils cleaned each day, suitable detergent used ( ), no cyanide or other poisonous compounds ( ) . . . . ( )
(10c) **Bactericidal treatment of eating and cooking utensils.**—Approved bactericidal treatment after cleaning: Immersed 2 minutes in 180° F. water, or 2 minutes in approved chlorine rinse ( ); cabinets have thermometer in coldest zone ( ); large utensils adequately treated with live steam, boiling water, or chlorine spray or swab ( ); dish-washing machine properly operated ( ). Utensils comply bacterial standard ( ); drying cloths, if used, kept clean and used for no other purpose ( ) . . . . (`
(11) **Storage and handling of utensils.**—Stored above floor in clean place protected from flies, splash, dust, etc., inverted or covered when practicable ( ); no handling of contact surfaces ( ); single-service cups, straws, etc., purchased in sanitary cartons, kept in clean dry place, and properly handled ( ); dispensing spoons, dippers kept in hot or running water ( ) . . . . ( )
(12) **Disposal of wastes.**—Liquid wastes into public sewer or as approved by State ( ); no back-siphonage into water supply from toilets, washing machines, sinks, etc. ( ); garbage stored in tight, non-absorbent, washable receptacles, covered pending removal ( ), removed frequently and receptacles washed to prevent nuisance ( ) . . . . ( )
(13) **Refrigeration.**—Readily perishable foods (including cream-filled pastry, meats, milk, etc.—see Code) stored at 50° F. or less ( ); ice stored and handled in approved manner ( ); drip enters open trapped drain or pan ( ) . . . . ( )
(14a) **Wholesomeness of food.**—Wholesome, clean, no spoilage ( ); prepared so safe for human consumption ( ); cream-filled pastry rebaked unless filling adequately cooked, and promptly cooled ( ) . . . . ( )
(14b) **Wholesomeness of milk products.**—Milk, fluid milk products, frozen desserts from approved sources ( ); milk, etc., served in original individual bottles or from approved bulk dispenser ( ) . . . . ( )

(14c) **Wholesomeness of shellfish.**—Shellfish from approved sources (   ); shucked shellfish kept in original containers (   ) . . . . (   )

(15a) **Storage of food and drink.**—No contamination by overhead leakage or submerging (   ); not on floors subject to flooding from sewage backflow (   ) . . . . (   )

(15b) **Display and serving of food and drink.**—Minimum manual contact with food and drink (   ); no open displays (   ); no animals or fowls (   ); flies, roaches, and rodents under control (   ); no un-colored poisonous insecticides or raticides (   ) . . . . (   )

(15c) **Ratproofing.**—Structure ratproofed . . . . (   )

(16) **Cleanliness of employees.**—Clean outer garments, used for no other purpose (   ); hands clean (   ); no spitting, no tobacco used where food prepared (   ); caps, hair nets (   ) . . . . (   )

(17) **Miscellaneous.**—Premises kept neat and clean (   ); no operations in living or sleeping rooms (   ); clean, adequate lockers for em-ployees' clothing, not in toilet rooms or kitchen (   ); soiled linens, coats, aprons kept in containers (   ) . . . . (   )

(Sec. 9) **Disease control.**—No person at work with any communicable disease, sores, or infected wounds (   ); section 907 posted in all toilets (   ); employees health certificates (   ) . . . . (   )

RECEIVED . . . .
Manager or Employee in Charge

REMARKS: . . . .
Date . . . .
Inspector.

NOTICE.—This report shall not be defaced or removed except by the health officer or his representa-tive.

1 Applicable only where grading ordinance is in effect. For violation of item 1, 2, 4, 5, or 17 degrade to grade B; for all other items to grade C.

2 The item numbers correspond to those for grade A in 1943 U. S. Public Health Service Restaurant Ordinance. For "itinerant restaurant" requirements see Code.

UTAH STATE DEPARTMENT OF HEALTH

Facilities Ownership:

Water Supply ....

Sewage System..

INSPECTION REPORT FOR
HOTELS AND MOTELS

Type ....

No. of Rooms.................................

No. of Units................................

....

City, County, or District

Name.. Address...

Owner.. Address...

Manager.. Address...

SIR: An inspection of your premises has this day been made, and you are notified of the defects marked below with a cross (x). Your prompt correction of any defects noted herein is respectfully requested.

1. **Guest Rooms Floor Area.** At least 100 square feet per room ( ) At least 60 square feet per bed ( ) At least 300 cubic feet per person ( ) .... ( )

2. **Floors.** Easily cleanable ( ) Good repair ( ) Clean ( ) Lobby ( ) Passageways ( ) Rooms ( ) .... ( )

3. **Walls and Ceilings.** Easily cleanable ( ) Good repair ( ) Clean ( ) Lobby ( ) Passageways ( ) Rooms ( ) .... ( )

4. **Furniture - Fixtures.** Suitable construction ( ) Clean ( ) Good repair ( ) Windows ( ) Shades ( ) Curtains ( ) Furniture ( ) Other Fixtures ( ) .... ( )

5. **Toilet, Wash and Bath Rooms.** Adequate ( ) Non-Absorbent floors or floor coverings ( ) Clean ( ) Good repair ( ) Walls and ceilings clean ( ) Good repair ( ) Fixtures and room ventilated ( ) Good repair ( ) Clean ( ) Well lighted ( ) .... ( )

6. **Eating and Drinking Utensils.** Clean ( ) Sanitized ( ) .... ( )

7. **Linen.** Towels adequate ( ) Pillow cases ( ) Under and over sheets ( ) Sheets of adequate size ( ) All bedding, mattresses, sheets, etc. clean ( ) Good repair ( ) .... ( )

8. **Plumbing - Lighting - Ventilation.** All plumbing properly installed ( ) Good repair ( ) Ventilation suitable ( ) Lighting suitable ( ) Guest room window area adequate ( ) Sufficient area openable to the outside air ( ) .... ( )

9. **Insects and Rodents.** Free of insects ( ) Rodents ( ) Self-closing screen doors ( ) Openable windows screened ( ) Building rodent proof ( ) Premises kept neat and clean ( ) .... ( )

10. **Water Supply.** Water supply approved ( ) Adequate ( ) Drinking fountains, approved type ( ) Common drinking cups not used ( ) .... ( )

11. **Sewage Disposal.** Sewage system approved ( )... ( )

12. **Garbage - Trash.** Tight non-absorbent metal containers ( ) Approved lids ( ) Covered pending removal ( ) Removed frequently to prevent nuisance ( ) .... ( )

REMARKS:..

....

.. ..

Date   **Sanitarian**

UTAH STATE DEPARTMENT OF HEALTH

Sanitation Inspection Report for

SCHOOLS

_____
City, County, or District

Name of School _____ Water Supply_____

Address _____ Sewage Disposal_____

Principal _____ Garbage Disposal _____
     An inspection of the School has this day been made, and you are notified of the
     deficiencies noted below with an (X). Your prompt attention to the correction of
     such defects noted herein is respectfully requested.

1. BUILDING: Proper location ( ) Adequate maintenance ( ) Properly constructed ( )_____( )

2. GROUNDS: Adequately drained ( ) Free of debris ( ) _____ ( )

3. WATER SUPPLY: Approved by USDOH ( ) Properly functioning ( )_____( )

4. DRINKING FOUNTAINS: Adequate number ( ) Conform to ASA ( ) Sufficient water flow ( ) Common cup eliminated ( )_____( )

5. SEWAGE DISPOSAL: Approved by USDOH ( ) Properly functioning ( )_____( )

6. GARBAGE DISPOSAL: Water-tight metal containers ( ) Proper lids ( ) Frequent collection ( ) Approved ( )_____( )

7. PLUMBING: Comply with Utah State and Local plumbing codes ( )_____( )

8. STORAGE: Adequate locker space ( ) Closets ( ) Other ( ) Locker rooms, closets, etc., clean ( ) Good repair ( )_____( )

9. SWIMMING POOLS: Approved by USDOH ( )( )

10. RODENTS & INSECTS: Absence of infesta- tion ( ) Flies ( ) Other insects ( )_____( )

11. FLOORS, WALLS AND CEILINGS: Easily cleanable construction ( ) Clean ( ) Good repair ( ) _____ ( )

12. HEATING AND VENTILATION: Adequate heating facilities ( ) Room thermometers ( ) Temperature of rooms ( ) Proper ventilation ( )_____ ( )

13. TOILETS AND LAVATORIES: Adequate toilet facilities ( ) Adequate hand washing facilities ( ) Clean ( ) Good repair ( ) _____ ( )

14. TOILET ROOMS: Impervious floors ( ) Walls and ceilings clean ( ) Good repair ( ) Ventilation to outside air ( ) Toilet paper ( ) Soap ( ) Warm and cold running water ( ) Towels ( ) Self- closing doors ( )_____( )

15. DRESSING ROOMS: Adequate ventila- tion ( ) Adequate lighting ( ) Floors easily cleanable ( ) Clean ( ) Good repair ( ) Disinfected regularly ( ) Walls and ceilings clean ( ) Good repair ( )_____( )

16. SHOWER ROOMS: Impervious floors ( ) Clean ( ) Good repair ( ) Prop- erly drained ( ) Disinfected regularly ( ) Adequate shower heads ( )_____( )

17. FOOT BATHS (OPTIONAL) Approved type ( ) Properly maintained ( )____( )

18. LUNCH FACILITIES: Comply with USDOH standards ( )_____( )

REMARKS_____

_____

_____

Date _____ Sanitarian _____

UTAH STATE DEPARTMENT OF HEALTH

Inspection Report for
Trailer Courts

_____
City, County, or District

Name of Court _____ Address _____

Owner (Or Manager) _____ Address _____

No. of Trailer Spaces, Total _____ Spaces Reserved for Overnight or Dependent
Coaches _____

* * * * * * * * * * * *

1. SITE PROVISIONS (Sec. IV) Trailer space boundary marked ( )   Driveway adequate, unob- structed ( ) 4' clearance between coach and property line ( )   8' other coaches ( ) 4' build- ings, adjoining trailer space, fence, etc. ( ) Trailer space adequate in width, length ( ) Vehicle parking adequate ( )   ( )

2. SERVICE BUILDINGS (Sec. V) Service building provided with sufficient toilets, lava- tories, showers, slop sinks, urinals, laundry facilities, etc. ( )   Clean, good repair ( ) Building properly constructed, maintained ( ) Not over 200 ft. from dependent coach ( ) Adequate heat, light, ventilation ( ) Easily cleanable ( ) Openings well screened ( ) ( )

3. WATER SUPPLY (Sec. VI) Supply ade- quate meets State standards ( )   Outlet for each trailer properly constructed ( ) Adequate hot and cold water in service building ( ) ( )

4. SEWAGE DISPOSAL (Sec. VII) All liquid waste in public sewer or approved private

system ( )   Trailer connection to sewer tight, trapped, properly constructed ( ) ( )

5. REFUSE DISPOSAL (Sec. VIII) Refuse containers adequate in number, construction, properly located ( )   Containers clean, cov- ered, no nuisance ( ) Refuse collected fre- quently ( )   Disposal of refuse adequate ( ) Premises clean, no litter, all refuse in con- tainers ( )   ( )

6. INSECT AND RODENT CONTROL (Sec. IX) Area free of breeding places ( )   Har- borage ( )   Rodents, flies, mosquitoes ( ) ( )

7. ELECTRICAL, PLUMBING, AND FIRE PROTECTION (Sec. X, XI, and XII). Local clearance on electrical, plumbing, and fire requirements ( )   ( )

8. ALTERATIONS, ANIMALS (Sec. XIII) No additions on trailers ( )   Only acceptable skirting ( )   Wheels attached to trailer ( ) Dogs, cats, etc., properly restricted ( ) ( )

REMARKS _____

_____

_____

_____

_____

Date _____   Sanitarian _____

5-59 Q.P.

Salt Lake City Board of Health

DIVISION OF FOODS AND SANITARY ENGINEERING
Sanitarian's Inspection Report
FOR CHILDREN'S CARE CENTERS   No. of Children.......................

Name of Home...Address...

Licensed Operator...Owner...

An inspection of the premises has this day been made, and you are notified of the defects marked below with a cross (X). Your prompt correction of any defects noted herein is hereby requested.

Item 1. ADMINISTRATION
Operator or qualified assistant
present .... ☐

Item 2. RECORDS
Important data and health certificate for
each child on file.. ☐

Item 3. FLOORS
Smooth, good repair, clean.............................. ☐

Item 4. WALLS AND CEILINGS
Good repair, clean... ☐

Item 5. DOORS AND WINDOWS
Effectively screened ☐ Outer screen doors
self-closing ☐ .... ☐

Item 6. TOILET FACILITIES
Ventilated to outside ☐ No direct
openings ☐ Comply with code ☐ Indi-
vidual towels available ☐ .... ☐

Item 7. LIGHTING, VENTILATION & HEATING
Adequate lighting ☐ Ventilation ☐
Heating ☐ ....:... ☐

Item 8. SAFE HOT AND COLD WATER
Safe from approved source............................... ☐

Item 9. SEWAGE DISPOSAL
In public sewer or as approved by
Board of Health.. ☐

Item 10. CONSTRUCTION OF UTENSILS & EQUIPMENT
Approved quality, easily cleanable and
in good repair.. ☐

Item 11. WASHING UTENSILS & EQUIPMENT
Washed, rinsed, sanitized — or washed and
sterilized in 170° water for two minutes.......... ☐

Item 12. GARBAGE — SURROUNDINGS
Garbage stored in clean covered approved
containers ☐ Surroundings neat and clean ☐ ☐

Item 13. FOOD AND EQUIPMENT STORAGE
Food from approved sources☐ Stored above
floor ☐ Perishable foods kept at 50° ☐
Utensils and equipment protected when
stored ☐ .... ☐

Item 14. STATE REGULATIONS
Must meet all State regulations........................ ☐

Item 15. BEDDING, LAUNDRY, SAFETY
Bedding and Clothing clean sanitized ☐
Properly stored ☐ Safety rails ☐
Medicine in locked cupboard ☐ .... ☐

Item 16. MISCELLANEOUS
Employees clean ☐ Current food handler's
card ☐ Recreation area clean and safe ☐
Yard free from hazards ☐ .... ☐

Received by...

REMARKS..
....
....
....

Date..   ....
                                                                                          Sanitarian

SALT LAKE CITY BOARD OF HEALTH
Division of Foods and Sanitary Engineering
115 South State Street

SANITARY INSPECTION FORM

Name of Establishment _____ Address _____

Owner _____ Address _____

Mgr., Operator _____ Address _____

BUSINESS ROOMS
1. Ceilings - - - - - - - - - - - ( )
2. Walls - - - - - - - - - - - - ( )
3. Floors- - - - - - - - - - - - ( )
4. Accumulation of Waste - - - ( )

SLEEPING ROOMS
5. Ceilings - - - - - - - - - - - ( )
6. Walls - - - - - - - - - - - - - ( )
7. Floors- - - - - - - - - - - - - ( )
8. Beds & Bedding - - - - - - - ( )

KITCHEN
9. Ceilings- - - - - - - - - - - ( )
10. Walls - - - - - - - - - - - - ( )
11. Floors (impervious)- - - - - ( )
12. Dishwater washer - - - - - ( )
13. (3) Compartment sink- - - ( )
14. Plumbing facilities - - - - - ( )
15. Utensils & equipment - - - - ( )
16. Disposal of Wastes - - - - - ( )

ORDINANCES
1146 Boarding Houses - - - - - ( )
3657 Massage Parlors - - - - - ( )
 621 Authorized said Inspection ( )

TOILETS
17. Ceilings - - - - - - - - - - - - -( )
18. Walls - - - - - - - - - - - - - - ( )
19. Floors (impervious)- - - - - - - ( )
20. Insufficient toilets - - - - - - ( )
21. Plumbing facilities - - - - - - ( )
22. Soap, tissue etc. - - - - - - - ( )
23. Hand washing facilities - - - - ( )
24. Ventilation - - - - - - - - - - - ( )
25. Self-closing doors - - - - - - - ( )
26. Location inconvenient - - - - - ( )

BASEMENT
27. Walls, ceilings & floors - - - - ( )
28. Improper storage - - - - - - - - ( )
29. Accessible to rats - - - - - - - ( )

GENERAL
30. Insects, & vermin - - - - - - - ( )
31. Garbage & Refuse - - - - - - - ( )
32. Condition of premises - - - - - ( )

PERSONNEL
33. Food Handlers Permit - - - - - ( )
34. Uniforms - - - - - - - - - - - - ( )
35. General appearance- - - - - - - ( )

Sir: An inspection of your establishment has this day been made, and you are notified
of the defects above with a cross (X):

REMARKS _____

_____

_____

_____

_____

DATE _____ SANITARIAN _____

SALT LAKE CITY BOARD OF HEALTH
DIVISION OF FOODS AND SANITARY ENGINEERING

Milk.................. ....   Ice Cream   ...   . **Type of Business**

Cream ....   Shellfish ... .

Name........................ ....   Address ....

Sir: An inspection of your premises has this day been made, and you are notified of the defects marked below with a cross (X). Your cooperation in correcting these defects is hereby requested.

1. **Floors.** Clean, smooth construction good repair ....( )

2. **Walls and Ceilings.** Clean, smooth, washable to level of splash ....( )

3. **Doors and Windows.** Screened, self-closing doors, fans, no flies ....( )

4. **Lighting.** Sufficient ....( )

5. **Ventilation.** Odor, moisture ....( )

6. **Toilet.** Adequate, convenient, clean, good repair, ventilated, no direct openings, self-closing door ....( )

7. **Water Supply.** Convenient, safe, easily accessible, adequate ....( )

8. **Lavatory Facilities.** Running Hot water, soap, approved sanitary towels, washing sign ....( )

9. **Construction of Utensils and Equipment.** Easily cleanable, good repair, no open seams, no corrosion ... .( )

10a. **Cleaning of Equipment and Utensils.** Clean cases, counters, shelves, tables, meat blocks, refrigerators, clean cloths used by employees, single service cartons, caps used only once; utensils thoroughly cleaned after each use .. ..( )

10b. **Bactericidal Treatment of Utensils.** Immersed 2 minutes in 180° F. water or in one-half minute in boiling water. Large utensils adequately treated with live steam, boiling water; drying cloths if used kept clean and used for no other purpose ....( )

11. **Storage and Handling of Utensils.** Stored above floor in clean place protected from flies, splash, dust etc., inverted or covered when practicable, no handling of contact surfaces; single-service cups, straws, etc., purchased in sanitary cartons, kept in clean dry place, and properly handled, dispensing spoons, dippers kept in hot or running water ....( )

12. **Disposal of Wastes.** Plumbing proper, good repair, approved disposal, no cross connection, back siphonage; tight, metal garbage cans, covered pending removal, adequate, clean ....( )

13. **Refrigeration.** Readily perishable foods (including cream-filled pastry) stored at 50° F. or less, ice stored and handled in approved manner, drip enters open trapped drain or pan ....( )

14. **Wholesomeness of Food and Drink.** Wholesome, no spoilage; milk, fluid milk products, frozen desserts from approved sources, shellfish from approved sources ....( )

15. **Storage and Display: Food & Drink.** No contamination by overhead leakage, submerging or unnecessary handling, not on floors, no animals, fowls, rodents, roaches, structure ratproof, etc., flies under control, no open displays, floor cleaning only after closing by dustless methods ....( )

16. **Cleanliness of employees.** Clean hands, outer garments, medical examinations, caps, hair nets ....( )

17. **Miscellaneous.** Premises, clean, dressing rooms — plumbing; no operations in living or sleeping rooms, soiled linens, etc. in containers ....( )

Received...
                                    Mgr. or Employee in Charge

REMARKS: ....

....

Date .... Inspector ....

Fundamentals of Nuclear Radiations

ATOM: Basic chemical unit of matter:

nucleus $\begin{cases} \text{protons—positive charge} \\ \text{neutrons—neutral charge.} \end{cases}$

electrons—negative charge, $\dfrac{1}{1,840}$ weight of proton or neutron.

nucleus—10^{-13} cm. diameter; atom 10^{-8} cm.

Number protons = number electrons in intact atoms.

Chemical reactions occur by interactions between electron shells, nuclear reactions by transformations within atomic nuclei.

ELEMENT—Matter composed of a single kind of atom.

ATOMIC NUMBER—sum of protons in a nucleus.

ATOMIC WEIGHT—sum of protons + neutrons in a nucleus.

ISOTOPES—Different forms of same element, differing by number of neutrons in the nucleus.

NUCLEAR RADIATION—That emitted when changes occur within atomic nucleus. Biologically harmful. Cannot be detected by human senses.

RADIOACTIVITY—Phenomenon associated with the emanation of nuclear radiation.

RADIOACTIVE SUBSTANCE—One which emits nuclear radiations.

RADIOACTIVE DECAY—Process which unstable (radioactive) nuclei undergo in achieving stability. This is represented by an observed decrease in radiation with time (from a given source).

HALF-LIFE—Time required for a quantity of a radioactive substance to lose half its activity: i.e., time required for half its atoms to decay. Constant for a given radioisotope.

ISOTOPES—1. Stable
    2. Unstable.
        a. Naturally occurring
        b. Artificially produced (induced)

INDUCED RADIOACTIVITY—Except in particle accelerators (cyclotrons, etc.), radioactivity is induced in stable atoms *only* by neutrons. Exposure of materials to other types of radiation will *not* cause the materials to be made radioactive.

FISSION—Neutron induced splitting of a large atomic nucleus into two smaller ones. Some mass is converted to energy in the process. Products are highly radioactive. This is the basic reaction in explosion of *atomic bombs,* also the one causing *atomic piles* and *nuclear reactors* to operate.

FUSION or THERMONUCLEAR REACTION—Coalescence of two small atoms to form a large one. Some mass is converted to energy in the process. Basis of the *hydrogen* bomb, as well as source of energy of the sun. Extremely high temperatures required to activate.

CURIE (c)—An amount of radioactive material that undergoes 3.7×10^{10} disintegrations per second. A measure of the strength of a radioactive source.

ROENTGEN (r)—Quantity or dose of radiation. Exact definition based on ionization produced in air by X or gamma radiation.

1 roentgen = 1,000 milliroentgens (mr)

ROENTGEN EQUIVALENT PHYSICAL (rep)

ROENTGEN EQUIVALENT MAN (rem)

Units devised to extend roentgen to include all types of radiations and their damage to body tissue.

There is no simple relation between curies and roentgens. A different conversion factor is necessary for each isotope.

DOSE = rate x time (for materials with half-lives long in relation to exposure time).

Rate in r/hr or mr/hr (speedometer, rate meter).

Dose in r or mr (mileage indicator, integrating instrument).

INVERSE SQUARE LAW**—Intensity of radiation from a *point source* decreases with the *square* of the distance from the source.

$$\frac{I_1}{I_2} = \frac{(d_2)^2}{(d_1)}$$

UNITS: CONVERSIONS AND DEFINITIONS

CURIE (c): Amount of radioactive material that undergoes 3.7×10^{10} disintegrations per second (d/s or dps).

$3.7 \times 10^{10} = 37$ billion $= 37,000,000,000$

MILLICURIE (mc): $\frac{1}{1,000}$ of a curie $= 3.7 \times 10^7$ dps.

MICROCURIE: $\frac{1}{1,000,000}$ of a curie $= 3.7 \times 10^4$ dps.

ROENTGEN (r): Quantity or dose of radiation. Exact definition based on amount of ionization produced.

ROENTGEN EQUIVALENT PHYSICAL (rep)

ROENTGEN EQUIVALENT MAN (rem)

Units devised to extend roentgen to include all types of nuclear radiation, and to signify the amount of ionization and damage caused in biological systems.

REM=RAD X RBE

MILLIROENTGEN (mr): $\dfrac{1}{1,000}$ of a roentgen.

TOTAL: Mileage indicator—dosimeter, film badge.

RATE: Speedometer—portable survey instruments.

Dose—rate × time (for materials with long half lives)

Rate in r/hr or mr/hr; dose in r or mr; time in hours.

A mgm. Radium = 1 millicurie = 8.4 r/hr at 1 cm.

INVERSE SQUARE LAW**—Intensity of radiation from a *point source* decreases with the *square* of the distance from the source.

For radium: r/hr = $\dfrac{1.3 \times \text{milligrams of radium (mc)}}{(\text{distance in inches})^2}$

Distance in inches from source for a given reading = $\sqrt{\dfrac{1.3 \times \text{mgm Ra (mc)}}{\text{r/hr you want}}}$

For Co^{60}: r/hr = $\dfrac{2.1 \times \text{activity in millicuries}}{(\text{distance in inches})^2}$

Distance in inches from source for a given reading = $\sqrt{\dfrac{2.1 \times \text{activity in mc}}{\text{r/hr you want}}}$

Student Semester Project

Choose a current major community health problem and discuss, using the following outline:

I. The Problem
1. Define the problem
2. Historical Aspects (footnote)
3. Compare the problem
   (a) local
   (b) state
   (c) nation
   (d) world
4. Where is the problem most acute?
5. Causes of the problem
6. Obstacles
7. Effect upon
   (a) infants
   (b) school age
   (c) adults
   (d) old age

II. Statistical Analysis of the Problem

III. Factors Involved in the Problem
1. Sociological Aspects

2. Psychological Aspects
3. Economical Aspects
4. Geographical Aspects
5. Rural-urban Aspects

IV. **Prevention and Control**
1. List the various agencies involved in prevention (local and state); services rendered; how financed.
2. List the various agencies involved in control (local and state); services rendered; how financed.
3. How is the program presently organized, administered, and financed?
4. Is the program coordinated? Does cooperation prevail?
5. How is the support of the public gained?
6. What is the role of the school, health department, voluntary agencies, and parents in attacking the problem?
7. Legislation—local and state.
8. What health education methods, techniques, and materials are utilized?
9. Community organization for health.

V. **Current Research and the Future** (footnote)
1. What research is being done to combat this problem?
2. List agencies giving research grants—amount of money alloted.
3. Theory behind research.
4. Writings in recent health journals.
5. The future.

VI. **Evaluation, interpretation, analysis, and recommendations.**

Index

339